PROPERTY OF:
Marilyn Krajicek, RN, EdD, FAAN
UCHSC, School of Nursing, Room 2951
303 (315-5026 or (303) 724-0650

D0961089

Health Literacy
A Prescription to End Confusion

Committee on Health Literacy

Board on Neuroscience and Behavioral Health

Lynn Nielsen-Bohlman, Allison M. Panzer, David A. Kindig, Editors

INSTITUTE OF MEDICINE
OF THE NATIONAL ACADEMIES

THE NATIONAL ACADEMIES PRESS
Washington, D.C.
www.nap.edu

THE NATIONAL ACADEMIES PRESS • 500 Fifth Street, NW • Washington, DC 20001

NOTICE: The project that is the subject of this report was approved by the Governing Board of the National Research Council, whose members are drawn from the councils of the National Academy of Sciences, the National Academy of Engineering, and the Institute of Medicine. The members of the committee responsible for the report were chosen for their special competences and with regard for appropriate balance.

Support for this project was provided by the American Academy of Family Physicians Foundation, California HealthCare Foundation, Commonwealth Fund, W.K. Kellogg Foundation, MetLife Foundation, National Cancer Institute, Pfizer Corporation, and the Robert Wood Johnson Foundation. The views presented in this report are those of the Institute of Medicine Committee on Health Literacy and are not necessarily those of the funding agencies.

Library of Congress Cataloging-in-Publication Data

Health literacy : a prescription to end confusion / editors, Lynn Nielsen-Bohlman ... [et al.] ; Committee on Health Literacy, Board on Neuroscience and Behavioral Health, [Institute of Medicine].
   p. ; cm.
Includes bibliographical references and index.
ISBN 0-309-09117-9 (hardcover)—ISBN 0-309-52926-3 (pdf)
1. Health education—United States. 2. Literacy—United States.
[DNLM: 1. Health Education—methods—United States. 2. Health Education—standards—United States. 3. Communication Barriers—United States. 4. Educational Status—United States. WA 590 H4362 2004] I. Nielsen-Bohlman, Lynn. II. Institute of Medicine (U.S.). Committee on Health Literacy.
RA440.H43 2004
613'.07'1073—dc22

                              2004004829

Additional copies of this report are available from the National Academies Press, 500 Fifth Street, NW, Lockbox 285, Washington, DC 20055; (800) 624-6242 or (202) 334-3313 (in the Washington metropolitan area); Internet, http://www.nap.edu.

For more information about the Institute of Medicine, visit the IOM home page at: **www.iom.edu**.

Copyright 2004 by the National Academy of Sciences. All rights reserved.

Printed in the United States of America.

COVER: Adapted from a design by Anne Quito, Academy for Educational Development.

The serpent has been a symbol of long life, healing, and knowledge among almost all cultures and religions since the beginning of recorded history. The serpent adopted as a logotype by the Institute of Medicine is a relief carving from ancient Greece, now held by the Staatliche Museen in Berlin.

"Knowing is not enough; we must apply.
Willing is not enough; we must do."
—Goethe

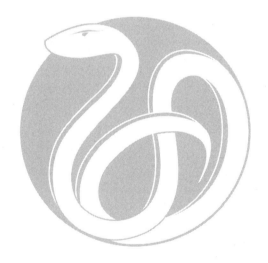

INSTITUTE OF MEDICINE
OF THE NATIONAL ACADEMIES

Adviser to the Nation to Improve Health

THE NATIONAL ACADEMIES
Advisers to the Nation on Science, Engineering, and Medicine

The **National Academy of Sciences** is a private, nonprofit, self-perpetuating society of distinguished scholars engaged in scientific and engineering research, dedicated to the furtherance of science and technology and to their use for the general welfare. Upon the authority of the charter granted to it by the Congress in 1863, the Academy has a mandate that requires it to advise the federal government on scientific and technical matters. Dr. Bruce M. Alberts is president of the National Academy of Sciences.

The **National Academy of Engineering** was established in 1964, under the charter of the National Academy of Sciences, as a parallel organization of outstanding engineers. It is autonomous in its administration and in the selection of its members, sharing with the National Academy of Sciences the responsibility for advising the federal government. The National Academy of Engineering also sponsors engineering programs aimed at meeting national needs, encourages education and research, and recognizes the superior achievements of engineers. Dr. Wm. A. Wulf is president of the National Academy of Engineering.

The **Institute of Medicine** was established in 1970 by the National Academy of Sciences to secure the services of eminent members of appropriate professions in the examination of policy matters pertaining to the health of the public. The Institute acts under the responsibility given to the National Academy of Sciences by its congressional charter to be an adviser to the federal government and, upon its own initiative, to identify issues of medical care, research, and education. Dr. Harvey V. Fineberg is president of the Institute of Medicine.

The **National Research Council** was organized by the National Academy of Sciences in 1916 to associate the broad community of science and technology with the Academy's purposes of furthering knowledge and advising the federal government. Functioning in accordance with general policies determined by the Academy, the Council has become the principal operating agency of both the National Academy of Sciences and the National Academy of Engineering in providing services to the government, the public, and the scientific and engineering communities. The Council is administered jointly by both Academies and the Institute of Medicine. Dr. Bruce M. Alberts and Dr. Wm. A. Wulf are chair and vice chair, respectively, of the National Research Council.

www.national-academies.org

COMMITTEE ON HEALTH LITERACY

DAVID KINDIG, (*Chair*), Wisconsin Public Health & Health Policy Institute, University of Wisconsin at Madison
DYANNE D. AFFONSO, Faculty of Nursing, University of Toronto
ERIC H. CHUDLER, University of Washington School of Medicine
MARILYN H. GASTON, Assistant Surgeon General of the United States, Retired
CATHY D. MEADE, University of South Florida College of Medicine H. Lee Moffitt Cancer Center & Research Institute
RUTH PARKER, Emory University School of Medicine
VICTORIA PURCELL-GATES, Michigan State University
IRVING ROOTMAN, University of Victoria
RIMA RUDD, Harvard University School of Public Health
SUSAN C. SCRIMSHAW, School of Public Health, University of Illinois at Chicago
BILL SMITH, Academy for Educational Development

Board on Neuroscience and Behavioral Health Liaisons

NANCY E. ADLER, Departments of Psychiatry and Pediatrics, University of California, San Francisco
RICHARD G. FRANK, Department of Health Care Policy, Harvard Medical School, Boston, MA

Board on Health Promotion and Disease Prevention Liaison

IRVING ROOTMAN, University of Victoria

Study Staff

LYNN NIELSEN-BOHLMAN, *Study Director*
ALLISON PANZER, *Research Assistant*
BENJAMIN N. HAMLIN, *Research Assistant*
ALLISON BERGER, *Program Assistant*

IOM Board on Neuroscience and Behavioral Health Staff

ANDREW M. POPE, *Director*
TROY PRINCE, *Administrative Assistant*
ROSA POMMIER, *Finance Officer*
JUDY ESTEP, *Senior Program Assistant*

Independent Report Reviewers

This report has been reviewed in draft form by individuals chosen for their diverse perspectives and technical expertise, in accordance with procedures approved by the National Research Council's (NRC's) Report Review Committee. The purpose of this independent review is to provide candid and critical comments that will assist the institution in making its published report as sound as possible and to ensure that the report meets institutional standards for objectivity, evidence, and responsiveness to the study charge. The review comments and draft manuscript remain confidential to protect the integrity of the deliberative process. We wish to thank the following individuals for their review of this report:

Moon Chen Jr., University of California, Davis School of Medicine
Linda C. Degutis, Yale University
Robert Graham, Agency for Healthcare Research and Quality
James Hyde, Tufts University School of Medicine
Irwin S. Kirsch, Educational Testing Service, Center for Global Assessment
Randall W. Maxey, National Medical Association
Alan R. Nelson, American College of Physicians of Internal Medicine
Joanne Nurss, Georgia State University, *Emeritus*
Yolanda Partida, University of Southern California
Debra Roter, Johns Hopkins University

Although the reviewers listed above have provided many constructive comments and suggestions, they were not asked to endorse the conclusions or recommendations nor did they see the final draft of the report before its release. The review of this report was overseen by **Daniel L. Azarnoff**, D.L. Azarnoff Associates, and **Kristine Gebbie**, Columbia University School of Nursing. Appointed by the NRC and the Institute of Medicine, they were responsible for making certain that an independent examination of this report was carried out in accordance with institutional procedures and that all review comments were carefully considered. Responsibility for the final content of this report rests entirely with the authoring committee and the institution.

Acknowledgments

The committee was aided in its deliberations by the testimony and advice of many knowledgeable and experienced individuals, and the efforts of a dedicated committee and staff. Consultants to the committee contributed ideas and report materials. The committee thanks consultants **Arlene Bierman**, Agency for Healthcare Research and Quality; **John Comings**, Harvard University; **Terry Davis**, Louisiana State University Health Sciences Center; **Julie Gazmararian**, Emory University; **David Howard**, Emory University; **Frank McClellan**, Temple University; **Scott Ratzan**, Johnson and Johnson; **Dean Schillinger**, University of California at San Francisco and San Francisco General Hospital Medical Center; **Steve Somers**, Center for Health Care Strategies; and **Barry Weiss**, University of Arizona.

The committee acknowledges with appreciation the testimony and other assistance of many individuals committed to improving health literacy. These individuals are **Paul S. Appelbaum**, University of Massachusetts Medical School; **Cynthia Baur**, U.S. Department of Health and Human Services; **Nancy Berkman**, RTI International; **Alvin Billie**, The Gathering Place; **Cindy Brach**, Agency for Healthcare Research and Quality; **L. Natalie Carroll**, National Medical Association; **Carolyn Clancy**, Agency for Healthcare Research and Quality; **Eduardo Crespi**, Centro Latino; **Barbara DeBuono**, Pfizer Pharmaceuticals Group; **Darren A. DeWalt**, University of North Carolina, Chapel Hill; **Janice A. Drass**, Centers for Medicare and Medicaid Services, DHHS; **Joyce Dubow**, AARP Public Policy Institute; **Lawrence J. Fine**, Office of Behavioral and Social Science Research, National Institutes of Health; **Heng L. Foong**, Pacific Asian Language Services for Health; **Robert Friedland**, Georgetown University and Center on an Aging Society; **Robert Graham**, Agency for Healthcare Research and Quality; **Rita Hargrave**, University of California, Davis, and Veterans Medical Center of Northern California System of Clinics; **Julie Hudman**, Henry J. Kaiser Family Foundation Commission on Medicaid and the Uninsured; **Marian James**, Agency for Healthcare Research and Quality; **Linda Johnston Lloyd**, Health Resources and Services Administration; **Lloyd J. Kolbe**, Centers for Disease Control; **Karen Lechter**, Center for Drug Evaluation and Research, U.S. Food and Drug Administration; **Estela Marin**, Louisiana State University Health Sciences Center; **Ed Martinez**, National Association of Public Hospitals and Health Systems; **Frank M. McClellan**, Temple University James E. Beasley School of Law; **Linda Morse**, New Jersey Office of Academic and Professional Standards; **Francisco Para**, Latino Health Access; **L. Gregory Pawlson**, National Committee for Quality Assurance; **Michael Pignone**, University of North Carolina at Chapel Hill; **Francis Prado**, Latino Health Access; **Sara Rosenbaum**, George Washington University; **Marisa Scala**, Center for Medicare Education, American Association of Homes and Services for the Aging; **Lauren Schwartz**, New York City Poison Control Center; **Joanne Schwartzberg**, American Medical Association; **Tetine Sentell**, University of California at Berkeley; **Judy A. Shea**, University of Pennsylvania School of Medicine; **Susan M. Shinagawa**, National Asian-American and Pacific Islander Cancer Survivors and Advocacy Network; **Colleen Sonosky**, George Washington University; **Anthony Tirone**, Joint Commission on Accreditation of Healthcare Organizations; **Tina Tucker**, American Foundation for the Blind; and **Marcia Zorn**, National Library of Medicine.

Special thanks to **K. Vish Viswanath** and **Patrick Weld** of the Division of Cancer Control and Population Sciences of the National Cancer Institute, **Scott Ratzan** of Johnson and Johnson, and to **Barbara DeBuono** and **Joel Rosenquist** of the Pfizer Pharmaceutical Group, for extra effort and repeated attention to the ongoing information needs and support of the study. The committee appreciates the efforts of **Terry C. Pellmar** for her dedication, effort, and commitment to moving this report from concept to reality in her role as Director of the Board on Neuroscience and Behavioral Health.

This report was made possible by the generous support of the American Academy of Family Physicians Foundation, California HealthCare Foundation, Commonwealth Fund, W.K. Kellogg Foundation, MetLife Foundation, National Cancer Institute, Pfizer Corporation, and the Robert Wood Johnson Foundation.

Foreword

Clear communication is critical to successful health care. Patients convey their symptoms and medical history to caregivers; health professionals issue orders, results, and recommendations to one another; and doctors, nurses, pharmacists, and others provide information and instructions to patients. Health professionals are trained to observe their patients keenly and to elicit a revealing history. Considerable effort and money are expended to automate reporting of test results and physician order entry so as to speed availability of clinical information and to reduce errors. However, comparatively little attention has been devoted to enabling patients to comprehend their condition and treatment, to make the best decisions for their care, and to take the right medications at the right time in the intended dose. As this report makes clear, *health literacy*—enabling patients to understand and to act in their own interest—remains a neglected, final pathway to high-quality health care.

Tens of millions of U.S. adults are unable to read complex texts, including many health-related materials. Arcane language and jargon that become second nature to doctors and nurses are inscrutable to many patients. Adults who have a problem understanding written materials are often ashamed and devise methods to mask their difficulty. They may be reluctant to ask questions for fear of being perceived as ignorant. If health professionals were able to take the time to ask their patients to explain exactly what they understand about their diagnoses, instructions, and bottle labels, the caregivers would find many gaps in knowledge, difficulties in understanding, and misinterpretations. These problems are exacerbated by language and cultural variation in our multicultural society, by technological complexity in health care, and by intricate administrative documents and requirements.

The Committee on Health Literacy here documents the problem and describes its origins, consequences, and solutions. The committee echoes the call of the Surgeon General and other health leaders on the import of health literacy, and it elaborates the cross-cutting priority for health literacy identified in the recent Institute of Medicine report on *Priority Areas for National Action in Quality Improvement.* Most importantly, the current report lays out a comprehensive strategy to improve health literacy in America. While this will be neither easy nor completed quickly, individuals, educators, community groups, health professionals, medical institutions, industry, and government agencies can all contribute, and this report tells how.

Health Literacy: A Prescription to End Confusion is a landmark report on an underappreciated challenge. I am grateful to the committee and its staff for their work and hope that their report receives the audience, attention, and action it deserves.

Harvey V. Fineberg, M.D., Ph.D.
President
Institute of Medicine

Preface

My understanding of the issues in health literacy was limited prior to taking on the role of Chair of this committee. From my expertise in defining and measuring population health and its determinants, I appreciated the importance of the social determinants of health. I had speculated about the role of health literacy as one pathway by which education might exert an independent effect on health outcomes. But until this rich and intense interaction with my colleagues from diverse fields such as literacy, biology, health communication, anthropology, epidemiology, medicine, nursing, and health policy, combined with poignant testimony from those affected and other experts, I had no idea of the importance and complexity of this topic.

I believe that what the United States puts into practice in medicine and health is much less than what is known. Only now do I know how profoundly the gap between knowledge and practice is widened by limited health literacy. Only now do I know why some refer to this as a "silent epidemic"—the lack of understanding by most professionals and policy makers of its extent and effect, and the individual shame associated with it that keeps it even more silent and hidden.

I hope that this report will produce several outcomes:

- It will become widely appreciated that 90 million adults with limited health literacy cannot fully benefit from much that the health and health-care system have to offer.
- It will become widely understood that efforts to improve quality, to

reduce costs, and to reduce disparities cannot succeed without simultaneous improvements in health literacy.

• It will become widely understood that health literacy is more than reading, but includes writing, numeracy, listening, speaking, and conceptual knowledge.

• It will be accepted that improving individual health literacy requires great effort from the public health and health-care systems, the education system, and society overall.

Chairing this committee was such a privilege and a challenge. We each struggled to overcome the limitations of our own knowledge and assumptions. We could not have completed this work without the many hours devoted by committee members, those providing testimony, and Institute of Medicine staff, and the financial support of our sponsors. As one firmly committed to the translation of research into policy and practice, I hope this report, containing the results of our efforts, will identify substantial new resources, not only for the research needed to establish causal relationships and evaluate effective interventions, but also to expand the many promising interventions identified here. The significance of the problem is too great to wait for complete understanding before we act.

David A. Kindig, M.D., Ph.D.
Chair

Contents

Tables, Figures, and Boxes

TABLES

FIGURES

BOXES

Executive Summary

Understanding is a two-way street. —*Eleanor Roosevelt*

ABSTRACT

I have a very good doctor. He takes the time to explain things and break it down to me. Sometimes, though, I do get stuff that can be hard—like when I first came home from the hospital and I had all these forms and things I had to read. Some words I come across I just can't quite understand (National Center for the Study of Adult Learning and Literacy, 2003).[1]

Nearly half of all American adults—90 million people—have difficulty understanding and acting upon health information. The examples below were selected from the many pieces of complex consumer health information used in America.

- *From a research consent form: "A comparison of the effectiveness of educational media in combination with a counseling method on smoking habits is being examined." (Doak et al., 1996)*

---

[1]All vignettes in shaded text in this report represent actual stories or materials. Names were omitted in most cases to protect the privacy of the author, and stories may have been edited for brevity and clarity. If not otherwise attributed, vignettes were drawn from the experiences of members of the committee.

• *From a consumer privacy notice: "Examples of such mandatory disclosures include notifying state or local health authorities regarding particular communicable diseases."*

• *From a patient information sheet: "Therefore, patients should be monitored for extraocular CMV infections and retinitis in the opposite eye, if only one infected eye is being treated."*

Forty million Americans cannot read complex texts like these at all, and 90 million have difficulty understanding complex texts. Yet a great deal of health information, from insurance forms to advertising, contains complex text. Even people with strong literacy skills may have trouble obtaining, understanding, and using health information: a surgeon may have trouble helping a family member with Medicare forms, a science teacher may not understand information sent by a doctor about a brain function test, and an accountant may not know when to get a mammogram.

This report defines health literacy as "the degree to which individuals have the capacity to obtain, process, and understand basic health information and services needed to make appropriate health decisions" (Ratzan and Parker, 2000). However, health literacy goes beyond the individual obtaining information. Health literacy emerges when the expectations, preferences, and skills of individuals seeking health information and services meet the expectations, preferences, and skills of those providing information and services. Health literacy arises from a convergence of education, health services, and social and cultural factors. Although causal relationships between limited health literacy and health outcomes are not yet established, cumulative and consistent findings suggest such a causal connection.

Approaches to health literacy bring together research and practice from diverse fields. This report examines the body of knowledge in this emerging field, and recommends actions to promote a health-literate society. Increasing knowledge, awareness, and responsiveness to health literacy among health services providers as well as in the community would reduce problems of limited health literacy. This report identifies key roles for the Department of Health and Human Services as well as other public and private sector organizations to foster research, guide policy development, and stimulate the development of health literacy knowledge, measures, and approaches. These organizations have a unique and critical opportunity to ensure that health literacy is recognized as an essential component of high-quality health services and health communication.

INTRODUCTION

> *A two-year-old is diagnosed with an inner ear infection and prescribed an antibiotic. Her mother understands that her daughter should take the prescribed medication twice a day. After carefully studying the label on the bottle and deciding that it doesn't tell how to take the medicine, she fills a teaspoon and pours the antibiotic into her daughter's painful ear (Parker et al., 2003).*

Modern health systems make complex demands on the health consumer. As self-management of health care increases, individuals are asked to assume new roles in seeking information, understanding rights and responsibilities, and making health decisions for themselves and others. Underlying these demands are assumptions about people's knowledge and skills.

National and international assessments of adults' ability to use written information suggest that these assumptions may be faulty. Current evidence reveals a mismatch between people's skills and the demands of health systems (Rudd et al., 2000a). Many people who deal effectively with other aspects of their lives may find health information difficult to obtain, understand, or use. While farmers may be able to use fertilizers effectively, they may not understand the safety information provided with the fertilizer. Chefs may create excellent dishes, but may not know how to create a healthy diet. Indeed, health literacy can be a hidden problem—because it is often not recognized by policy makers and health care providers, and because people with low literacy skills or who are confused about health care may be ashamed to speak up about problems they encounter with the increasingly complex health system (Baker et al., 1996; Parikh et al., 1996). Without improvements in health literacy, the promise of scientific advances for improving health outcomes will be diminished.

The Institute of Medicine (IOM) convened the Committee on Health Literacy, composed of experts from a wide range of academic disciplines and backgrounds, to assess the problem of limited health literacy and to consider the next steps in this field. The committee addressed the following charge:

1. Define the scope of the problem of health literacy. The intent is to clarify the root problems that underlie health illiteracy. This would include identifying the affected populations and estimating the costs for society. Develop a set of basic indicators of health literacy to allow assessment of the extent of the problem at the individual, community, and national levels.

2. Identify the obstacles to a creating a health-literate public. These are likely to include the complexity of the health care system, the many and often contradictory health messages, rapidly advancing technologies, limits within public education to promote literacy of adults as well as children, etc.

3. Assess the approaches that have been attempted to increase health literacy both in the United States and abroad. Identify the gaps in research and programs that need to be addressed. The focus should be on public health interventions attempting to increase health literacy of the public rather than on improving health provider/primary care interactions.

4. Identify goals for health literacy efforts and suggest approaches to overcome the obstacles to health literacy in order to reach these goals. These might include research or policy initiatives, interventions, or collaborations that would promote health literacy.

WHAT IS HEALTH LITERACY?

In this report, the committee accepted the definition of health literacy presented by the National Library of Medicine (Selden et al., 2000) and used in *Healthy People 2010* (HHS, 2000):

> The degree to which individuals have the capacity to obtain, process, and understand basic health information and services needed to make appropriate health decisions (Ratzan and Parker, 2000).

Health literacy is a shared function of social and individual factors. Individuals' health literacy skills and capacities are mediated by their education, culture, and language. Equally important are the communication and assessment skills of the people with whom individuals interact regarding health, as well as the ability of the media, the marketplace, and government agencies to provide health information in a manner appropriate to the audience.

The committee developed a framework for health literacy which identifies three major areas of potential intervention and forms the organizational principle of this report (see Figure ES-1). This framework illustrates the potential influence on health literacy as individuals interact with educational systems, health systems, and cultural and social factors, and suggests that these factors may ultimately contribute to health outcomes and costs. The proposed framework is a model, because available research supports only limited conclusions about causality. However, the cumulative effect of a body of consistent evidence suggests that causal relationships may exist between health literacy and health outcomes. Research is needed to establish the nature of the causal relationships between and among the various factors portrayed in the framework.

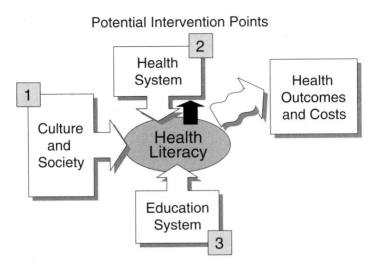

FIGURE ES-1 Potential points for intervention in the health literacy framework.

The committee reviewed the strengths and limitations of currently available measures of literacy and health literacy. Health literacy involves a range of social and individual factors, and includes cultural and conceptual knowledge, listening, speaking, arithmetical, writing, and reading skills. However, most of the tools currently available to measure health literacy primarily measure reading skills, and do not include other critical skills. Furthermore, adults' reading abilities are often estimated with a "grade level" measure, an estimate that is imprecise at best. Advancement of the field of health literacy requires the development of new measures which can be used to establish baseline levels and monitor change over time.

Finding 2-1 Literature from a variety of disciplines is consistent in finding that there is strong support for the committee's conclusion that health literacy, as defined in this report, is based on the interaction of individuals' skills with health contexts, the health-care system, the education system, and broad social and cultural factors at home, at work, and in the community. The committee concurs that responsibility for health literacy improvement must be shared by these various sectors. The committee notes that the health system does carry significant but not sole opportunity and responsibility to improve health literacy.

Finding 2-2 The links between education and health outcomes are strongly established. The committee concludes that health literacy may be one pathway explaining the well-established link between education and health, and warrants further exploration.

Finding 2-3   Health literacy, as defined in this report, includes a variety of components beyond reading and writing, including numeracy, listening, speaking, and relies on cultural and conceptual knowledge.

Finding 2-4   While health literacy measures in current use have spurred research initiatives and yield valuable insights, they are indicators of reading skills (word recognition or reading comprehension and numeracy), rather than measures of the full range of skills needed for health literacy (cultural and conceptual knowledge, listening, speaking, numeracy, writing, and reading). Current assessment tools and research findings cannot differentiate among (a) reading ability, (b) lack of background knowledge in health-related domains, such as biology, (c) lack of familiarity with language and types of materials, or (d) cultural differences in approaches to health and health care. In addition, no current measures of health literacy include oral communication skills or writing skills and none measure the health literacy demands on individuals within different health contexts.

THE EXTENT AND ASSOCIATIONS OF
LIMITED HEALTH LITERACY

Studies of health literacy or of literacy in health contexts suggest that limited health literacy skills, as measured by current assessment tools, are common, with significant variations in prevalence depending on the population sampled (see Chapter 3). People of all literacy levels may be able to manage texts that they frequently encounter and use for everyday activities, but will often face problems with difficult and confusing types of text (Kirsch et al., 1993).

Findings from the National Adult Literacy Survey (NALS) and International Adult Literacy Surveys (IALS) indicate that a large percentage of adults lack the literacy skills needed to meet the demands of twenty-first century society. More than 47 percent, or 90 million, of U.S. adults have difficulty locating, matching, and integrating information in written texts with accuracy and consistency. Of the 90 million with limited literacy skills, about 40 million can perform simple and routine tasks using uncomplicated materials. An additional 50 million adults can locate information in moderately complicated texts, make inferences using print materials, and integrate easily identifiable pieces of information. However, they find it difficult to perform these tasks when complicated by distracting information and complex texts (Kirsch, 2001; Kirsch et al., 1993).

These findings have serious implications for the health sector. Over 300 studies, conducted over three decades and assessing various health-related materials, such as informed consent forms and medication package inserts, have found that a mismatch exists between the reading levels of the materials and the reading skills of the intended audience. In fact, most of the assessed materials exceed the reading skills of the average high school graduate (Rudd et al., 2000a).

Studies suggest that while individuals with limited health literacy come from many walks of life, the problem of limited health literacy is often greater among older adults, people with limited education, and those with limited English proficiency (e.g., Beers et al., 2003; Gazmararian et al., 1999; Williams et al., 1995). For individuals whose native language is not English, issues of health literacy are compounded by issues of basic communication and the specialized vocabulary used to convey health information.

Associations with Health Knowledge, Behavior, and Outcomes

Research linking limited health literacy as it is currently measured to health knowledge, health behaviors, and health outcomes is accumulating. Patients with limited health literacy and chronic illness have less knowledge of illness management than those with higher health literacy (Kalichman et al., 2000; Schillinger et al., 2002; Williams et al., 1998a, b). Compared to those with adequate health literacy, patients with limited health literacy have decreased ability to share in decision-making about prostate cancer treatment (Kim et al., 2001), lower adherence to anticoagulation therapy (Lasater, 2003; Win and Schillinger, 2003), higher likelihood of poor glycemic control (Schillinger et al., 2002), and lower self-reported health status (Arnold et al., 2001; Baker et al., 2002; Kalichman and Rompa, 2000; Kalichman et al., 2000; Williams et al., 1998a, b).

Financial Associations of Limited Health Literacy

The limited amount of data available suggests that there is an association between health literacy, health-care utilization, and health-care costs. Baker and others (2002) found that public hospital patients with limited health literacy had higher rates of hospitalization than those with adequate health literacy. This increased hospitalization rate may be associated with greater resource use. Another analysis (Friedland, 1998) concluded that the additional health expenditure attributable to inadequate reading skills (as identified by the NALS) in 1996 was $29 billion. This estimate would increase to $69 billion if as few as half the individuals with marginal reading skills were also not health literate. Weiss and Palmer (2004) reported on a direct measure of cost in a small sample of Medicaid patients in

Arizona. Patients with reading levels at or below third grade had mean Medicaid charges $7,500 higher than those who read above the third grade level.

For this report, David Howard examined the expenditure data collected in association with the Baker and colleagues (2002) utilization study (see Appendix B). He found that predicted inpatient spending for a patient with inadequate health literacy was $993 higher than that of a patient with adequate reading skills. A difference of $450 remained after controlling for health status, although the causality of the associations between health status and health-care cost could not be determined. In both analyses, higher emergency care costs were incurred by individuals with limited health literacy compared to those with marginal or adequate health literacy as measured by the Test of Functional Health Literacy in Adults (TOFHLA), while pharmacy expenses were similar and outpatient expenditures lower.

Although a robust estimate for the effect of limited health literacy on health expenditures is lacking, the magnitudes suggested by the few studies that are available underscore the importance of addressing limited health literacy from a financial perspective.

Finding 3-1   About 90 million adults, an estimate based on the 1992 NALS, have literacy skills that test below high school level (NALS Level 1 and 2). Of these, about 40–44 million (NALS Level 1) have difficulty finding information in unfamiliar or complex texts such as newspaper articles, editorials, medicine labels, forms, or charts. Because the medical and public health literature indicates that health materials are complex and often far above high school level, the committee notes that approximately 90 million adults may lack the needed literacy skills to effectively use the U.S. health system. The majority of these adults are native-born English speakers. Literacy levels are lower among the elderly, those who have lower educational levels, those who are poor, minority populations, and groups with limited English proficiency such as recent immigrants.

Finding 3-2   On the basis of limited studies, public testimony, and committee members' experience, the committee concludes that the shame and stigma associated with limited literacy skills are major barriers to improving health literacy.

Finding 3-3   Adults with limited health literacy, as measured by reading and numeracy skills, have less knowledge of disease management and of health-promoting behaviors, report poorer health status, and are less likely to use preventive services.

Finding 3-4 Two recent studies demonstrate a higher rate of hospitalization and use of emergency services among patients with limited literacy. This higher utilization has been associated with higher health-care costs.

THE CONTEXTS OF HEALTH LITERACY AND OPPORTUNITIES FOR INTERVENTION

Culture and Society

The ho'ola said Mom should confess to me and before God Jehovah. She did. She asked me to forgive her and I did. I wasn't angry. . . . And later Mom's sickness left her. Of course, she still had diabetes, but the rest—being so confused and miserable—all that left her (Shook, 1985: 109).

Culture is the shared ideas, meanings, and values that are acquired by individuals as members of a society. Culture is socially learned, continually evolves, and often influences us unconsciously. We learn culture through interactions with others, as well as through the tangible products of culture such as books and television (IOM, 2002). Culture gives significance to health information and messages, and can shape perceptions and definitions of health and illness, preferences, language and cultural barriers, care process barriers, and stereotypes. These culturally influenced perceptions, definitions, and barriers can affect how people interact with the health care system and help to determine the adequacy of health literacy skills in different settings.

The fluid nature of culture means that health-care encounters are rich with differences that are continuously evolving. Differing cultural and educational backgrounds between patients and providers, as well as between those who create health information and those who use it, may contribute to problems in health literacy. Culture, cultural processes, and cross-cultural interventions have been discussed in depth in several recent IOM reports and represent possible nexuses of culture and health literacy (IOM, 2002, 2003a).

It is important to understand how people obtain and use health information in order to understand the potential impact of health literacy. Information about health is produced by many sources, including the government and the food and drug industries, and is distributed by the popular media. Commercial and social marketing of health information, products, and services is a multibillion dollar industry. People are frequently and repeatedly exposed to quick, often contradictory bits of information. This inundation with information has increased as the Internet has become an increasingly important source of health information. Socioeconomic status, education level, and primary language all affect whether consumers will seek out health information, where they will look for the information, what type of information they prefer, and how they will interpret that information. Limited health literacy decreases the likelihood that health-related information will be accessible to all (Houston and Allison, 2002).

Finding 4-1   Culture gives meaning to health communication. Health literacy must be understood and addressed in the context of culture and language.

Finding 4-2   More than 300 studies indicate that health-related materials far exceed the average reading ability of U.S. adults.

Finding 4-3   Competing sources of health information (including the national media, the Internet, product marketing, health education, and consumer protection) intensify the need for improved health literacy.

Finding 4-4   Health literacy efforts have not yet fully benefited from research findings in social and commercial marketing.

The Educational System

Adult education is an important resource for individuals with limited literacy or limited English proficiency. A major source of support for American adult education programs in literacy is the U.S. adult basic education and literacy (ABEL) system. ABEL programs provide classes in topics that support health literacy including basic literacy and math skills, English language, and high school equivalence, and predominantly serve students with literacy and math skills in NALS Levels 1, 2, or the low end of NALS Level 3. Sadly, these programs serve far fewer than the millions of Americans who could benefit.

Both childhood literacy education and childhood health education can provide a basis for health literacy in adulthood. Although most elementary, middle, and high schools require students to take health education, the sequence of coursework is not coordinated. The percentage of schools that require health education increases from 33 percent in kindergarten to 44 percent in grade 5, but then falls to 10 percent in grade 9, and 2 percent in grade 12. The absence of a coordinated health education program across grade levels may impede student learning of needed health literacy skills. Furthermore, only 9.6 percent of health education classes have a teacher who majored in health education or in combined health and physical education (Kann et al., 2001).

In 1995, the Joint Committee on National Health Standards published the *National Health Education Standards* with the subtitle *Achieving Health Literacy*. These standards describe the knowledge and skills essential for health literacy, and detail what students should know and be able to do in health education by the end of grades 4, 8, and 11. They provide a framework for curricula development and student assessment. Unfortunately, these standards have not been widely met.

Finding 5-1   Significant obstacles and barriers to successful health literacy education exist in K-12 education programs.

Finding 5-2   Opportunities for measuring literacy skill levels required for health knowledge and skills, and for the implementation of programs to increase learner's skill levels, currently exist in adult education programs and provide promising models for expanding programs. Studies indicate a desire on the part of adult learners and adult education programs to form partnerships with health communities.

Finding 5-3   Health professionals and staff have limited education, training, continuing education, and practice opportunities to develop skills for improving health literacy.

Health Systems

Health systems in the United States are complex and often confusing. Their complexity derives from the nature of health care and public health itself, the mix of public and private financing, and the variations across states and between types of delivery settings. An adult's ability to navigate these systems may reflect this systemic complexity in addition to individual skill levels. Even highly skilled individuals may find the systems too complicated to understand, especially when these individuals are made more vulnerable by poor health. Directions, signs, and official documents, including informed consent forms, social services forms, public health information, medical instructions, and health education materials, often use jargon and technical language that make them unnecessarily difficult to use (Rudd et al., 2000b). In addition, cultural differences may affect perceptions of health, illness, prevention, and health care. Lack of mutual understanding of health, illness and treatments, and risks and benefits has implications for behavior for both providers and consumers, and legal implications for providers and health systems. Imagine having to face this complexity if you are one of the 90 million American adults who lack the functional literacy skills in English to use the U.S. health care system.[2]

Health literacy permeates all areas of the provider–consumer information exchange, and provides a common pathway for the successful transfer of information. A number of emerging areas are likely to increase the burden of limited health literacy on those entering and using the health-care system. These include demands inherent in chronic disease management, increased use of new technologies, decreased time for patient/provider discussions, and legal and regulatory requirements.

Many different interventions and approaches that may hold promise for addressing limited health literacy are being attempted across health-care systems, professional organizations, federal and state agencies, educational institutions, and community and advocacy groups across the United States and in other countries. Those profiled in the report are indicators of the creativity and promise for future improvements in countering the effects of limited health literacy. However, few of these approaches have been formally evaluated, and most are fragmented single approaches rather than part of a systematic approach to health literacy. In order for progress to be made, many more systematic demonstrations must be funded and rigorously evaluated.

Finding 6-1   Demands for reading, writing, and numeracy skills are intensified due to health-care systems' complexities, advancements in scientific discoveries, and new technologies. These demands exceed the health-literacy skills of most adults in the United States.

Finding 6-2   Health literacy is fundamental to quality care, and relates to three of the six aims of quality improvement described in the IOM Quality Chasm Report: safety, patient-centered care, and equitable treatment. Self-management and health literacy have been identified by IOM as cross-cutting priorities for health-care quality and disease prevention.

Finding 6-3   The readability levels of informed consent documents (for research and clinical practice) exceed the documented average reading levels of the majority of adults in the United States. This has important ethical and legal implications that have not been fully explored.

VISION FOR A HEALTH-LITERATE AMERICA

The evidence and judgment presented in this report indicate that heath literacy is important to improving the health of individuals and popula-

---

[2]See Finding 3-1.

tions. This is supported by the conclusions and statements of others. Health literacy was one of two cross-cutting factors that affect health care identified by the IOM in its recent report *Priority Areas for National Action in Quality Improvement* (IOM, 2003b). The Surgeon General recently stated that "health literacy can save lives, save money, and improve the health and well being of millions of Americans . . . health literacy is the currency of success for everything I am doing as Surgeon General" (Carmona, 2003).

More needs to be known about the causal pathways between education and health, the role of literacy, and the discrete contribution of health literacy to health. With this knowledge we will be able to understand which interventions and approaches are the most appropriate and effective. This Committee believes that a health-literate America is an achievable goal. We envision a society within which people have the skills they need to obtain, interpret, and use health information appropriately and in meaningful ways. We envision a society in which a variety of health systems structures and institutions take responsibility for providing clear communication and adequate support to facilitate health-promoting actions based on understanding. We believe a health-literate America would be a society in which:

- Everyone has the opportunity to improve their health literacy.
- Everyone has the opportunity to use reliable, understandable information that could make a difference in their overall well-being, including everyday behaviors such as how they eat, whether they exercise, and whether they get checkups.
- Health and science content would be basic parts of K-12 curricula.
- People are able to accurately assess the credibility of health information presented by health advocate, commercial, and new media sources.
- There is monitoring and accountability for health literacy policies and practices.
- Public health alerts, vital to the health of the nation, are presented in everyday terms so that people can take needed action.
- The cultural contexts of diverse peoples, including those from various cultural groups and non-English-speaking peoples, are integrated in to all health information.
- Health practitioners communicate clearly during all interactions with their patients, using everyday vocabulary.
- There is ample time for discussions between patients and health-care providers.
- Patients feel free and comfortable to ask questions as part of the healing relationship.
- Rights and responsibilities in relation to health and health care are presented or written in clear, everyday terms so that people can take needed action.

•   Informed consent documents used in health care are developed so that all people can give or withhold consent based on information they need and understand.

While achieving this vision is a profound challenge, we believe that significant progress can and must be made over the coming years, so that the potential for optimal health can benefit all individuals and populations in our society.

Recommendation 2-1   The Department of Health and Human Services and other government and private funders should support research leading to the development of causal models explaining the relationships among health literacy, the education system, the health system, and relevant social and cultural systems.

Recommendation 2-2   The Department of Health and Human Services and public and private funders should support the development, testing, and use of culturally appropriate new measures of health literacy. Such measures should be developed for large ongoing population surveys, such as the National Assessment of Adult Literacy Survey, Medical Expenditure Panel Survey, and Behavioral Risk Factor Surveillance System, and the Medicare Beneficiaries Survey, as well as for institutional accreditation and quality assessment activities such as those carried out by the Joint Commission on Accreditation of Healthcare Organizations and the National Committee for Quality Assurance. Initially, the National Institutes of Health should convene a national consensus conference to initiate the development of operational measures of health literacy which would include contextual measures.

Recommendation 3-1   Given the compelling evidence noted above, funding for health literacy research is urgently needed. The Department of Health and Human Services, especially the National Institutes of Health, Agency for Healthcare Research and Quality, Health Resources and Services Administration, the Centers for Disease Control and Prevention, Department of Defense, Veterans Administration, and other public and private funding agencies should support multidisciplinary research on the extent, associations, and consequences of limited health literacy, including studies on health service utilization and expenditures.

Recommendation 4-1   Federal agencies responsible for addressing disparities should support the development of conceptual frameworks on the intersection of culture and health literacy to direct in-depth theoretical explorations and formulate the conceptual underpinnings that can guide interventions.
  4-1.a   The National Institutes of Health should convene a consensus conference, including stakeholders, to develop methodology for the incorporation of health literacy improvement into approaches to health disparities.
  4-1.b   The Office of Minority Health and Agency for Healthcare Research and Quality should develop measures of the relationships between culture, language, cultural competency, and health literacy to be used in studies of the relationship between health literacy and health outcomes.

Recommendation 4-2 The Agency for Healthcare Research and Quality, the Centers for Disease Control and Prevention, the Indian Health Service, the Health Resources and Services Administration, and the Substance Abuse and Mental Health Services Administration should develop and test approaches to improve health communication that foster healing relationships across culturally diverse populations. This includes investigations that explore the effect of existing and innovative communication approaches on health behaviors, and studies that examine the impact of participatory action and empowerment research strategies for effective penetration of health information at the community level.

Recommendation 5-1 Accreditation requirements for all public and private educational institutions should require the implementation of the National Health Education Standards.

Recommendation 5-2 Educators should take advantage of the opportunity provided by existing reading, writing, reading, oral language skills, and mathematics curricula to incorporate health-related tasks, materials, and examples into existing lesson plans.

Recommendation 5-3 The Health Resources and Services Administration and the Centers for Disease Control and Prevention, in collaboration with the Department of Education, should fund demonstration projects in each state to attain the National Health Education Standards and to meet basic literacy requirements as they apply to health literacy.

Recommendation 5-4 The Department of Education in association with the Department of Health and Human Services should convene task forces comprised of appropriate education, health, and public policy experts to delineate specific, feasible, and effective actions relevant agencies could take to improve health literacy through the nation's K-12 schools, 2-year and 4-year colleges and universities, and adult and vocational education.

Recommendation 5-5 The National Science Foundation, the Department of Education, and the National Institute of Child Health and Human Development should fund research designed to assess the effectiveness of different models of combining health literacy with basic literacy and instruction. The Interagency Education Research Initiative, a federal partnership of these three agencies, should lead this effort to the fullest extent possible.

Recommendation 5-6 Professional schools and professional continuing education programs in health and related fields, including medicine, dentistry, pharmacy, social work, anthropology, nursing, public health, and journalism, should incorporate health literacy into their curricula and areas of competence.

Recommendation 6-1 Health care systems, including private systems, Medicare, Medicaid, the Department of Defense, and the Veterans Administration should develop and support demonstration programs to establish the most effec-

Continued

tive approaches to reducing the negative effects of limited health literacy. To accomplish this, these organizations should:

- Engage consumers in the development of health communications and infuse insights gained from them into health messages.
- Explore creative approaches to communicate health information using printed and electronic materials and media in appropriate and clear language. Messages must be appropriately translated and interpreted for diverse audiences.
- Establish methods for creating health information content in appropriate and clear language using relevant translations of health information.
- Include cultural and linguistic competency as an essential measure of quality of care.

Recommendation 6-2 The Department of Health and Human Services should fund research to define the needed health literacy tasks and skills for each of the priority areas for improvement in health care quality. Funding priorities should include participatory research which engages the intended populations.

Recommendation 6-3 Health iteracy assessment should be a part of healthcare information systems and quality data collection. Public and private accreditation bodies, including Medicare, the National Committee for Quality Assurance, and the Joint Commission on Accreditation of Healthcare Organizations should clearly incorporate health literacy into their accreditation standards.

Recommendation 6-4 The Department of Health and Human Services should take the lead in developing uniform standards for addressing health literacy in research applications. This includes addressing the appropriateness of research design and methods and the match among the readability of instruments, the literacy level, and the cultural and linguistic needs of study participants. In order to achieve meaningful research outcomes in all fields:

- Investigators should involve patients (or subjects) in the research process to ensure that methods and instrumentation are valid and reliable and in a language easily understood.
- The National Institutes of Health should collaborate with appropriate federal agencies and institutional review boards to formulate the policies and criteria to ensure that appropriate consideration of literacy is an integral part of the approval of research involving human subjects.
- The National Institutes of Health should take literacy levels into account when considering informed consent in human subjects research. Institutional Review Boards should meet existing standards related to the readability of informed consent documents.

REFERENCES

Arnold CL, Davis TC, Berkel HJ, Jackson RH, Nandy I, London S. 2001. Smoking status, reading level, and knowledge of tobacco effects among low-income pregnant women. *Preventive Medicine.* 32(4): 313–320.

Baker DW, Parker RM, Williams MV, Pitkin K, Parikh NS, Coates W, Imara M. 1996. The health care experience of patients with low literacy. *Archives of Family Medicine.* 5(6): 329–334.

Baker DW, Gazmararian JA, Williams MV, Scott T, Parker RM, Green D, Ren J, Peel J. 2002. Functional health literacy and the risk of hospital admission among Medicare managed care enrollees. *American Journal of Public Health.* 92(8): 1278–1283.

Beers BB, McDonald VJ, Quistberg DA, Ravenell KL, Asch DA, Shea JA. 2003. Disparities in health literacy between African American and non-African American primary care patients. Abstract. *Journal of General Internal Medicine.* 18(Supplement 1): 169.

Carmona RH. 2003. *Health Literacy in America: The Role of Health Care Professionals.* Prepared Remarks given at the American Medical Association House of Delegates Meeting. Saturday, June 14, 2003. [Online]. Available: http://www.surgeongeneral.gov/news/speeches/ama061403.htm [accessed: August, 2003].

Doak LG, Doak CC, Meade CD. 1996. Strategies to improve cancer education materials. *Oncology Nursing Forum.* 23(8): 1305–1312.

Friedland R. 1998. New estimates of the high costs of inadequate health literacy. In: *Proceedings of Pfizer Conference "Promoting Health Literacy: A Call to Action."* October 7–8, 1998, Washington, DC: Pfizer, Inc. Pp. 6–10.

Gazmararian JA, Baker DW, Williams MV, Parker RM, Scott T, Greemn DCFSN, Ren J, Koplan JP. 1999. Health literacy among Medicare enrollees in a managed care organization. *Journal of the American Medical Association.* 281(6): 545–551.

HHS (U.S. Department of Health and Human Services). 2000. *Healthy People 2010: Understanding and Improving Health.* Washington, DC: U.S. Department of Health and Human Services.

Houston TK, Allison JJ. 2002. Users of Internet health information: Differences by health status. *Journal of Medical Internet Research.* 4(2): E7.

IOM (Institute of Medicine). 2002. *Speaking of Health: Assessing Health Communication Strategies for Diverse Populations.* Washington, DC: The National Academies Press.

IOM (Institute of Medicine). 2003a. *Unequal Treatment: Confronting Racial and Ethnic Disparities in Health Care.* Smedley BD, Stith AY, Nelson AR, Editors. Washington, DC: The National Academies Press.

IOM (Institute of Medicine). 2003b. *Priority Areas for National Action: Transforming Healthcare Quality.* Adams K, Corrigan JM, Editors. Washington, DC: The National Academies Press.

Kalichman SC, Rompa D. 2000. Functional health literacy is associated with health status and health-related knowledge in people living with HIV-AIDS. *Journal of Acquired Immune Deficiency Syndromes and Human Retrovirology.* 25(4): 337–344.

Kalichman SC, Benotsch E, Suarez T, Catz S, Miller J, Rompa D. 2000. Health literacy and health-related knowledge among persons living with HIV/AIDS. *American Journal of Preventive Medicine.* 18(4): 325–331.

Kann L, Brener ND, Allensworth DD. 2001. Health education: Results from the School Health Policies and Programs Study 2000. *Journal of School Health.* 71(7): 266–278.

Kim SP, Knight SJ, Tomori C, Colella KM, Schoor RA, Shih L, Kuzel TM, Nadler RB, Bennett CL. 2001. Health literacy and shared decision making for prostate cancer patients with low socioeconomic status. *Cancer Investigation.* 19(7): 684–691.

Kirsch IS. 2001. *The International Adult Literacy Survey (IALS): Understanding What Was Measured.* Princeton, NJ: Educational Testing Service.

Kirsch IS, Jungeblut A, Jenkins L, Kolstad A. 1993. *Adult Literacy in America: A First Look at the Results of the National Adult Literacy Survey (NALS)*. Washington, DC: National Center for Education Statistics, U.S. Department of Education.

Lasater L. 2003. Patient literacy, adherence, and anticoagulation therapy outcomes: A preliminary report. Abstract. *Journal of General Internal Medicine*. 18(Supplement 1): 179.

National Center for the Study of Adult Learning and Literacy. (Harvard School of Public Health, Department of Society, Human Development and Health). 2003. *Voices from Experience*. [Online]. Available: http://www.hsph.harvard.edu/healthliteracy/voices.html [accessed: December 4, 2003].

Parikh NS, Parker RM, Nurss JR, Baker DW, Williams MV. 1996. Shame and health literacy: The unspoken connection. *Patient Education and Counseling*. 27(1): 33–39.

Parker RM, Ratzan SC, Lurie N. 2003. Health literacy: A policy challenge for advancing high-quality health care. *Health Affairs*. 22(4): 147.

Ratzan SC, Parker RM. 2000. Introduction. In: *National Library of Medicine Current Bibliographies in Medicine: Health Literacy*. NLM Pub. No. CBM 2000-1. Selden CR, Zorn M, Ratzan SC, Parker RM, Editors. Bethesda, MD: National Institutes of Health, U.S. Department of Health and Human Services.

Rudd R, Moeykens BA, Colton TC. 2000a. Health and literacy. A review of medical and public health literature. In: *Annual Review of Adult Learning and Literacy*. Comings J, Garners B, Smith C, Editors. New York: Jossey-Bass.

Rudd RE, Colton T, Schacht R. 2000b. *An Overview of Medical and Public Health Literature Addressing Literacy Issues: An Annotated Bibliography*. Report #14. Cambridge, MA: National Center for the Study of Adult Learning and Literacy.

Schillinger D, Grumbach K, Piette J, Wang F, Osmond D, Daher C, Palacios J, Sullivan GaD, Bindman AB. 2002. Association of health literacy with diabetes outcomes. *Journal of the American Medical Association*. 288(4): 475–482.

Selden CR, Zorn M, Ratzan SC, Parker RM. 2000. *National Library of Medicine Current Bibliographies in Medicine: Health Literacy*. NLM Pub. No. CBM 2000-1. Bethesda, MD: National Institutes of Health, U.S. Department of Health and Human Services.

Shook EV. 1985. *Ho'oponopono: Contemporary Uses of a Hawaiian Problem-Solving Process*. Honolulu, HI: East-West Center, University of Hawaii Press.

Weiss BD, Palmer R. 2004. Relationship between health care costs and very low literacy skills in a medically needy and indigent Medicaid population. *Journal of the American Board of Family Practice*. 17(1): 44–47.

Williams MV, Parker RM, Baker DW, Parikh NS, Pitkin K, Coates WC, Nurss JR. 1995. Inadequate functional health literacy among patients at two public hospitals. *Journal of the American Medical Association*. 274(21): 1677–1682.

Williams MV, Baker DW, Honig EG, Lee TM, Nowlan A. 1998a. Inadequate literacy is a barrier to asthma knowledge and self-care. *Chest*. 114(4): 1008–1015.

Williams MV, Baker DW, Parker RM, Nurss JR. 1998b. Relationship of functional health literacy to patients' knowledge of their chronic disease. A study of patients with hypertension and diabetes. *Archives of Internal Medicine*. 158(2): 166–172.

Win K, Schillinger D. 2003. Understanding of warfarin therapy and stroke among ethnically diverse anticoagulation patients at a public hospital. Abstract. *Journal of General Internal Medicine*. 18(Supplement 1): 278.

1

Introduction

A two-year-old is diagnosed with an inner ear infection and prescribed an antibiotic. Her mother understands that her daughter should take the prescribed medication twice a day. After carefully studying the label on the bottle and deciding that it doesn't tell how to take the medicine, she fills a teaspoon and pours the antibiotic into her daughter's painful ear (Parker et al., 2003).

Health consumers face numerous challenges as they seek health information, including the complexity of the health systems, the rising burden of chronic disease, the need to engage as partners in their care, and the proliferation of consumer information available from numerous and diverse sources. Individuals are asked to assume new roles in seeking information, advocating for their rights and privacy, understanding responsibilities, measuring and monitoring their own health and that of their community, and making decisions about insurance and options for care. Underlying these complex demands are the varying and sometimes inadequate levels of, first, consumer knowledge and, second, skills for using and applying a wide range of health information.

In their work, health care educators and providers make assumptions about an individual's ability to comprehend health information. However over 300 studies have shown that health information cannot be understood by most of the people for whom it was intended, suggesting that the assumptions regarding the recipient's level of health literacy made by the creators of this information are often incorrect. Over the past decade, concerns related to literacy skills and health provided a wake-up call to many in the health fields. *Health literacy*, a newly emerging field of inquiry and practice, focuses on literacy concerns within the context of health. The committee defines health literacy as "the degree to which individuals have the capacity to obtain, process, and understand basic health information and services needed to make appropriate health decisions" (Ratzan and Parker, 2000), and views health literacy as a shared function of social and individual factors. This chapter will provide an overview of health literacy and this report in a broad societal context; please refer to Chapter 2 for an in-depth discussion of the definition and conceptual basis of health literacy.

SOCIAL AND ECONOMIC FACTORS AND HEALTH

Epidemiologists have been able to document links between socioeconomic status and health, and links between educational attainment and health. A 1998 report from the U.S. Department of Health and Human Services offered evidence from accumulated studies that health, morbidity, and mortality are related to income and education factors (Pamuk et al., 1998). For example, life expectancy is related to family income. So too are death rates from cancer and heart disease, incidences of diabetes and hypertension, and use of health services. Similarly, death rates for chronic disease, communicable diseases, and injuries as reported in 1998 were inversely related to education: those with lower education achievement are more likely to die of a chronic disease than are those with higher education achievement. In essence, the lower your income or educational achievement, the worse your health.

Some researchers have suggested that education provides a key to understanding these relationships. Grossman and Kaestner (1997) asserted that "Years of formal schooling completed is the most important correlate of good health." House and colleagues (1994) noted that "A causal impact of education on health is highly plausible." However, research has not yet fully examined other aspects or measures of education beyond years in school such as knowledge and skills. Literacy is one set of skills related to education. National literacy assessments indicate that literacy is a set of measurable skills (Kirsch, 2001) that includes reading, writing, listening, speaking, and arithmetical skills. Chapter 3 discusses the research that exists on the relationship between literacy and health.

Culture and ethnicity also influence health, and Chapter 4 of this report includes a discussion of their relationship with health literacy. Culture and ethnicity are often blended into categories of race which may not represent scientifically sound classifications. As discussed in a recent Institute of Medicine (IOM) report, *Speaking of Health* (IOM, 2002), race is not a meaningful biological classification system for human populations, and even ethnicity can be interpreted too rigidly. This IOM report drew on current anthropological thinking to suggest that both individuals and populations should be assessed in terms of the influences on their lives and cultural histories, or "experiential identity." This experiential identity may include influences from multiple cultures and languages, sometimes within the same family, but more often from life experiences. People's knowledge and understanding of their health, and their health literacy, are based on a composite of these life experiences. In this report, the terms race and ethnicity will be used in the discussions of population studies.

LIVING IN A SOCIETY WITH HIGH LITERACY DEMANDS

Every day, millions of adults must make decisions and take actions on issues that protect not only their own well-being, but also that of their family members and communities. These actions are not confined to traditional health-care settings such as doctors and dentists' offices, hospitals, and clinics. They take place in homes, at work, in schools, and in community forums across the country. Health-related activities are part of the daily life of adults, whether they are sick or well.

At home, parents may have to calculate a child's weight and age to determine the correct dosage of an over-the-counter medicine. People are also expected to follow directions from health-care providers, presented verbally or in writing, during recovery from an illness or the management of a chronic disease. At work, employees may need to determine correct workstation placement or safe use of toxic chemicals. Safety warnings are posted in the community, and at work, and are discussed in newspapers and on television. Many health-related decisions are made in the marketplace. When reading nutritional information on food labels, for example, consumers are expected to understand that calculation of sugar content must include the sugar listed on the snack food label as well as the fructose and corn syrup. In the pharmacy, consumers must differentiate between a cough syrup that is an expectorant and one that is a suppressor.

Examples of language taken from actual product and warning labels

- *Topical antiseptic bactericide/viricide for degerming skin and mucus membranes*
- *Non-potable water*
- *Notify appropriate authorities*

In medical care settings, health-care providers expect patients to provide accurate health histories and descriptions of their symptoms, as well as listen to and comprehend verbal instructions (Roter et al., 1998).

> Sometimes the doctors and pharmacy use the type of words that are sometimes hard. I mean sometimes there's some word that, it's there, but you don't know what it means. They are using those fine words, those college words, that are hard for people like me to understand and read (Rudd and DeJong, 2000).

Adults need to meet the demands of bureaucracies and institutions to access health programs and services. For example, adults are asked to fill out insurance forms, understand their rights and responsibilities, provide medical history, and provide informed consent for medical procedures. The documents required for some of these activities often contain legal and scientific terms unfamiliar to many individuals.

Signs and directions posted for employees and visitors outside and within institutions are often inadequate. As Baker and colleagues noted in a study based on patient focus groups at two public hospitals, many of the patients did not benefit from signs indicating that the nephrology unit was straight ahead. The nephrologists, however, most likely knew where to go (Baker et al., 1996; Rudd, 2002).

An inability to speak English at all or an ability to speak with only limited proficiency presents additional obstacles to understanding health information and accessing health care. These obstacles are compounded when written translations and trained translators are not available (Carrasquillo et al., 1999; Flores et al., 2003; IOM, 2003a; Sarver and Baker, 2000).

> When I started six months ago, it was a new job and it was transporting patients. So we got a dispatcher. We had to call back to the floor and get the orders where to take the patients. I went looking for about 30 minutes. The patient and I were lost (Rudd and DeJong, 2000).

The presentation of health information is often unnecessarily complex. Findings from three decades of early medical and public health studies examining the reading level of print materials developed for patient education and for procedures and processes in the health-care setting (Rudd et al., 2000) established that most health materials fall into reading level ranges requiring high school, college, or graduate degrees. Overall, the literacy demands of health materials exceeded the reading abilities of the average American adult.

In addition, the language typically used by those working in health and medicine is filled with scientific jargon. This increases the difficulty for the average consumer. References are made to biological systems (e.g., endocrine) and anatomy (e.g., atrial valve) as well as to groupings of diseases and disorders (e.g., renal, cardiovascular, neurological, respiratory) that are not typically used in everyday conversation. Furthermore, they are scientific terms not typically taught in the K-12 school system. For example, many people do not know that they have bronchi or where they are located; yet those with asthma will be presented with the very critical information that this chronic disease involves inflammation of the bronchi and that a particular type of medicine helps. A person's ability to understand health, medical issues, and directions is related to the clarity of the communication.

After being diagnosed with recurrent aphthous stomatitis involving the epithelium of the buccal mucosa, Winston did what he thought was necessary.

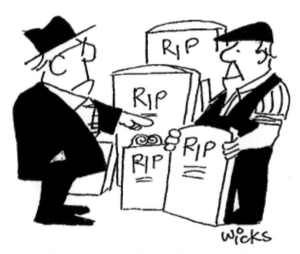

Which is a funny thing to do for a canker.

SOURCE: Canadian Public Health Association, Plain Language Service. Reprinted with permission.

Of course, literacy demands differ by setting and by circumstance. The types of health information a person is exposed to changes as a person's life changes. Sociological and anthropological research has documented that literacy practices are inextricably intertwined and shaped by life circumstances (Barton and Hamilton, 1998; Purcell-Gates et al., 2000; Street,

2001). For example, a woman is more likely to receive information about hormone replacement therapy after menopause rather than when she is a teenager. Purcell-Gates documented how literacy demands changed in the lives of adult education students because of life events such as a new living situation or a change in a family member's health. For example, the adults in this study reported that new health literacy demands arose with the birth of their children. They were required to fill out health history forms, maintain vaccination records, and keep track of their children's appointments with health-care workers. They needed to read and understand dosage instructions on over-the-counter and prescription medications for their infants. They were required to install car seats by following printed directions. Those with school-aged children needed to read and sign materials sent home from school related, for example, to lunch programs or field trips.

Changes in their own or a family member's health were often reported as initiating a change in literacy practice. A commonly reported change was the beginning of, or increase in, reading associated with medicines: print on medicine bottles, prescriptions, and directions from doctors. Many reported a need to read the print on food containers for the first time as part of the vigilance required in managing a chronic illness like diabetes. Following a health change that necessitated repeated doctor visits, people found and read medical reference books, and began to use personal calendars and appointment books (Purcell-Gates et al., 2000).

Demands on an individual's literacy skills can create a barrier to the use and understanding of health tools and information. In many ways, literacy serves as a social determinant of health when a mismatch exists between the skills of the individual and the literacy skill demands of the health context. Poor communication, whether it be based on faulty assumptions, inappropriate language, incomplete disclosures, or hidden confusion, does a disservice to clients as well as to health-care professionals. When words get in the way, the communication process fails, leading to confusion, loss of dignity, and unhealthful outcomes.

Another result of this failure of communication is that limited health literacy is often undetected, in part because individuals with limited literacy skills may feel ashamed. People may not be at ease acknowledging reading difficulties or vocabulary limitations. Consequently, they may feel shame or mask these difficulties in order to maintain dignity (Baker et al., 1996; Parikh et al., 1996).

Identifying the extent of limited health literacy is also problematic because individuals tend not to tell their health-care providers about literacy problems that they encounter in the increasingly complex health system, including trouble understanding both printed materials and the meaning of discussions with providers. Also of concern is the possibility that people may perceive their skills to be adequate when they are not. For example, data from the 1992 National Adult Literacy Survey (NALS) show that among those scoring in the lowest level on the prose literacy scale, only 29 percent reported they did not read well and only 34 percent reported they did not write well. The majority of those performing at this level perceive their reading and writing skills to be adequate. Among those in the next highest level the results were even more surprising, as only 3 percent said they couldn't read well and 6 percent said they couldn't write well (Kirsch et al., 1993; see Chapter 2 for more information on the NALS).

To Err Is Human: Building a Safer Health System is a widely publicized IOM study on the quality of health care that examined factors to medical errors (IOM, 2000). One study cited in this report found that 10 percent of adverse drug events were linked to errors in the use of the drug as a result of communication failure (Leape et al., 1993). The report noted that management of complex drug therapies, especially in elderly patients, is extremely difficult and requires special attention to the ability of the patient to understand and remember the amount and timing of dose, as well as behavioral modifications required by the regimen (e.g., dietary restrictions) (IOM, 2000). The ability of patients and consumers to manage their own health and medical care can be improved through better provider–patient communication and greater inclusion of the patient in treatment decisions, as discussed in Chapter 6 (Hausman, 2001; Hayes-Bautista, 1976; Hulka et al., 1975, 1976; Miller, 1975; Snyder et al., 1976).

HEALTH LITERACY AS A PUBLIC CONCERN

In its report Healthy People 2010, the U.S. Department of Health and Human Services included improved consumer health literacy as Objective 11-2, and identified health literacy as an important component of health communication, medical product safety, and oral health (HHS, 2000). The importance of health literacy has also been recognized globally. The World Health Organization has included health literacy as a key factor in health promotion (WHO, 2000), and the U.S. Agency for International Development (U.S. AID) has recognized health literacy as an important contributor in the move towards a healthier society (U.S. Agency for International Development, 2001). Much of the pioneering work in health literacy arose from the fields of health education and health communication in the 1970s and 1980s (Rudd et al., 2000).

Health literacy is intimately linked to many issues of critical importance to the nation and to our health policies. The public health mandate of protecting the health of the nation relies on communication strategies for issues as different as obesity and bioterrorism. Health literacy is of concern to people addressing worker health and safety, product labeling, environmental health, patient rights and responsibilities, quality of care, or access to information, insurance, and services (Hausman, 2001; Hayes-Bautista, 1976; Hulka et al., 1975, 1976; Rudd et al., 2003; Snyder et al., 1976).

Crossing the Quality Chasm: A New Health System for the 21st Century (IOM, 2001) proposed a reorganization of the complex health system practices that decrease patient safety. The report stressed that the "patient-centered" approach should be implemented to ensure that patients have a full understanding of all of their options (IOM, 2001). Limited health literacy is often unreported by patients, unappreciated by policy makers and health-care workers, and unappreciated by the general public. Without improvements in health literacy, the promise of many scientific advances to improve health outcomes will be diminished. Consequently, the IOM has identified improving health literacy as one of two cross-cutting issues in health care needing attention in its recent report, *Priority Areas for National Action: Transforming Healthcare Quality* (IOM, 2003b). This report called for increased attention to culturally and socially sensitive communication to improve the overall quality of health care and the health of minority and lower-income patients.

CHARGE TO THE COMMITTEE

Although a greater appreciation for the potential consequences of limited health literacy has been developing over recent years, the health field has lacked a comprehensive yet concise summary of what is known about health literacy and what needs to be done. Watters (2003) suggests that an interdisciplinary literacy model that addresses health, literacy, and culture could successfully guide development, diffusion, and adoption of appropriate information.

In 2002 the IOM convened the Committee on Health Literacy for a project sponsored by the American Association of Family Physicians Foundation, the California HealthCare Foundation, the Commonwealth fund, the Kellogg Foundation, the Metlife Foundation, the National Cancer Institute, the Pfizer Corporation, and the Robert Wood Johnson Foundation. Committee membership included individuals with expertise in public health, primary medical care, health communication, sociology, nursing, anthropology, adult literacy education, and K-12 education. As reflected by the composition of the committee, many academic fields can inform health literacy inquiries, and have contributed to our understanding of the area. The committee was carefully selected to ensure that it possessed appropriate expertise for assessing past efforts to promote health literacy and for providing options to overcome the obstacles to health literacy in future endeavors. Furthermore, the committee represents a balance of intellectual perspectives and experiences, ranging from practical experience in promoting health literacy to research and theoretical experience in the closely related fields such as anthropology, psychology, and education. The chair brought to the study experience with health-care systems and population health determinants as well as with committee processes. For further information regarding the backgrounds of the members of the committee, the reader is directed to the short biographies presented in Appendix D. The committee was asked to assess the problem of health literacy and come to consensus on the next steps, addressing the following charge:

- Define the scope of the problem of health literacy. The intent is to clarify the root problems that underlie health illiteracy. This would include identifying affected populations and estimating the costs for society. Develop a set of basic indicators of health literacy to allow assessment of the extent of the problem at the individual, community, and national levels.
- Identify the obstacles to a creating a health-literate public. These are likely to include the complexity of the health-care system, the many and often-contradictory health messages, rapidly advancing technologies, limits within public education to promote literacy of adults as well as children, etc.
- Assess the approaches that have been attempted to increase health literacy both in the United States and abroad. Identify the gaps in research and programs that need to be addressed. The focus should be on public health interventions attempting to increase health literacy of the public as well as on improving health provider/primary care interactions. Identify activities that could improve health literacy with special attention to Medicaid and Medicare patients.
- Identify goals for health literacy efforts and suggest approaches for overcoming obstacles to health literacy in order to reach these goals. Approaches might include research or policy initiatives, interventions, or collaborations that would promote health literacy.

SCOPE OF THE REPORT

This report explores what is known about the epidemiology of limited health literacy and promising approaches for increasing health literacy. It offers a conceptual framework for thinking about how society, culture, and the health and education systems contribute to the problem and to possible solutions. Throughout, the report seeks to put a human face on the problem of limited health literacy. Each chapter aims to provide new directions and blend knowledge from divergent areas of inquiry. Overarching recommendations are presented at the end of the report.

Chapter 2 clarifies the concept of health literacy by discussing its definition and delineating literacy and functional literacy within the context of health. A conceptual model of health literacy is presented with a visual framework that makes clear that health literacy is a function of the interaction between individuals and the health contexts to which they are exposed. In addition, the committee outlines limitations to the conceptualization and measures of health literacy. By these means, the strengths and weaknesses of existing measures of literacy and health literacy are examined, with a view toward continued development of health literacy assessment, including population indicators and measures of health literacy within health systems.

Although the charge to the committee included the development of a set of basic indicators of health literacy, the committee determined that to do so within the context and limitations of the current knowledge and available measures would be premature and inappropriate. Development of population-level public health indicators cannot precede the development of adequate individual-level measures. The committee limited its findings and recommendations to suggestions that could promote the development of improved measures and new basic indicators of health literacy, rather than developing the indicators themselves. The committee hopes that future research will enable the development of these indicators.

Chapter 3 reviews the extent and associations of limited health literacy as currently measured, exploring the broad social effect of disparities between health literacy needs and demands. This chapter provides insight into the relationship of the health consumer and health literacy. Current research related to the associations of limited health literacy is summarized, both in terms of individual health behaviors and outcomes, and in terms of the financial, legal, and regulatory consequences in health contexts. This chapter contains extensive tables on the epidemiology of health literacy skills in various populations and the characteristics and associations of limited health literacy.

Chapter 4 explores the web of culture and health literacy, and how these encompass patient perspectives and quality of care, with attention to clinical uncertainty, patient safety, and the building of health literacy into standard health care. The interrelationships among culture, language and meaning, and health literacy measures are discussed as well as culturally based approaches to improving health literacy.

Chapter 5 explores health literacy within the context of educational systems and seeks to understand the roles that K-12, university, adult, and health professional education systems can take to improve health literacy. In particular, the chapter addresses difficulties encountered by educators in the K-12 system, and explores possible approaches to improving health literacy by integrating health into curricula.

Chapter 6 discusses health literacy within the context of the health-care system, including providers, insurers, administrators, national agencies that guide health policy, and others. Current issues facing health care are discussed as they relate to health literacy. The chapter also reviews various types of approaches that may help to address the problem of limited health literacy when applied in health care settings.

Chapter 7 presents the committee's vision for a health literate society.

REFERENCES

Baker DW, Parker RM, Williams MV, Pitkin K, Parikh NS, Coates W, Imara M. 1996. The health care experience of patients with low literacy. *Archives of Family Medicine.* 5(6): 329–334.

Barton D, Hamilton M. 1998. *Local Literacies: Reading and Writing in One Community.* New York: Routledge.

Carrasquillo O, Orav EJ, Brennan TA, Burstin HR. 1999. Impact of language barriers on patient satisfaction in an emergency department. *Journal of General Internal Medicine.* 14(2): 82–87.

Flores G, Laws MB, Mayo SJ, Zuckerman B, Abreu M, Medina L, Hardt EJ. 2003. Errors in medical interpretation and their potential clinical consequences in pediatric encounters. *Pediatrics.* 111(1): 6–14.

Grossman M, Kaestner R. 1997. The effects of education on health. In: *The Social Benefits of Education.* Behermean R, Stacey N, Editors. Ann Arbor, MI: University of Michigan Press. Pp. 69–123.

Hausman A. 2001. Taking your medicine: Relational steps to improving patient compliance. *Health Marketing Quarterly.* 19(2): 49–71.

Hayes-Bautista DE. 1976. Modifying the treatment: Patient compliance, patient control and medical care. *Social Science & Medicine.* 10(5): 233–238.

HHS (U.S. Department of Health and Human Services). 2000. *Healthy People 2010: Understanding and Improving Health.* Washington, DC: U.S. Department of Health and Human Services.

House JS, Lepkowski JM, Kinney AM, Mero RP, Kessler RC, Herzog AR. 1994. The social stratification of aging and health. *Journal of Health & Social Behavior.* 35: 213–234.

Hulka BS, Kupper LL, Cassel JC, Mayo F. 1975. Doctor-patient communication and outcomes among diabetic patients. *Journal of Community Health.* 1(1): 15–27.

Hulka BS, Cassel JC, Kupper LL, Burdette JA. 1976. Communication, compliance, and concordance between physicians and patients with prescribed medications. *American Journal of Public Health.* 66(9): 847–853.

IOM (Institute of Medicine). 2000. *To Err Is Human: Building a Safer Health System.* Washington, DC: National Academy Press.

IOM. 2001. *Crossing the Quality Chasm: A New Health System for the 21st Century.* Washington, DC: National Academy Press.

IOM. 2002. *Speaking of Health: Assessing Health Communication Strategies for Diverse Populations.* Washington, DC: The National Academies Press.

IOM. 2003a. *Unequal Treatment: Confronting Racial and Ethnic Disparities in Health Care.* Smedley BD, Stith AY, Nelson AR, Editors. Washington, DC: The National Academies Press.

IOM. 2003b. *Priority Areas for National Action: Transforming Healthcare Quality.* Adams K, Corrigan JM, Editors. Washington, DC: The National Academies Press.

Kirsch IS. 2001. *The International Adult Literacy Survey (IALS): Understanding What Was Measured.* Princeton, NJ: Educational Testing Service.

Kirsch IS, Jungeblut A, Jenkins L, Kolstad A. 1993. *Adult Literacy in America: A First Look at the Results of the National Adult Literacy Survey (NALS)*. Washington, DC: National Center for Education Statistics, U.S. Department of Education.

Leape LL, Lawthers AG, Brennan TA, Johnson WG. 1993. Preventing medical injury. *Quality Review Bulletin*. 19(5): 144–149.

Miller WD. 1975. Drug usage: Compliance of patients with instructions on medication. *Journal of the American Osteopathic Association*. 75(4): 401–404.

Pamuk E, Makuc D, Heck K, Rueben C, Lochner K. 1998. *Socioeconomic Status and Health Chartbook. Health, United States, 1998*. Hyattsville, MD: National Center for Health Statistics.

Parikh NS, Parker RM, Nurss JR, Baker DW, Williams MV. 1996. Shame and health literacy: The unspoken connection. *Patient Education and Counseling*. 27(1): 33–39.

Parker RM, Ratzan SC, Lurie N. 2003. Health literacy: A policy challenge for advancing high-quality health care. *Health Affairs*. 22(4): 147.

Purcell-Gates V, Degener S, Jacobson E, Soler M. 2000. Affecting Change in Literacy Practices of Adult Learners: Impact of Two Dimensions of Instruction. NCSALL Report No. 17. Boston, MA: National Center for the Study of Adult Learning and Literacy.

Ratzan SC, Parker RM. 2000. Introduction. In: *National Library of Medicine Current Bibliographies in Medicine: Health Literacy*. Selden CR, Zorn M, Ratzan SC, Parker RM, Editors. NLM Pub. No. CBM 2000-1. Bethesda, MD: National Institutes of Health, U.S. Department of Health and Human Services.

Roter DL, Rudd RE, Comings J. 1998. Patient literacy: A barrier to quality of care. *Journal of General Internal Medicine*. 13(12): 850–851.

Rudd, R. 2002. *Health and Literacy: Recalibrating the Norm*. Paper presented at the American Public Health Association Annual Conference, Philadelphia, PA.

Rudd R, Moeykens BA, Colton TC. 2000. Health and literacy: A review of medical and public health literature. In: *Annual Review of Adult Learning and Literacy*. Comings J, Garners B, Smith C, Editors. New York: Jossey-Bass.

Rudd RE, DeJong W. 2000. *In Plain Language: The Need for Effective Communication in Medicine and Public Health* [Video]. Cambridge, MA: Harvard University.

Rudd RE, Comings JP, Hyde J. 2003. Leave no one behind: Improving health and risk communication through attention to literacy. *Journal of Health Communication, Special Supplement on Bioterrorism*. 8(Supplement 1): 104–115.

Sarver J, Baker DW. 2000. Effect of language barriers on follow-up appointments after an emergency department visit. *Journal of General Internal Medicine*. 15(4): 256–264.

Snyder D, Lynch JJ, Gruss L. 1976. Doctor-patient communications in a private family practice. *Journal of Family Practice*. 3(3): 271–276.

Street B. 2001. *Literacy and Development: Ethnographic Perspectives*. New York: Routledge.

U.S. Agency for International Development. 2001. *DRAFT "Communication activity authorization document."*

Watters EK. 2003. Literacy for health: An interdisciplinary model. *Journal of Transcultural Nursing*. 14(1): 48–54.

WHO (World Health Organization). 2000. *Health Promotion. Report by the Secretariat*. World Health Organization.

2

What Is Health Literacy?

A 29-year-old African-American woman with three days of abdominal pain and fever was brought to a Baltimore emergency department by her family. After a brief evaluation she was told that she would need an exploratory laparotomy. She subsequently became agitated and demanded to have her family take her home. When approached by staff, she yelled "I came here in pain and all you want is to do is an exploratory on me! You will not make me a guinea pig!" She refused to consent to any procedures and later died of appendicitis.

DEFINITION OF HEALTH LITERACY

Health literacy is of concern to everyone involved in health promotion and protection, disease prevention and early screening, health care and maintenance, and policy making. Health literacy skills are needed for dialogue and discussion, reading health information, interpreting charts, making decisions about participating in research studies, using medical tools for personal or familial health care—such as a peak flow meter or thermometer—calculating timing or dosage of medicine, or voting on health or environmental issues. This report makes use of the operational definition of health literacy developed for the National Library of Medicine and used by *Healthy People 2010*:

The degree to which individuals have the capacity to obtain, process, and understand basic health information and services needed to make appropriate health decisions (Ratzan and Parker, 2000).

The capacity of the individual is a substantial contributor to health literacy. The term "capacity" refers to both the innate potential of the individual, as well as his or her skills. An individual's health literacy capacity is mediated by education, and its adequacy is affected by culture, language, and the characteristics of health-related settings. In this report, the committee has captured the range of environments and situations related to health in the term "health context". The health context includes the media, the marketplace, and government agencies, as well as those individuals and materials a person interacts with regarding health—all must be able to provide basic health information in an appropriate manner (Rudd, 2003). This health context is of equal importance to individuals' health literacy skills, as the impact of health literacy arises from the interaction of the individual and the health context (Rudd, 2003; Rudd et al., 2003). Health literacy, then, is a shared function of cultural, social, and individual factors. Both the causes and the remedies for limited health literacy rest with our cultural and social framework, the health and education systems that serve it, and the interactions between these factors.

A Conceptual Framework for Health Literacy

Figures 2-1 and 2-2 provide visual frameworks for considering health literacy. Figure 2-1 places literacy as the foundation of health literacy and health literacy as the active mediator between individuals and health contexts. Individuals bring specific sets of factors to the health context, including cognitive abilities, social skills, emotional state, and physical conditions such as visual and auditory acuity. Literacy provides the skills that enable individuals to understand and communicate health information and concerns. Literacy is defined as a set of reading, writing, basic mathematics, speech, and speech comprehension skills (Kirsch, 2001a). Health literacy is the bridge between the literacy (and other) skills and abilities of the individual and the health context. This interaction is explored in Chapter 3, where associations between health literacy and health-related outcomes are discussed in detail.

Figure 2-2 illustrates the three key sectors that should assume responsibility for health literacy, and within which health literacy skills can be built. The sectors that constitute the contexts of health literacy are culture and society, the health system, and the education system. These sectors also provide intervention points that are both challenges and opportunities for improving health literacy.

Health Literacy Framework

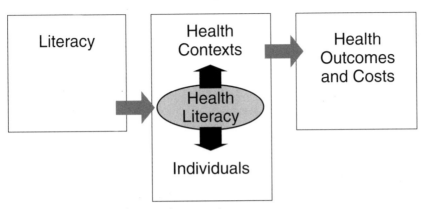

FIGURE 2-1   Health literacy framework.

Figure 2-2 illustrates the interaction of individuals with education systems, health systems, and societal factors as they relate to health literacy. It is not a causal model. It is likely that the determinants of health literacy are as varied and complex as those of the most refractory problems now facing the health fields. Although causal relationships between limited health literacy and health outcomes are not yet established, cumulative and consistent findings suggest such a causal connection. Research is needed to establish the nature of the causal relationships between and among these factors. Mapping this web of causation should be a goal of research, but it is important to note that current knowledge can serve as the basis for changing practice and policy. Below, we introduce the role each of the sectors plays in supporting or impairing health literacy. The opportunities for and obstacles to health literacy in these three sectors will be discussed in detail in Chapters 4, 5, and 6.

Culture and Society

The term "culture" in this report primarily refers to the shared ideas, meanings, and values acquired by individuals as members of society. Cultural, social, and family influences are of critical importance in shaping attitudes and beliefs. In this way, they influence how people interact with the health system and help determine the adequacy of health literacy skills in different settings. People know humanity, deal with the world they live in, and understand their place in the universe through cultural processes. Conditions over which the individual has little or no control but which

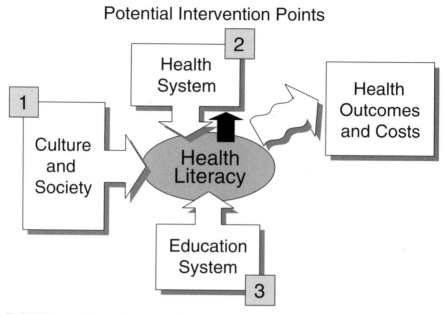

FIGURE 2-2   Potential points for intervention in the health literacy framework.

affect the ability to participate fully in a health-literate society comprise social determinants of health. Included are native language, socioeconomic status, gender, race, and ethnicity, along with influences of mass media as represented by news publishing, advertising, marketing, and the plethora of health information sources available through electronic sources. Culture is crucial for understanding, thinking, and responding to human experiences and world events. American culture is formed from historical, racial-ethnic, social, political, psychological, educational, and economic forces that are woven into the context of American lifestyles. Because they are pathways to understanding American life, cultural contexts should be harnessed in the quest for a health-literate America.

The Education System

The education system in the United States consists of the K-12 system, adult education programs, and higher education. K-12 education is charged with the development of literacy and numeracy skills in English, which cumulatively form the foundation for more complex skills involving comprehension and application in the later grades. Adult education programs provide opportunities for individuals who drop out of K-12 education for academic or social reasons, for those who completed high school but did not acquire strong skills, for elders who did not have full schooling opportunities, and for adult immigrants who may never have had access to education and/or wish to learn to speak, read, and write English. Individuals with college-level education or higher frequently have adequate literacy skills, and generally are not discussed in this report. Formative and continuing education for health professionals is also considered within the context of education.

The Health System

Within the many components of health-care systems, health-related messages and action plans are crafted, rights and responsibilities are shaped, research initiatives are begun, health-promoting recommendations are developed and supported, access is monitored, and regulations are enforced. In this report, we use the term health system to refer to all people performing these activities, including those working in hospitals, clinics, physician's offices, home health care, public health agencies, accreditation groups, regulatory agencies, and insurers. Published reviews of the literature (for example, see Kerka, 2000; Rudd et al., 2000) and the committees research into the literature from a range of related fields, including health communication and social marketing, provide consistent evidence supporting the notion that health literacy affects the interaction of individuals with health contexts and the health-care system, and may further affect health status and outcomes.

Finding 2-1 Literature from a variety of disciplines is consistent in finding that there is strong support for the committee's conclusion that health literacy as defined in this report is based on the interaction of individuals' skills with health contexts, the health-care system, the education system, and broad social and cultural factors at home, at work, and in the community. The committee concurs that responsibility for health literacy improvement must be shared by these various sectors. The committee notes that the health system does carry significant but not sole opportunity and responsibility to improve health literacy.

Finding 2-2 The links between education and health outcomes are strongly established. The committee concludes that health literacy may be one pathway explaining the well-established link between education and health, and warrants further exploration.

The Scope of Health Literacy

If people who promote health care, create policy, and develop health materials have a clear understanding of the problem of health literacy, procedures, policies, and programs can be developed to meet the health literacy needs of the average American adult. A clear understanding of health literacy can guide the health system of public health practitioners, care providers, insurers, and community agencies toward adopting definitions and policies that resolve incompatibilities between the needs of individuals and the demands of health systems. The committee believes that both a commonly accepted definition and a conceptual framework will contribute to the clear understanding of health literacy. In choosing the definition and developing the framework in this report the committee examined the existing definitions and concepts of health literacy. The committee believes the definition and framework in this report incorporate aspects essential to the understanding of health literacy, and allow for a flexibility of response within the framework of a widely accepted definition.

Health literacy is a newly emerging concept and field of inquiry, so it is not surprising that the scope of health literacy varies according to how it is defined. For example, in 1999, the Ad Hoc Committee on Health Literacy of the American Medical Association defined health literacy as the "constellation of skills, including the ability to perform basic reading and numerical tasks required to function in the health care environment," and included everyday health functions such as the "ability to read and comprehend prescription bottles, appointment slips, and other essential health-related materials" (American Medical Association, 1999). This definition captures important components of health care, but confines the scope of health literacy to the health-care sector. This committee extends the concept of health literacy beyond health-care settings to include the variety of contexts (such as in the community and at work) in which individuals make health-related decisions.

Another concept of health literacy is found in the definition used by the Joint Committee on National Health Education Standards: "the capacity of individuals to obtain, interpret and understand basic health information and services and the competence to use such information and services in ways which enhance health" (Joint Committee on National Health Education Standards, 1995). This definition does move beyond the health-care setting; however, this and similar definitions (e.g., Kickbusch, 1997) maintain a focus on the capacity of individuals and emphasize the characteristics, knowledge, and skills of individuals without attention to the complexity of various health contexts, the tasks involved, or the materials in use.

The committee chose to adopt the definition used in *Healthy People 2010* for purposes of measurement and clarity in this report. As previously noted, *Healthy People 2010*, the document that reports the federal government's national health objectives, defines health literacy as "the degree to which individuals have the capacity to obtain, process, and understand basic health information and services needed to make appropriate health decisions" (HHS, 2000; Ratzan and Parker, 2000). This definition is useful because it encompasses the variety of contexts within which individuals may confront and interact with health issues. As with a number of the other definitions discussed above, however, it focuses attention on and appears to limit the problem of health literacy to the capacity and competence of the individual. This limitation is acknowledged and addressed in the action plan for the *Healthy People 2010* health literacy objective, which expands the definition to include system-level contributions (Rudd, 2003). Recognizing the limitations of this definition, the committee acknowledges the need for future development of definitions and measures that address the critical role that society, the health system, and the education system play in creating a truly health-literate America.

DEFINITION OF LITERACY

Educators do not associate literacy with reading alone, but often consider literacy to represent a constellation of skills including reading, writing, basic mathematical calculations, and speech and speech comprehension skills (Kirsch, 2001a). Speech and speech comprehension are collectively termed oral literacy, while reading and writing are referred to as print literacy. For our discussion in this report, we further differentiate among the following terms: basic print literacy, literacy for different types of text, and functional literacy. Basic print literacy ability means the ability to read, write, and understand written language that is familiar and for which one has the requisite amount of background knowledge. Reading or text literacy is related to characteristics of the text being read such as complexity and format. Functional literacy is the use of literacy in order to perform a particular task. We note that health literacy has been variously defined, but as currently used and measured, often consists of reading or text literacy (see below for further discussion). Figure 2-3 below illustrates the relationships between the different contributors to literacy.

As illustrated above in Figure 2-3, a consideration of health literacy must include component parts directly related to the broad concept of literacy. Literacy, as noted earlier, is context specific. For example, literacy could be placed within the multiple health contexts noted earlier. In this case, the construct includes cultural and conceptual knowledge that could include an understanding of health and illness and a conceptualization of risks and benefits. Listening and speaking skills are essential for public health communication, the commercial sector's advertising goals, and for

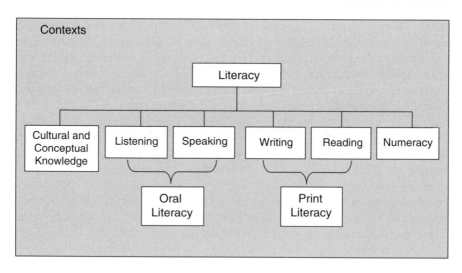

FIGURE 2-3   Components of literacy.

practitioner–patient interactions, such as for the presentation of symptoms critically needed for diagnosis. Writing and reading skills, often called print literacy, are needed for tasks related to the use of the printed word, whether the words are found on labels in the market, in health education brochures, on medicine bottles or in informed consent documents. Numeracy skills are needed to calculate nutrition labels, calibrate temperature, and compare benefit packages, and for determining the proper dosage and timing of medicines. The committee recognizes that these skills are essential components of health literacy. However, most literature focused on health literacy issues has focused predominantly on assessments of materials and on measures of people's skills based on their ability to read a sample of these materials. Thus, print literacy has dominated the discussion in health literacy so far. At the same time, the focus on print literacy has yielded profound insights into difficulties and barriers linking literacy skills to health outcomes.

Finding 2-3   Health literacy, as defined in this report, includes a variety of skills beyond reading and writing, including numeracy, listening, and speaking, and relies on cultural and conceptual knowledge.

Basic Print Literacy

As mentioned earlier, basic print literacy ability means the ability to read, write, and understand written language that is familiar and for which one has the requisite amount of background knowledge. It includes the ability to decode letters and sound out words, but also includes the ability to understand the meaning of the printed text. Some people with limited skills may know how to decode letters into sounds and pronounce words but may not be able to understand the meaning of a sentence formed by these words. However, as many new readers build on these skills, they learn how to read words in sentence sequence and accumulate levels of fluency for reading and writing. Fluency in reading includes accuracy, rate, and appropriate phrasing and intonation. Fluent reading "sounds" natural rather than halting and effortful. Basic print literacy is what is referred to when someone inquires, "can he read?" People who are termed "illiterate" have few, if any, of the skills needed for basic print literacy. The terms "low literate" or "limited" reading skills refer to difficulty with reading and comprehending materials written beyond very simple levels.

Literacy for Different Types of Text

Possessing the skills needed for basic literacy does not guarantee that one can read and comprehend all types of written text. Readers must know and understand the individual words and terms used in the text and be familiar with the concepts addressed in the text. They must understand how to "read" the structure of the text. For example, a prescription label has a unique structure and the reader must be able to use that structure to understand the directions that follow. The reader may be helped or hindered by various text features such as font size, layout and design, syntax, or use of graphs. Not all texts are equally readable and comprehensible to every person, regardless of that person's reading ability. The same literate person who can read the daily newspaper, the Bible, novels, or a manual at work may not be able to figure out instructions for connecting a DVD player to a television, directions for taking medicine, a blueprint for a new skyscraper, or the bias in an editorial. Thus, the readability of different texts depends on the skills and background knowledge of individual readers, factors in the text, and the purpose for which readers use the materials.

All Literacy is Functional

Texts serve specific functions, and readers come to them in order to accomplish specific tasks. At times, the task at hand may be clear; for example, a person is most likely to read a bus schedule in order to determine when the bus is arriving at a certain place. In other cases, the task may be less clear; a person is most likely to read a novel for pleasure. In both examples, however, the person is applying literacy skills to perform a function.

The content and structure of a bus schedule is meant to be a reflection of the function it serves to help a traveler plan an excursion. A bus schedule generally lists the routes and stops of different buses—often identified with numbers—for people who need to plan their transportation and arrive at a particular destination at a specific time. More complicated schedules include variations based on days of the week or holiday exceptions. Similarly, the content and structure of a label on a pediatric over-the-counter medicine is designed to provide the parent with information about the medicine and a mechanism for calculating the appropriate dose based on the child's age and weight. This information is often present in a table format that requires special reading skills that many people do not have.

An individual's ability to apply his or her literacy skills changes with the challenges of the task (Kirsch, 2001b; Kirsch et al., 1993). The example below, the text of an actual letter sent by a doctor to a patient, captures a very complicated message. Although the patient in this case holds a graduate degree, his anxiety was greatly increased as a result of a confusing message. He asked, "How can I have a recurrence of thyroid cancer if my thyroid was removed?"

Dear Mr. Smith,

The May thyroid tests showed TSH 2.794 µU/ml, which, though "normal," is too high for someone who has had prior thyroid carcinoma. Keeping TSH between 0.1 – 0.3 µU/ml minimizes recurrence of thyroid cancer. Free T4 1.60 mg% is a high-normal level.

I suggest you increase L-thyroxine from 150 mcg 7 days a week to 150 mcg 5 days a week and 225 mcg (1½ tablets) Wednesdays and Sundays weekly. Have a repeat TSH, free T4 and total T3 in 8 weeks. I should also on that occasion like you to have a serum plasma metanephrine level.

Two weeks after having those tests, please see me for a consultative office visit.

Sincerely yours,
John Doe, M.D.
Endocrinology

LITERACY IN HEALTH CONTEXTS

Health-related activities take place in a wide variety of settings (home, work, community health-care institutions) and can involve a wide range of activities related to family, community, economics, leisure, and safety issues. The parent taking a child's temperature, the worker reading about proper procedures for handling materials, the shopper calculating the difference in salt content on the labels of two brands of canned vegetables, the patient reading about dental options, and the elder filling out an application for Medicare are all engaged in health-related tasks, in different environments, for different purposes, and with different types of materials. All are applying literacy skills to printed health information.

This report uses the term "health contexts" to reflect the many situations and activities relating to health. Health contexts are unusual, compared to other contexts, because of an ever-present or underlying stress or fear factor. Various exposures, products, or actions might enhance health, safeguard health, harm health, or lead to very dire consequences. In addition, health-care settings can involve unique conditions such as the physical or mental impairment experienced by a patient due to illness, stress, or fear (Alexander, 1990; Dumas, 1966). Health-care settings also involve specialized vocabulary, use of jargon, legal forms, complex procedures and processes, as well as differences in power and access to information.

Literacy Skill Demands of Health Contexts

A complex array of health literacy skills are needed for functioning in a variety of health contexts. These skills include reading, writing, mathematics, speaking, listening, using technology, networking, and rhetorical skills associated with requests, advocacy, and complaints. Table 2-1 presents some brief (and incomplete) examples to provide a sense of the complexity of skills needed for health.

While many of the examples presented in Table 2-1 emphasize the skills of individuals, the skills of those communicating also contribute to health literacy. We must consider a health-care provider's ability to use common words and to perceive whether a patient is understanding a discussion or not. A media developer needs the skills to shape a message that consumers can understand. Manufacturers need skills to design clear product labels. Educators need skills to engage students in health-related issues and to incorporate health messages into science, language, and math curricular materials. The example below represents the level of confusion created by a lack of clear information, even for the most educated consumer.

TABLE 2-1   Examples of Skills Needed for Health

Health-Related Goal	Sample Tasks and Skills Needed
Promote and protect health and prevent disease	• read and follow guidelines for physical activity • read, comprehend, and make decisions based on food and product labels • make sense of air quality reports and modify behavior as needed • find health information on the internet or in periodicals and books
Understand, interpret, and analyze health information	• analyze risk factors in advertisements for prescription medicines • determine health implications of a newspaper article on air quality • determine which health web sites contain accurate information and which do not • understand the implications of health-related initiatives in order to vote
Apply health information over a variety of life events and situations	• determine and adopt guidelines for increased physical activity at an older age • read and apply health information regarding childcare or eldercare • read and interpret safety precautions at work; choose a health-care plan
Navigate the health-care system	• fill out health insurance enrollment or reimbursement forms • understand printed patient rights and responsibilities • find one's way in a complicated environment such as a busy hospital or clinical center
Actively participate in encounters with health-care professionals and workers	• ask for clarification • ask questions • make appropriate decisions based on information received • work as a partner with care providers to discuss and develop an appropriate regimen to manage a chronic disease
Understand and give consent	• comprehend required informed consent documents before procedures or for involvement in research studies
Understand and advocate for rights	• advocate for safety equipment based on worker right-to-know information • request access to information based on patient rights documents • determine use of medical records based on the privacy act • advocate on behalf of others such as the elderly or mentally ill to obtain needed care and services

> A highly publicized, large-scale study of combination estrogen-progestin hormone therapy by the Women's Health Initiative came to a sudden end in the summer of 2002 when researchers noticed higher levels of heart disease, blood clots and breast cancer in the group taking hormones.
>
> According to Wyeth spokeswoman Natalie DeVane, 15 million American women were taking some form of hormone treatment before the study was stopped. This past June, she said, the number was 9.2 million.
>
> Rep. Rosa L. DeLauro (D-Conn.) led the effort to mandate an FDA education effort on hormone therapies. "I'm pretty well-informed about these things, and I didn't know what to do," she said. "In the absence of clear information, it can get pretty scary for women." (Kaufman, 2003)

MEASURES USED IN HEALTH LITERACY RESEARCH

Measures of literacy are needed to allow us to assess people's literacy competence and to suggest promising intervention points and strategies. However, we must recognize that assessment of literacy ability (as for any assessment) depends on how literacy is defined and how assessment results are to be used. Literacy assessment has evolved over the years and takes several different forms, resulting in the necessity to interpret and use the results accordingly.

Literacy Surveys

Assessments of adult literacy conducted since the late 1980s have focused on functional literacy and numeracy as outlined by the National Literacy Act of 1991.[1] This act defines literacy as "the ability to read, write, and speak in English, and compute and solve problems at levels of proficiency necessary to function on the job and in society, to achieve one's goals, and develop one's knowledge and potential." This definition was applied to the development of the national assessments of adult literacy in the United States and other industrialized nations. The surveys measured three of the five accepted components of literacy: reading, writing, and mathematical calculations (or numeracy). Oral language skills, including speaking and listening, were not assessed for the national studies, in part because of time constraints and a possible burden on participants (Kirsch,

---

[1]P.L. 102-73, The National Literacy Act of 1991. 102nd Congress, 1st Session. H.R. 751.

2001a). The Young Adult Literacy Survey (performed in 1985) (Kirsch and Jungeblut, 1986), the Department of Labor Survey (1990) (Kirsch and Jungeblut, 1992), the National Adult Literacy Survey (NALS) (1992) (Campbell et al., 1992), and the International Adult Literacy Survey (IALS) (the initial study was performed in 1994–1998) (Kirsch, 2001a) all focus on the ability to use print materials to accomplish a task. These task-oriented assessments differ in complexity from basic literacy assessments that focus on the ability to recognize or pronounce words, or to read and comprehend text written specifically for test purposes.

Materials for these surveys were drawn from six contexts in order to represent literacy tasks from everyday life: home and family, health and safety, community and citizenship, consumer economics, work, and leisure and recreation. Materials included both continuous and noncontinuous texts. Continuous texts or prose, which is the term used in these large-scale assessments, are typically composed of sentences that are, in turn, organized into paragraphs. These paragraphs are used to form larger structures such as stories, newspaper or magazine articles, and even sections or chapters in a book. A common way of organizing continuous texts is by their rhetorical structure. These might include: narratives, exposition, description, argumentation, instructions, or a document and record. Noncontinuous texts or documents as they are referred to involve the display of information using other structures or formats. These might include tables, charts, graphs, entry forms, maps, and diagrams. They have been described by Mosenthal and Kirsch (1998) and Kirsch (2001b). These materials range in both length and complexity. Some prose materials are very short such as a brief sports article or letter. Others are more lengthy and complex such as an editorial. Documents, too, range in length and complexity such as a social security card on which someone has to enter their signature to a complex table showing the results of a survey or an embedded bus schedule.

NALS scores were based on people's ability to accomplish tasks using printed texts. The difficulty of each task was related to three variables: type of match, type of information, and plausibility of distracting information (Kirsch, 2001a). Four types of matching strategies were identified: locating, cycling, integrating, and generating.

The tasks, in ascending order of difficulty, included:

• Locating—requires the reader to find information based on conditions or features specified in the text or document.
• Cycling—requires the reader to engage in a series of matching or locating operations that involve the strategy of locating.
• Integrating—requires the reader to pull together pieces of information from a text or document often times having to compare or contrast this information.

- Generating—requires the reader to produce a response either by making a text-based inference or by drawing on their background knowledge.
- Formulating and Calculating—requires the reader to identify both the numbers or quantities and the operation that must be performed. If more than one operation is required, the reader must determine the appropriate order of the operations.

Tasks were further identified by specific characteristics: type of match, type of information requested, plausibility of distracters, type of calculation, and operation specificity. Detailed discussions of how these factors contributed to scoring may be found in the *International Adult Literacy Survey: Understanding What Was Measured* (Kirsch, 2001b).

Findings reported participants' ability to complete these tasks with 80 percent accuracy and consistency for three types of literacy: prose (tasks involving materials using full sentences in paragraph format), document (tasks involving materials consisting of lists, graphs, and charts), and numeracy (quantitative literacy; tasks involving the application of basic mathematical processes). Assessments were scored on a 0 to 500 scale and findings were reported by score for various population groups and by levels:

- Level 1 (score of 0 to 225): Many adults at this level can perform tasks involving brief and uncomplicated texts and documents. Adults at this level can generally locate a piece of information in a news story or on a form such as a social security card.
- Level 2 (score of 226 to 275): Adults at this level of proficiency are generally able to locate information in text, make low-level inferences using printed materials, and integrate easily identifiable pieces of information.
- Level 3 (score of 276 to 325): Adults at this level are able to integrate information from relatively long or dense texts or documents, determine appropriate arithmetic operations based on information contained in the directive, and identify quantities needed to perform the operation.
- Levels 4 (score of 326 to 375) and 5 (score of 376 to 500): Adults at these levels demonstrate proficiencies associated with long and complex documents and text passages.

Grade-Level Measures of Literacy

One of the most familiar terms associated with the assessment of reading levels is that of *grade level*. This term is used in two different ways. First, individual scores on assessments of reading achievement are often reported in terms of grade level, for example, *He scored a Grade Equivalent (GE) of 5.2.* The second way that grade level is used is to indicate the readability level of a text, for example, *the story was written at a fifth grade level.* The two uses of the term grade level, while related, do not mean the same thing. The first refers to a norm-referenced score on a norm-referenced reading achievement test and applies to individuals. The second is the result of applying a formula for reading ease to written materials and applies to texts.

Grade-Level Ability for Individual Readers

Within the area of assessment and psychometrics, the construct of grade level indicates relative placement of an individual or group score on a norm-referenced test, that is, a test designed so that an individual's score can be established by comparison to the test scores of a representative sample of persons. Grade level is one type of transformed score. Others include *percentiles, stanines,* and *standard scores.* While these other transformed scores indicate specific locations on a bell-shaped normal curve of scores of a sample of previously tested individuals (the norm sample), grade-level scores do not, and therefore the potential for their misinterpretation is higher. Statistically, the grade-level score is derived from the mean score on a norm-referenced test. This means that the average raw score on a norm-reference achievement test for a given grade is transformed into the grade-level score for that grade. For example, if the average score attained by fifth graders in the norm sample on a norm-referenced reading achievement test, taken in the second month of fifth grade, is 75 (out of, say 100), then the score of 75 will be assigned a grade-level score of 5.2 (fifth year, second month). Therefore, one can say with accuracy that a student who scores on grade level is achieving, according to this test, on average. All other scores, both lower and higher, on this test are transformed into grade-level scores through a process of mathematical extrapolation. Thus, a grade-level score (GE; grade equivalency) of 3.5 for a fifth grader on this test indicates a certain distance below the average score; a GE of 7.2 correspondingly indicates a certain distance above the average score. The appropriate interpretation of the on-grade-level, or average, score is as a measure of the student's ability to read material at his or her current grade level. Above- and below-grade-level scores are less reliable due to the extrapolation involved. This is due to their extrapolation from raw scores.

Studies that examined the reading ability of the intended audience, performed in the 1980s and early 1990s, frequently assessed reading ability with short-word recognition tests, Cloze tests (in which random words from a passage are deleted; Taylor, 1953), or other reading comprehension tests. These types of assessments of literacy typically result in the assignment of a grade-level score, and are frequently used by adult educators to place adult students in appropriate level classes. One of these assessments, the reading recognition subtest of the Wide Range Achievement Test-Revised (WRAT-R) requires participants to read aloud lists of words that become increasingly difficult. The test is stopped when 10 words have been consecutively mispronounced (Jastak and Wilkinson, 1984). The Instrument for Diagnosis of Reading, also known as the Instrumento Para Diagnostical Lecturas (IDL), is another test commonly used to assess reading ability. Although the IDL is lengthy, taking more than 20 minutes to administer, it is useful because it was developed in the Spanish language and provides a comprehensive assessment of reading comprehension in Spanish (Blanchard et al., 1989). A shortened form is available that takes about 7 minutes to administer.

Grade-Level Measures of Materials

Well over 300 articles in public health and medical journals focus on the assessment of various types of health-related materials (Roter et al., 2001; Rudd, 2003; Rudd et al., 2000). Many researchers used readability score to indicate text complexity. A commonly used formula for readability score is the Simplified Measure of Gobbledygook (SMOG) which is based on calculations of the number of polysyllabic words in a set number of sentences. Consequently, the SMOG focuses on sentence and word length, both of which are associated with reading ease or difficulty (McLaughlin, 1969). Other commonly used assessment measures include the Fry Readability Scale (Fry, 1977) and the Flesch-Kincaid Reading Grade Level (Flesch, 1974). Measures of reading levels probably required to understand different materials have contributed to the research agenda in health literacy by providing initial indications of text complexity, based on words and sentence length. These determinations of reading level are valuable when considered in light of the audiences for the material.

Measures of Health Literacy

Assessments of print literacy in the context of health were initially developed in the 1990s. Two frequently used assessments that have been described in detail are the Rapid Estimate of Adult Literacy in Medicine (REALM; Davis et al., 1993) and the Test of Functional Health Literacy in Adults (TOFHLA; Parker et al., 1995).

The REALM is a medical-word recognition and pronunciation test for screening adult reading ability in medical settings. It can be administered and scored in under 3 minutes by personnel with minimal training, making it easy to use in clinical settings. Participants read from a list of 66 common medical terms that patients may be expected to be able to read in order to participate effectively in their own health care. The words are arranged in three columns according to the number of syllables and pronunciation difficulty. Each correctly read and pronounced word increases the participant's score by 1. Scores (0–66 words read and pronounced correctly) can be converted into four reading grade levels: grades 0–3 (0–18 words), grades 4–6 (19–44 words), grades 7–8 (45–60 words), and grade 9 and above (61–66 words). The REALM's criterion validity is established through correlation with other standardized reading tests: Peabody Individual Achievement Test-Revised, 0.97 (Markwardt, 1989), Slosson Oral Reading Test-Revised, 0.96 (Slosson, 1990), and WRAT-R, 0.88 (Davis et al., 1993, 1998; all correlations p < 0.0001). The REALM also reports high intra-subject reliability (0.97). The REALM has been developed in English only. A Spanish-language version is not possible because reading tests based on pronunciation are not valid in Spanish. This is due to the regular phoneme–grapheme correspondence of Spanish, in which there is usually a one-to-one correspondence between letters and sounds, making it relatively easy to pronounce unfamiliar words even for readers with limited literacy skills (Nurss et al., 1995).

The TOFHLA includes a 17-item test of numerical ability and a 50-item test of reading comprehension, as measured by a Cloze procedure (see Appendix C for examples of items from the TOFHLA). The TOFHLA draws on materials commonly used in health-care settings at the time the test was developed. Reading passages were selected from instructions for preparation for an upper gastrointestinal series, the patient "Rights and Responsibilities" section of a Medicaid application, and a standard informed consent form. The numeracy items on the TOFHLA test a patient's ability to understand monitoring blood glucose, keep a clinic appointment, obtain financial assistance, and understand directions for taking medicines using an actual pill bottle.

Total scores for the TOFHLA are divided into three criterion levels: inadequate, marginal, and adequate. Those with inadequate health literacy scores often misread medication dosing instruction, appointment slips, and instructions for the upper gastrointestinal tract radiographic procedure. Those with marginal health literacy scores perform better on those tasks, but often misread information on prescription bottles and have trouble understanding the Medicaid "Rights and Responsibilities" passage. Those who score in the adequate range do well on these tasks, but may have some difficulty comprehending the more difficult tasks like determining financial eligibility and the informed consent document (Parker et al., 1995). The TOFHLA takes up to 22 minutes to administer and has good criterion validity, with correlation coefficients of r = 0.74 with the WRAT-R and r =

0.84 with the REALM, and a high reliability (Cronbach's alpha = 0.98; Parker et al., 1995).

For time considerations, the TOFHLA was reduced to an abbreviated version called the S-TOFHLA that takes 12 minutes or less to administer (Baker et al., 1999). It consists of a reading comprehension section containing a 36-item test using the initial two passages in the reading comprehension section of the full TOFHLA—instructions for preparation for an upper gastrointestinal series and the patient "Rights and Responsibilities" section of a Medicaid application. It also contains a shortened 4-item measure of numeracy. The S-TOFHLA has been shown to have good internal consistency reliability (Cronbach's alpha = 0.98 for all items combined) and concurrent validity compared to the long version of the TOFHLA (r = 0.91) and the REALM (r = 0.80). Both the TOFHLA and the S-TOFHLA are available in English and in Spanish. The Spanish and English versions were developed simultaneously and use the same standard of measurement.

Additional measures continue to be developed, including a measure of health literacy in Veterans Administration hospital populations based on the S-TOFHLA (Chew and Bradley, 2003), a literacy test for patients with diabetes (Nath et al., 2001), and a functional test of ability to maintain a medication regimen (Edelberg et al., 1998, 1999, 2001).

The use of these tests of literacy for printed material in the health context has enabled medical researchers to explore differences among various health-related outcomes for patients based on approximations of patients' health literacy as indicated by patients' reading skills for health materials. As a result, a growing body of research has shown that limited reading and/or numeracy skills reduce access to health information and preventive services, reduce understanding of illness and disease, regimens and medications, and increase outcomes such as hospitalization or decrease outcomes such as disease management markers. This research is discussed in detail in Chapter 3.

Limitations of Existing Measures

Functional Literacy Measures

Education scholars consider literacy a changing set of skills, knowledge, and strategies that adults build throughout their lives. As noted earlier, this set of skills includes reading, writing, speaking, listening, and numeracy (Kirsch, 2001b). However, available assessments of adult literacy (NALS, IALS, National Assessment of Adult Literacy [NAAL]) do not fully measure all these aspects of literacy because measurements of oral literacy skills (including speech and speech comprehension) were considered beyond the scope of what was feasible at the time these surveys were carried out.

Oral language skills are of critical concern for public health and health care. Public health and risk communication rely on a variety of channels and media, including oral communication, to convey health promotion and protection information, as well as for local and national alerts. Health-care encounters rely on a dialogue between patient and provider that allow the provider to understand symptoms, follow the course of an illness or disease as experienced by the patient, and provide diagnosis and treatment options. Patients are expected to tell their stories, describe their experiences, provide explanations, and obtain help with needed action. Given the importance of speech and speech comprehension skills to health literacy, the current measures of health literacy that are modeled on previous functional literacy assessment tools do not tap the full scope of health literacy.

Grade-Level Scores

Grade-level scores are problematic because they require an interpretation of assessments for the level of ability for individual readers. The use of grade level as a meaningful norm-referenced score is so problematic that the International Reading Association recommended that it not be used for K-12 (Joint Task Force on Assessment, 1994). Its use in adults for whom there are no "grades" from which to extrapolate from a mean score on a norm-referenced test is even more inaccurate.

Health Literacy Measures

Although useful for assessment in clinical and community settings, from a psychometric perspective neither the REALM nor the TOFHLA capture the full complexity of the construct of health literacy. They are both measures of basic print literacy using health-related terms, and to some degree, texts. To this degree, they provide a valid picture of basic print literacy ability within health contexts. While the TOFHLA also includes a measure of numeracy, a full range of text types are not included. However, health literacy includes more than word recognition, text comprehension, and numeracy skills. Furthermore, health tasks are not limited to the health-care system but instead comprise a broad spectrum of activities in a variety of contexts. Therefore, we do not yet possess a measure that takes into account the full set of skills and knowledge associated with health literacy as defined in this report. The results of such measures as the REALM and the TOFHLA must be interpreted in this light.

The TOFHLA includes passages with readability levels on the Gunning Fog index of grades 4.3, 10.4, and 19.5. However, the TOFHLA, unlike the NALS, did not examine the complexity of the materials or the difficulty of tasks involved in the use of the materials. Although both the TOFHLA and the S-TOFHLA include numeracy tasks, the REALM does not examine numeracy, and none of these assessments examine writing. The contents of the REALM and the TOFHLA focus on medical terms or materials found in medical settings and do not represent the broad spectrum of health literacy materials and processes that occur outside the clinical setting, limiting the conclusions that can be drawn. As discussed above, neither considers oral language skills.

Researchers using existing measures of health literacy have been able to establish differences in health-related outcome measures for patients based on differences in test scores. While the existing measures do not fully capture the construct of health literacy, they have provided information about vulnerable populations. Although the existing body of research is revealing and suggestive, generalization of results to large populations is limited. Each study focuses on a specific population, which differs from others along relevant dimensions such as age, socioeconomic status, ethnicity, and primary languages. Also many studies use different measurement tools and in some cases the researchers modified the scoring of these tools. Better measures are needed if we are to be able to align our understanding of the distribution of health literacy with the development of intervention strategies.

Finding 2-4 While health literacy measures in current use have spurred research initiatives and yield valuable insights, they are indicators of reading skills (word recognition or reading comprehension and numeracy), rather than measures of the full range of skills needed for health literacy (cultural and conceptual knowledge, listening, speaking, numeracy, writing and reading). Current assessment tools and research findings cannot differentiate among (1) reading ability, (2) lack of background knowledge in health-related domains, such as biology, (3) lack of familiarity with language and types of materials, and (4) cultural differences in approaches to health and health care. In addition, no current measures of health literacy include oral communication skills or writing skills and none measure the health literacy demands on individuals within different health contexts.

NEEDS AND OPPORTUNITIES

Links between socioeconomic status and health outcomes are well established (Adler et al., 1999; Berkman and Kawachi, 2000; Pamuk et al., 1998; Williams, 1990). Socioeconomic status is generally measured by income, educational attainment, and occupation. Epidemiological studies indicate a strong inverse relationship between health and education. Incidence rates of chronic diseases, communicable diseases, and injuries are all inversely related to education, as are disease prevention actions (Pamuk et al., 1998). The pathways by which educational attainment and health outcomes affect each other have yet to be established (Grossman and Kaestner, 1997). The component parts of educational attainment, such as literacy skills, also have not yet been examined in full.

Reliable and valid measures of health literacy will enable researchers to establish and monitor the magnitude of the issue, changes over time, the links between health literacy and health outcomes, factors that lead to health literacy, and the effectiveness of health literacy interventions. Robust health literacy indicators are needed to move this field of inquiry forward. Although the committee is not in a position to develop such measures, it has identified some potentially worthwhile directions to move towards.

The first is conceptual. As noted above, several definitions of health literacy are in current use. Consensus is needed to develop an operationally defined construct of health literacy. This can be accomplished through a national consensus conference, bringing together stakeholders from a wide array of health contexts and researchers in health, education, and psychometrics to address the issue of developing operational measures of health literacy at population levels. Such a conference could build on the work of this committee by adopting the definition recommended here and concentrating on the measurement issues identified by the committee.

Conference participants might consider a process similar to that undertaken for the development of the national and international assessments of functional literacy, but with a unique focus on health contexts. Such a focus would build on this report to develop a detailed and consistent theoretical model delineating health contexts and articulating the inherent demands and assumptions within each context. Researchers could be charged with rigorously collecting health-related texts and tasks used in and outside of health-care settings. These researchers then could conduct a purposive sampling to adequately represent the broad array of health activities in appropriate contexts. Numerous text types would have to be represented for each context area. Both the materials and the tasks associated with them would have to be carefully calibrated for levels of complexity and difficulty.

Furthermore, such materials and tasks must consider the role of oral language skills in health literacy. As noted above, oral language skills, including both speaking and listening comprehension, were not assessed by national literacy assessments such as the NALS or IALS. Further explorations are needed, in partnership with scholars in health communication, education, and linguistics, to develop meaningful measures of oral exchange skills that are so vital to health contexts.

Causal relationships are another area for future exploration. The National Institutes of Health (NIH), foundations, and for-profit organizations that support health research, particularly on health disparities and inequalities, could address the interrelationships between limited health literacy and cultural and socioeconomic factors by encouraging research to develop and test causal models. Establishing causality could help identify intervention points. Factors to be considered in the exploration of causality include the relationships between and among health literacy, socioeconomic status, health status, educational achievement, geographic location, and culture. These relationships should be considered in the design of large population surveys.

Links between health literacy and health outcomes initially could be made through data collection of a number of illustrative public health, medical, and dental indicators. These might include data relevant to immunization, cancer screening, cardiovascular disease prevention, and on-going measures of physical activity and nutritional practices. Other opportunities might include measures of tobacco use, substance use, or injury. Of critical concern would be access to care and insurance status. In addition, monitoring mechanisms for literacy-related access barriers and supportive factors in hospitals, physician practices, pharmacies, and workplaces are sorely needed.

National government and statistical agencies could incorporate measures of health literacy into their work on an ongoing basis. This would include on-going national surveys of adult literacy such as the NAAL, designed to follow the 1992 NALS. NAAL has broadened the representation of health tasks and items in the current survey and the results will include a separate "health literacy score" derived from questions which assess how well adults apply literacy skills to understand health-related materials (National Center for Education Statistics, 2003). Health literacy measures could be incorporated into other ongoing national surveys such as the Health Interview Survey (HIS), the Medical Expenditure Panel Survey (MEPS), Medicare Beneficiary Survey (MBS), and the Behavioral Health Risk Factor Surveillance System (BHRFSS). The status of health literacy can be gauged, quantified, and monitored at timely intervals with such indicators if they are developed through partnerships with national institutions charged with ongoing data collection for health, education, and labor.

Simple measures of health literacy that better reflect the entire literacy skill set in the context of health are needed for use in intervention research studies. Researchers in a variety of settings would benefit from simple and unobtrusive measures to explore the links between individuals' literacy-related skills and a variety of outcome measures. Further development of assessments that differentiate between and among measures of basic literacy, print literacy for health-related texts and purposes, and health literacy as a whole would provide greater insight into the factors underlying limited health literacy. More rigorous work is needed to develop appropriate, reliable, and valid measures.

For current practice in health-care settings, practitioners could consider the use of informal assessment measures to gauge health literacy. For example, this may involve asking such questions as "How do you learn best?" or "What would help you most as you learn about your illness and how to take care of yourself? or "What help do you need for taking this medicine properly?" Health educators could explore where and how people access health information and the kinds of visual, oral, or printed materials people are most comfortable and familiar with. Such informal assessment techniques can be coupled with more formal but easy-to-administer literacy assessment methods to create a health literacy profile and promote more meaningful exchanges of information (Doak CC et al., 1998; Doak LG et al., 1996; Meade, 2001).

A variety of evaluation measures can be infused into the dialogue between patients and care providers. Doak CC et al. (1996) provide a series of helpful questions that verify understanding of information. For example, the care provider might ask "Can you tell me in your own words what the purpose of this medical test is and how you will prepare for it?" to quickly identify any communication mismatches or misunderstandings and allow for clarifications. Approaches to limited health literacy that focus on changes in clinical practices are discussed in detail in Chapter 5. Research directions would benefit from considering the strengths and weaknesses of current practice, so that the most reliable and effective approaches can be identified.

Finding 2-1 Literature from a variety of disciplines is consistent in finding that there is strong support for the committee's conclusion that health literacy, as defined in this report, is based on the interaction of individuals' skills with health contexts, the health-care system, the education system, and broad social and cultural factors at home, at work, and in the community. The committee concurs that responsibility for health literacy improvement must be shared by various sectors. The committee notes that the health system does carry significant but not sole opportunity and responsibility to improve health literacy.

Finding 2-2 The links between education and health outcomes are strongly established. The committee concludes that health literacy may be one pathway explaining the well-established link between education and health, and warrants further exploration.

Finding 2-3 Health literacy, as defined in this report, includes a variety of components beyond reading and writing, including numeracy, listening, speaking, and relies on cultural and conceptual knowledge.

Finding 2-4 While health literacy measures in current use have spurred research initiatives and yield valuable insights, they are indicators of reading skills (word recognition or reading comprehension and numeracy), rather than measures of the full range of skills needed for health literacy (cultural and conceptual knowledge, listening, speaking, numeracy, writing and reading). Current assessment tools and research findings cannot differentiate among (1) reading ability, (2) lack of background knowledge in health-related domains, such as biology, (3) lack of familiarity with language and types of materials, and (4) cultural differences in approaches to health and health care. In addition, no current measures of health literacy include oral communication skills or writing skills and none measure the health-literacy demands on individuals within different health contexts.

Recommendation 2-1 The Department of Health and Human Services and other government and private funders should support research leading to the development of causal models explaining the relationships among health literacy, the education system, the health system, and relevant social and cultural systems.

Recommendation 2-2 The Department of Health and Human Services and public and private funders should support the development, testing, and use of culturally appropriate new measures of health literacy. Such measures should be developed for large ongoing population surveys, such as the NAAL Survey, the MEPS, the BHRFSS, and the MBS, as well as for institutional accreditation and quality assessment activities such as those carried out by the Joint Commission on Accreditation of Healthcare Organizations and the National Committee for Quality Assurance. Initially, NIH should convene a national consensus conference to initiate the development of operational measures of health literacy that would include contextual measures.

REFERENCES

Adler NE, Ostrove JM. 1999. Socioeconomic status and health: What we know and what we don't. *Annals of the New York Academy of Sciences.* 896: 3–15.

Alexander M. 1990. Informed consent, psychological stress and noncompliance. *Humane Medicine.* 6(2): 113–119.

American Medical Association. 1999. Health literacy: Report of the Council on Scientific Affairs. Ad Hoc Committee on Health Literacy for the Council on Scientific Affairs, American Medical Association. *Journal of the American Medical Association.* 281(6): 552–557.

Baker DW, Williams MV, Parker RM, Gazmararian JA, Nurss J. 1999. Development of a brief test to measure functional health literacy. *Patient Education and Counseling.* 38: 33–42.

Berkman LF, Kawachi IO. 2000. *Social Epidemiology.* Oxford: Oxford University Press.

Blanchard JS, Garcia HS, Carter RM. 1989. *Instrumento Para Diagnosticar Lecturas (Español-English): Instrument for the Diagnosis of Reading.* Dubuque, IA: Kendall-Hunt.

Campbell A, Kirsch IS, Kolstad A. 1992. *Assessing Literacy: The Framework for the National Adult Literacy Survey.* Washington, DC: National Center for Education Statistics, U.S. Department of Education.

Chew LD, Bradley KA. 2003. Brief questions to detect inadequate health literacy among VA patients. Abstract. *Journal of General Internal Medicine.* 18(Supplement 1): 170.

Davis TC, Long SW, Jackson RH, Mayeaux EJ, George RB, Murphy PW, Crouch MA. 1993. Rapid estimate of adult literacy in medicine: A shortened screening instrument. *Family Medicine.* 25(6): 391–395.

Davis TC, Michielutte R, Askov EN, Williams MV, Weiss BD. 1998. Practical assessment of adult literacy in health care. *Health Education and Behavior.* 25(5): 613–624.

Doak CC, Doak LG, Root J. 1996. *Teaching Patients with Low Literacy Skills.* 2nd edition. New York: Lippincott.

Doak CC, Doak LG, Friedell GH, Meade CD. 1998. Improving comprehension for cancer patients with low literacy skills: Strategies for clinicians. *Ca: A Cancer Journal for Clinicians.* 48(3): 151–162.

Doak LG, Doak CC, Meade CD. 1996. Strategies to improve cancer education materials. *Oncology Nursing Forum.* 23(8): 1305–1312.

Dumas RG. 1966. Utilization of stress as a therapeutic nursing measure. Utilization of a concept of stress as a basis for nursing practice. *ANA Clinical Sessions.* 193–212.

Edelberg HK, Shallenberger E, Hausdorff JM, Wei JY. 1998. Application of the DRUGS tool to assess function in ambulatory elderly. Abstract. *Journal of the American Geriatrics Society.* 46(9): S103.

Edelberg HK, Shallenberger E, Wei JY. 1999. Medication management capacity in highly functioning community-living older adults: Detection of early deficits. *Journal of the American Geriatrics Society.* 47(5): 592–596.

Edelberg HK, Rubin RN, Palmieri JJ, Leipzig RM. 2001. Preliminary validation of the Drug Regimen Unassisted Grading Scale (DRUGS) in community dwelling older adults. *Journal of the American Geriatrics Society.* 49(4): S65–S66.

Flesch R. 1974. *The Art of Readable Writing.* New York: Harper and Row.

Fry EB. 1977. *Elementary Reading Instruction.* New York: McGraw-Hill.

Grossman M, Kaestner R. 1997. The effects of education on health. In: *The Social Benefits of Education.* Behermean R, Stacey N, Editors. Ann Arbor, MI: University of Michigan Press. Pp. 69–123.

HHS (U.S. Department of Health and Human Services). 2000. *Healthy People 2010: Understanding and Improving Health.* Washington, DC: U.S. Department of Health and Human Services.

Jastak S, Wilkinson GS. 1984. *Wide Range Achievement Test–Revised (WRAT-R).* Jastak Assessment Systems.

Joint Committee on National Health Education Standards. 1995. *National Health Education Standards: Achieving Health Literacy.* Atlanta, GA: American Cancer Society.

Joint Task Force on Assessment, International Reading Association and National Council of Teachers of English. 1994. *Standards for the Assessment of Reading and Writing.* Newark, DE: International Reading Association.

Kaufman M. 2003, September. FDA Offers Guidance on Hormone Therapy. *The Washington Post.*

Kerka S. 2000. *Health and Adult Literacy.* Practice Application Brief No. 7. Columbus, OH: ERIC Clearinghouse on Adult, Career, and Vocational Education.

Kickbusch I. 1997. Think health: What makes the difference? *Health Promotion International.* 12: 265–272.

Kirsch IS. 2001a. The framework used in developing and interpreting the International Adult Literacy Survey (IALS). *European Journal of Psychology of Education.* 16(3): 335–361.

Kirsch IS. 2001b. *The International Adult Literacy Survey (IALS): Understanding What Was Measured.* Princeton, NJ: Educational Testing Service.

Kirsch IS, Jungeblut A. 1986. *Literacy: Profiles of America's Young Adults.* Princeton, NJ: Educational Testing Service.

Kirsch IS, Jungeblut A. 1992. *Profiling the Literacy Proficiencies of JTPA and ES/UI Populations: Final Report to the Department of Labor.* Washington, DC: Employment and Training Administration.

Kirsch IS, Jungeblut A, Jenkins L, Kolstad A. 1993. *Adult Literacy in America: A First Look at the Results of the National Adult Literacy Survey (NALS).* Washington, DC: National Center for Education Statistics, U.S. Department of Education.

Markwardt FS. 1989. *Peabody Individual Achievement Test–Revised.* Circle Pines, MN: American Guidance Service.

McLaughlin GH. 1969. SMOG grading: A new readability formula. *Journal of Reading.* 12(8): 639–646.

Meade CD. 2001. Community health education. In: *Community Health Nursing: Promoting the Health of Aggregates.* 3rd edition. Nies M, McEwen M, Editors. Philadelphia: W.B. Saunders Co.

Mosenthal PB, Kirsch IS. 1998. A new measure for assessing document complexity: The PMOSE/IKIRSCH document readability formula. *Journal of Adolescent and Adult Literacy.* 41(8): 638–657.

Nath CR, Sylvester ST, Yasek V, Gunel E. 2001. Development and validation of a literacy assessment tool for persons with diabetes. *Diabetes Educator.* 27(6): 857–864.

National Center for Education Statistics. 2003. *NAAL 2003: Overview.* [Online]. Available: http://nces.ed.gov/naal/design/about02.asp [accessed: December, 2003].

Nurss JR, Baker D, Davis T, Parker R, Williams M. 1995. Difficulty in functional health literacy screening in Spanish-speaking adults. *Journal of Reading.* 38: 632–637.

Pamuk E, Makuc D, Heck K, Rueben C, Lochner K. 1998. *Socioeconomic Status and Health Chartbook. Health, United States, 1998.* Hyattsville, MD: National Center for Health Statistics.

Parker RM, Baker DW, Williams MV, Nurss JR. 1995. The Test of Functional Health Literacy in Adults: A new instrument for measuring patients' literacy skills. *Journal of General Internal Medicine.* 10(10): 537–541.

Ratzan SC, Parker RM. 2000. Introduction. In: *National Library of Medicine Current Bibliographies in Medicine: Health Literacy.* Selden CR, Zorn M, Ratzan SC, Parker RM, Editors. NLM Pub. No. CBM 2000-1. Bethesda, MD: National Institutes of Health, U.S. Department of Health and Human Services.

Roter DL, Stashefsky-Margalit R, Rudd R. 2001. Current perspectives on patient education in the U.S. *Patient Education and Counseling.* 44(1): 79–86.

Rudd R. 2003. Objective 11-2: Improvement of health literacy. In: *Communicating Health: Priorities and Strategies for Progress.* Washington, DC: Office of Disease Prevention and Health Promotion, U.S. Department of Health and Human Services.

Rudd RE, Colton T, Schacht R. 2000. *An Overview of Medical and Public Health Literature Addressing Literacy Issues: An Annotated Bibliography. Report #14.* Cambridge, MA: National Center for the Study of Adult Learning and Literacy.

Rudd RE, Comings JP, Hyde J. 2003. Leave no one behind: Improving health and risk communication through attention to literacy. *Journal of Health Communication, Special Supplement on Bioterrorism.* 8(Supplement 1): 104–115.

Slosson RJL. 1990. *Slosson Oral Reading Tests—Revised*. East Aurora, NY: Slosson Educational Publishers.

Taylor WL. 1953. "Cloze procedure": A new tool for measuring readability. *Journalism Quarterly*. 30: 415–433.

Williams DR. 1990. Socioeconomic differentials in health: A review and redirection. *Social Psychology Quarterly*. 53: 81–99.

3

The Extent and Associations of Limited Health Literacy

This report has already noted that an individuals' health literacy level is the product of a complex set of skills and interactions on the part of the individual, the health-care system, the education system, and the cultural and societal context. It has also been noted that most individuals will encounter health literacy barriers at some point. High educational attainment may not be sufficient to negotiate medical and technical language and meanings. The following chapters discuss in more detail some of the barriers and potential approaches to health literacy in the various contexts. Here, the focus is on the individual, and particularly, on the individual who has limited literacy skills. This chapter provides an overview of how limited health literacy may restrict an individual's participation in health contexts and activities. Look at Figure 3-1 on the following page and put yourself in the shoes of a patient with limited literacy skills. How would you feel, what would you do, where would you go, to whom would you turn if this medication is prescribed for you by your doctor? How compliant could you be about taking your medications correctly?

Navigating modern life in America with very limited literacy can be like trying to find a hotel in another land, armed with a map of the city but unable to decipher the letters on the street signs. Everyone—not just those with limited literacy skills—is increasingly faced with difficult and confusing text at work, at home, in institutional settings such as schools, banks, social service organizations, and within health-care settings. People of all literacy levels might be able to manage texts that they frequently encounter

Kedai Ubat Sunshine
123 Jalan Main, Los Angeles, CA 90015

Nama Paskit:
John Lin

Nama Ubat:
Crixivan (empat ratus mg)

Arahan:
Telan dua biji, tiga kali sehari.
Jangan makan dua jam sebelum
dan satu jam selepas anda makan
ubat ini.

Mustahak! Sila baca:
Ubat ini mungkin
menyebabkan cirit birit,
loya kagatalan kulit,
kekeringan kulit, sakit
kepala, atau sakit perut.
Pesakit dinasihatkan
supaya minum banyak air
untuk mengelakkan
pembentukan batu
karang.

FIGURE 3-1 Mock-up prescription medication instructions in Bahasa Malaysia,
the written language of Malaysia.
SOURCE: Shinagawa and Foong (2003). Reprinted with permission.

and use for everyday activities, but will often face problems with unfamiliar
types of text. For example, a woman who has never lived near a public
transportation system may find herself unable to interpret a bus schedule.
Directions for operating a particle accelerator, filing income tax returns, or
choosing between health insurance plans may be similarly indecipherable
for most adults, regardless of literacy skills in other contexts.

As discussed in detail in Chapter 2, current measures of health literacy
rely primarily on print in the health context and not on the broad array of
skills needed for true health literacy. However, since skills with the written
word are linked to skills with the spoken word, we can use information
from these measures as a starting point to make reasonable assumptions
about the average health literacy skill level of adults in the United States.
The following section examines the extent of the problem of health literacy,
estimated from existing measures of literacy based on the National Adult
Literacy Survey (NALS) and from assessments of health literacy.

LITERACY IN AMERICA

About 90 million (47 percent) U.S. adults cannot accurately and consistently locate, match, and integrate information from newspapers, advertisements, or forms (Kirsch et al., 1993). These adults can perform a variety of

straightforward tasks using printed materials; however, they are unlikely to perform, with accuracy and consistency, more challenging tasks using long or dense texts. These findings have been compared to those in 22 industrialized nations that participated in the International Adult Literacy Surveys. The U.S. scores are very similar to those in Canada, higher than those in England or Ireland, but lower than those in the Scandinavian countries (Organization for Economic Co-operation and Development and Statistics Canada, 2000). U.S. and international education and workforce researchers note that the average skill levels are barely sufficient for full participation in the civic and economic sectors of current industrialized societies (Sum et al., 2002). About 90 million adults have skills that are inadequate for many needed tasks.

Of the 90 million adults with limited literacy skills, about 42 million demonstrated skills in NALS Level 1. Of these, a small percentage had such limited English literacy skills that they were unable to respond to much of the survey. Most people performing at Level 1 can perform simple and routine tasks using uncomplicated materials. They can, for example, locate a single piece of information in a short and simple piece of text. However, they have trouble with tasks requiring them to locate or match several pieces of information in moderately complicated texts. Adults performing at NALS Level 1 can solve simple math problems when the numbers and the operations are provided but find it difficult to solve the same problems when they must locate the numbers and the operations in a piece of text (Kirsch, 2001; Kirsch et al., 1993). A package of over-the-counter pediatric cold medicine can be used as an example. An adult performing at NALS Level 1 would likely be able to locate the words *child, children, pediatric* on a package of cold medicine for children. However, one would not expect an adult with NALS Level 1 skills to be able to read a chart in order to identify "how much . . . syrup is recommended for a child who is 10 years old and weighs 50 pounds?" What makes this task so much more complex and difficult is the fact that the structure of the chart is in columns starting with age, then typical weights associated with age, then dosage by type including drops, syrup, chewable 80 mg, and chewable 160 mg. The typical reader would look down the column to find the age of the child and then over the row to the column for syrup. In very small print outside the chart itself there is a conditional statement that tells the reader "if child is significantly under- or overweight, dosage may need to be adjusted accordingly . . . ." This level task would fall at NALS level 4 or 5 (Rudd et al., 2003).

Of the 90 million adults with limited literacy skills, 50 million adults nationwide demonstrated skills at NALS Level 2. Those adults who scored at NALS Level 2 can locate information in moderately complicated text, make low-level inferences using print materials, and integrate easily identifiable pieces of information. They can solve simple math problems when the numbers and operations are found in familiar and uncomplicated materials. However, adults at Level 2 find it difficult to perform these operations in difficult text and to perform operations that are complicated by distracting information and complex texts (Morse, 2002). In addition, they will find the demands of the chart to determine dosage for children's cold medicine difficult and, according to studies assessing informed consent documents, will find the process of informed consent arduous and most likely not possible.

Most of the adults in NALS Levels 1 and 2 are "literate"; however, adults in Level 1 are at a severe disadvantage and adults in Level 2 are disadvantaged, in relation to the demands of twenty-first century life. These findings have serious implications for the health sectors. Rudd, Kirsch, and Yamamoto, in a reanalysis of the NALS with a focus on health-related tasks only, report similar findings (Rudd et al., 2003). The 1992 NALS survey provides the most recent nationally representative population survey data on literacy skills of adults in the United States. The committee believes that levels of American literacy have not improved over the past decade and that health systems have become more complex. The committee looks forward to the publication of the National Assessment of Adult Literacy[1] (NAAL), conducted in 2003, which contains health-related literacy tasks. The committee believes that the NAAL will significantly expand our understanding of literacy and health literacy in America, and regrets that the data are not yet available. In addition, a representative sample of American adults is included in the new international Adult Literacy & Lifeskills Survey (ALL).[2] Linked to the NAAL framework, the ALL also contains health-related literacy tasks. These two surveys have the potential to provide detailed information on the extent of limited health literacy in America.

Demographic Associations with Limited Literacy

The largest proportion of American adults with limited literacy are native-born Caucasian speakers of English. Over half of the people with NALS Level 1 skills are Caucasians, and about 57 million Caucasian Americans have limited literacy skills (NALS Levels 1 and 2) (Kirsch et al., 1993). However, many groups with higher rates of limited literacy than would be predicted from population estimates alone were identified by the NALS. Groups with lower average proficiency scores include those who are poor, members of ethnic and cultural minorities, those who live in the southern

---

[1]For more information, see the NAAL on the National Center for Education Statistics web site: http://nces.ed.gov/naal/.

[2]For more information, see ALL on the Educational Testing Service web site: http://www.ets.org/all.

and western regions of the United States, those with less than a high school degree or GED, and those who are above the age of 65. It is important to keep in mind that the NALS was performed only in English, and that clear differentials for literacy proficiencies can be seen within each population group on the basis of nativity, education, and access to economic resources (Kirsch et al., 1993). Table 3-1 displays the percentage of persons overall and various demographic groups that have NALS Level 1 or 2 literacy skills, the lowest of five skill levels. Each of these groups is discussed briefly below in order to highlight those that could potentially benefit from interventions aimed at improving health literacy.[3]

Adults over the age of 65 have more limited literacy proficiency than younger, working adults, according to the NALS data. However, cross-tabulations indicate that scores for elders vary by education level and access to financial resources (Kirsch et al., 1993). Hispanics, African Americans, Pacific Islanders, and Native Americans are also (including Alaska Natives) over-represented in the numbers of adults with lower literacy proficiency scores, as indicated by the NALS data (Kirsch et al., 1993). These populations have increased in number since 1992, when the NALS was performed, and as a group represent a larger proportion of the U.S. population (U.S. Census Bureau, 2002). Hispanic and Asian populations in particular have increased at a greater rate than other U.S. populations. While more recent literacy data is not yet available, these population increases may represent an increase in the number of individuals, and the percentage of American adults, affected by limited health literacy.

Individuals without a high school diploma or GED have lower levels of literacy proficiency than do those with a high school diploma or education beyond high school. Nearly all adults who did not finish eighth grade scored at Level 1 or 2 on the NALS, and 77 percent of these individuals scored at Level 1. Similarly, among individuals who entered high school but did not graduate, 81 percent scored at NALS Levels 1 or 2, while only 55 percent of high school graduates scored at those levels (Kirsch et al., 1993). Since between 400,000 and 500,000 students drop out of high school each year in the United States (Young, 2002), high school dropouts constitute a large population likely living without adequate literacy skills.

Overall, more than 70 percent of immigrants tested on the NALS scored at Levels 1 or 2. The NALS was conducted in English only. Thus the finding that 25 percent of those scoring in the lowest levels of literacy proficiency were immigrants to the United States might be expected, since many of

---

[3]The information in this section is drawn in part from the background paper "Outside the Clinician-Patient Relationship: A Call to Action For Health Literacy," commissioned by the committee from Barry D. Weiss, M.D. The committee appreciates his contributions. The full text of the paper can be found in Appendix B.

TABLE 3-1 Percentage of Adult Population Groups with Literacy Skills at NALS Levels 1, 2, or 3–4

Group	Percent Respondents at Skill Level		
	Level 1	Level 2	Levels 3–4
All NALS Respondents	22	28	50
Age			
16–54 years	15	28	57
55–64 years	28	33	39
65 years and older	49	32	19
Highest Education Level Completed			
0–8 years	77	19	4
9–12 years (no high school graduation)	44	37	19
High school diploma/GED (no college study)	18	37	45
Racial/Ethnic Group			
White	15	26	59
American Indian/Alaska Native	26	38	36
Asian/Pacific Islander	35	25	40
Black	41	36	23
Hispanic (all groups)	52	26	22
Immigrants to US (various countries of origin)			
0–8 years of education prior to arrival in US	60	31	9
9+ years of education prior to arrival in US	44	27	29
Disability			
Any mental or emotional condition	48	26	27
Learning disability	59	22	19
Hearing difficulty	35	34	32
Speech disability	54	27	19
Visual difficulty	55	26	19

SOURCE: Unadjusted averages of prose and document literacy scores on the NALS as reported on Tables 1.1A, 1.1B, 1.2A, 1.2B, 1.8, and Figure 1.10 in Kirsch et al. (1993) and on Table B3.13 in the U.S. Department of Education's report *English Literacy and Language Minorities in the United States* (2001).

those immigrants might have just begun to learn English. In addition, 91 percent of those who did not complete a high school education in their country of origin scored at the lowest levels of proficiency (see Table 3-1). A high proportion of people entering the United States from non-English-speaking nations come from non-industrialized areas of the world in which there are limited educational opportunities. For example, more than half of adults who emigrate to the United States from Spanish-speaking countries had not finished high school in their country of origin (Greenberg et al., 2001).

Individuals who described themselves as having a physical or mental condition which prevented them from participating fully in normal activities tended to score at the lowest levels of proficiency. More than half the individuals with vision, speech, or learning disabilities performed at NALS Level 1, as did 48 percent of individuals reporting a mental or emotional condition. In contrast, 35 percent of individuals reporting a hearing difficulty performed at NALS Level 1.

Approximately 7 of 10 prisoners surveyed by the NALS demonstrated limited literacy proficiency. Individuals who did not finish school are overrepresented among prison inmates, so in many cases, prisoners represent the same individuals as those with limited education. NALS investigators studied nearly 1,150 inmates in 80 federal and state prisons that had been randomly selected to represent penal institutions across the country (Haigler, 1994).

Several other groups, not specifically studied in the NALS, are also known to have limited literacy skills. These groups include the persons who are poor and/or homeless, and military recruits. As discussed in Chapter 2, social factors affect literacy. Poverty is intertwined with many sociodemographic variables (Balsa and McGuire, 2001), which, in turn, are associated with limited literacy. Although the causal relationships are not known, individuals with limited incomes/access to resources are also more likely than those with higher incomes/access to resources to have lower literacy proficiency (Kirsch et al., 1993). Homeless individuals, who may also be affected by limited literacy and poverty, are the audience recipients of a variety of state programs developed to enhance literacy skills (Profiles of State Programs, 1990). Weiss and colleagues used Medicaid enrollment as a proxy for low income and administered the Instrument for the Diagnosis of Reading/Instrumento Para Diagnosticar Lectura (IDL) as a measure of literacy. They found that the majority of low-income individuals involved in their study had limited reading skills, with the average score at the fifth-grade level (Weiss et al., 1994). In addition, reading and mathematics skills of potential military recruits are assessed, and enlistment in the military requires passing these tests. As many recruits cannot adequately perform the high school level reading tasks they face in the military, all branches of the military operate educational programs to increase the literacy skills of their members (Hegerfeld, 1999).

THE EPIDEMIOLOGY OF LIMITED HEALTH LITERACY

Ninety million people—approximately one-half of our adult population—lack the basic literacy skills required for full participation in American society (Comings et al., 2001; Sum et al., 2002). Basic literacy skills that can be applied in the context of health are required for health literacy. As discussed in Chapter 2, there are no assessment tools that fully measure health literacy, and consequently, no population-based study to date has directly examined the relationship of literacy to health literacy or of health literacy, as fully defined, to health. However, correlations between measures of literacy and measures of reading in the health context such as the Rapid Estimate of Adult Literacy in Medicine (REALM) and the Short Test of Functional Health Literacy in Adults (S-TOFHLA) suggest a strong association (Davis et al., 1993; Parker et al., 1995).

Routine health and health-care tasks are often complicated and may require more literacy skills than those needed to meet the demands of everyday life. To date, no researcher has fully delineated tasks needed for the full range of health-related activities nor has anyone fully calibrated the levels of complexity of the various types of materials used in health contexts. However, a review of health literature indicates that research findings over three decades place a wide variety of assessed materials (based primarily on reading level analyses) at levels that exceed the reading skills of most high school graduates (Rudd et al., 2000a). The substantial volume of literature focused on assessments of health-related materials.

Health literacy may also be more reliant on domains of literacy such as oral (speaking) ability and aural (listening) comprehension that are not measured by NALS, or the tools currently used to measure health literacy (discussed in Chapter 2 of this report). Recognizing that basic literacy skills are required for health literacy, it is reasonable to conclude that individuals with limited literacy—the 90 million individuals that scored in Levels 1 and 2 of NALS—probably also have limited health literacy. These individuals likely lack the necessary literacy skills in English needed to effectively obtain and understand much of the health-related information they will interact with at home, at work, or in their communities. Furthermore, limited health literacy probably affects more than just those with limited literacy. Individuals with adequate literacy may be affected by the complex literacy demands of the health-care context, and some individuals may continue to be affected despite attempts to reduce these demands. These findings, combined with the average NALS scores of U.S. adults, offer a strong argument that 90 million U.S. adults are severely disadvantaged as they attempt to function in health-care contexts. The committee considers health literacy to be a reciprocal function of the health context and the individual. Therefore, any person, no matter what literacy skills he or she possesses, may well have limited health literacy once he or she enters complex health-care contexts.

I am a nurse with advanced degrees. I read on a college level. Yet, I am a total health illiterate. How can this be? Well, I've been diagnosed with an unusual type of autoimmune disease that has extended into several other diseases, one of which—lymphoma—might be fatal. Yet despite my healthcare background, my ability to understand the written word at a high grade level, and the many resources at my immediate disposal, I still don't understand everything I need to know about my condition. I am writing this to share with you that it is difficult to piece together all the various components of the healthcare system even when you have a knowledgeable support system and excellent reading ability. I am sharing my personal health situation with you because even with all the supposed advantages I have as mentioned above, I still don't understand my condition and prognosis (Mayer, 2003).

Finding 3-1 About 90 million adults, an estimate based on the 1992 NALS, have literacy skills that test below high school level (NALS Levels 1 and 2). Of these, about 40–44 million (NALS Level 1) have difficulty finding information in unfamiliar or complex texts such as newspaper articles, editorials, medicine labels, forms, or charts. Because the medical and public health literature indicates that health materials are complex and often far above high school level, the committee notes that approximately 90 million adults may lack the needed literacy skills to effectively use the U.S. health system. The majority of these adults are native-born English speakers. Literacy levels are lower among the elderly, those who have lower educational levels, those who are poor, minority populations, and groups with limited English proficiency such as recent immigrants.

Studies of Limited Health Literacy

In this section, we examine the extent of limited health literacy by examining peer-reviewed studies that provide evidence about the epidemiology, or relative rates, of health literacy skills using currently available measures in different demographic groups. The conclusions that can be drawn about health literacy from this research are limited because in most cases, the studies below identify individuals and groups in which only the print component of health literacy skills is measured (see Chapter 2).

Studies described in this and the following section represent a sample of the English-language peer-reviewed studies that measure literacy or use the REALM or TOFHLA among patients or consumers in a health context. We note that these measures are, for the most part, assessments of print literacy in the health context. While these measures all tap into some aspect of health literacy, the studies do not necessarily use the same standard for identifying people with limited skills. It is even the case that any two tests both claiming to use grade-level scores would not identify the same students as being below a selected standard because their norming samples most likely were not the same. Thus the percentages falling below a particular standard are not directly comparable, but do clearly point to where problems exist.

Studies were identified by searching the Medline (1966–2003), PsycInfo (1974–2003), ERIC[4] (1963–2003), Sociological Abstracts (1963–2003), and CINAHL[5] (1982–2003) databases through the OVID web gateway for the indicated years with the following terms as keyword searches: "health literacy," "literacy and health," and "reading and health." To be included, the study had to define the health or health-care population cohort, the literacy measurement tool, and the result of the literacy screening assessment. Additional studies for inclusion were identified through testimony to the committee by experts in the field (see Appendix A), and the available bibliographies (Greenberg, 2001; Rudd et al., 2000b; Zobel et al., 2003).

Table 3-2 summarizes identified studies containing information on the rates of health literacy skills as currently measured among various study populations. Results are given as percentages of the study participants with (1) marginal and inadequate health literacy as measured by the TOFHLA (Parker et al., 1995) or its shorter version (S-TOFHLA; Baker et al., 1999); or (2) inadequate health literacy as indicated by a score below grade 9 on the REALM (Davis et al., 1993); or (3) what the authors reported if a standard measure was not used or if a standard measure was modified. Table 3-2 also identifies the reported demographic characteristics of the study participants that were reported to be associated with limited health literacy.

Studies noted in Table 3-2 document the prevalence of limited health-literacy skills as measured by the REALM or TOFHLA among patients in general medical and pediatric clinics; specialty care clinics including those for asthma, HIV, family planning, obstetrics, and oncology; and community-based sites including retirement homes and social service agencies. The studies show that limited health literacy skills, as measured by current assessment tools, are common, with significant variations in prevalence depending on the population sampled (Williams et al., 1998b). In many cases, however, education was not controlled for, and in some cases differences based on health literacy assessments were no longer significant when education was controlled for.

Two large multisite studies of convenience samples that provide esti-

---

[4]Educational Resources Information Center.
[5]Cumulative Index to Nursing and Allied Health Literature.

mates of the prevalence of limited health literacy among users of urban public hospitals showed variation in prevalence in different geographic locations. In one study, Williams and colleagues (1995) administered the TOFHLA in either English or Spanish to patients presenting for acute care at public hospitals in Atlanta and Los Angeles. The study participants included 1,892 English speakers from Atlanta or Los Angeles, and 767 Spanish-speaking individuals from Los Angeles only. Almost half (47.4 percent) of the participants in Atlanta had inadequate (34.7 percent) or marginal (12.7 percent) health literacy scores on the TOFHLA, while in Los Angeles the rates of limited and marginal health literacy scores were 12.5 percent and 9.5 percent for English speakers and 41.9 percent and 19.8 percent for Spanish speakers. Spanish-speaking participants (tested in Spanish) had higher rates of limited health literacy scores than did English-speaking participants, but these differences were not significant after controlling for years of education.

A more recent multisite study used the S-TOFHLA to assess new enrollees in a Medicare managed care organization in four different geographic areas: Cleveland, Houston, Tampa, and an area of southern Florida including Fort Lauderdale and Miami (Gazmararian et al., 1999b). Participants were 304 Spanish-speaking and 2,956 English-speaking enrollees. The prevalence of inadequate and marginal health literacy scores on the S-TOFHLA among English speakers was 23.5 percent and 10.4 percent, respectively, while among Spanish speakers prevalence rates were 34.2 percent and 19.7 percent. Results varied by city, with the participants in Cleveland showing the highest rate of inadequate health literacy scores among English speakers at 34.1 percent, and those in Tampa showing the lowest rate at 16.6 percent. The geographic variation between Spanish-speaking populations was even more striking; 60 percent of those in Tampa had inadequate health literacy scores compared with 21.2 percent of those in Houston. The authors of this study indicated that the geographic variation between study sites might reflect differences in the interrelated characteristics of race, language, and socioeconomic status. However, when these variables were controlled for, participants in Cleveland continued to show the highest rates of limited health literacy scores among English speakers. Factors mediating geographic differences in skills remain unknown and warrant further investigation. Increased awareness of these variations could lead to regionally tailored health literacy interventions.

Studies shown in Table 3-2 suggest that the segments of the U.S. population that could be considered at greatest risk for limited health literacy are those that were reported to have higher rates of limited literacy in the NALS study and other sources. As with limited literacy reported in the NALS (Kirsch et al., 1993), limited health literacy as currently measured is more prevalent among the elderly (Beers et al., 2003; Benson and Forman, 2002;

TABLE 3-2   The Epidemiology of Health Literacy Skills Among Various
Populations

Citation	Population	Participation Rate	Study Design	Setting
Arnold et al., 2001	N = 600 Pregnant women 296 African American 303 Caucasian Mean age: 23 years	96%	Convenience sample	Obstetric clinics, Louisiana
Beers et al., 2003. Published Abstract	N = 1805 58% African American 66% male (Health Literacy and Patient Satisfaction Study)	—	—	Primary care clinics, VA medical center and university hospital
Bennett et al., 1998	N = 212 African American, 103 Mean age: 70.8 years	96%	Convenience sample	Prostate clinics in Shreveport, LA, and Chicago, IL
Benson and Forman, 2002	N = 93 71 women Mean age: 83 years	52%	Convenience sample	Affluent retirement community in Albuquerque, NM

Measure	Reported Demographic Associations with Low Health Literacy	Prevalence of Literacy Levels

REALM	African American race	African American women
		  3rd and below: 9%
		  4th–6th: 19%
		  7th–8th: 41%
		  9th and above: 31%
		Caucasian women
		  3rd and below: 4%
		  4th–6th: 5%
		  7th–8th: 26%
		  9th and above: 66%

REALM	African American race
	Older age
	Lower education level
	Association with age was no longer significant when stratified by education level
	Association with race remained significant when stratified by education level
		REALM
		  3rd and below: 2%
		  4th–6th: 8%
		  7th–8th: 31%
		  9th and above: 59%

REALM	African American race
	Geographic location (Louisiana site)
		African American men
		  6th and below: 52.3%
		Caucasian men:
		  6th and below: 8.7%
		Chicago, IL:
		  6th and below: 12.3%
		Shreveport, LA:
		  6th and below: 38.1%

TOFHLA	Older age Fewer years of education	74% or less on TOFHLA: 30%

Continued

TABLE 3-2 Continued

Citation	Population	Participation Rate	Study Design	Setting
Davis et al., 1994	N = 396 Parents or other caretakers accompanying pediatric outpatients Mean age: 30 years	96%	—	Pediatric clinic in a public hospital, Louisiana
Fortenberry et al., 2001	N = 1035 Mean age: 26.36	78%	—	Clinics, community-based organizations, and by street intercept in 4 sites (CO, IN, NY, and AL)
Gazmararian et al., 1999b	N = 3260 New Medicare enrollees 2,956 English speakers, 304 Spanish speakers Age distribution: 65–69 years: 37% 70–74 years: 27.3% 75–79 years: 19.3% 80–84 years: 11% 85 years: 5.4%	39% 3,260 participated out of 8,409 identified for study	Cohort	Prudential Medicare Managed Care Study 4 sites: Cleveland, OH, Houston, TX, south Florida, and Tampa, Florida

Measure	Reported Demographic Associations with Low Health Literacy	Prevalence of Literacy Levels	
REALM and WRAT-R	—	REALM 3rd and below: 11% 4th–6th: 16% 7th–8th: 37% 9th and above: 35% WRAT Less than 4th: 31% Less than 7th: 55% Less than 9th: 73%	
REALM	—	8th and below: 35% 9th and above: 65%	

S-TOFHLA	African American race
	Older age
	Fewer years of school completed
	History of blue collar occupations
	Older age was strongly associated with lower health literacy, and this association remained after adjusting for years of school completed and cognitive impairment
		Total
		English
		  Inadequate: 23.5%
		  Marginal: 10.4%
		  Adequate: 66.1%
		
		Cleveland, OH
		English
		  Inadequate: 34.1%
		  Marginal: 9.9%
		  Adequate: 56.0%
		
		Houston, TX
		English
		  Inadequate: 28.0%
		  Marginal: 9.4%
		  Adequate: 62.6%
			Spanish
			  Inadequate: 34.2%
			  Marginal: 19.7%
			  Adequate: 46.1%
			
			Spanish
			  Inadequate: 21.2%
			  Marginal: 19.2%
			  Adequate: 59.6%

Continued

TABLE 3-2 Continued

Citation	Population	Participation Rate	Study Design	Setting
Gazmararian et al., 1999a	N = 406 Women enrolled in a Medicaid managed care plan Age distribution: 19–24 years: 144 25–29 years: 86 30 years: 175	19% 406 participated out of 2,197 identified for study	Cohort	Medicaid managed care plan in Memphis, Tennessee
Kalichman et al., 2000	N = 228 HIV-infected adults Mean age: 39.7 years	—	Convenience sample	HIV clinics, AIDS service organizations, social service agencies
Kalichman et al., 1999	N = 182 HIV-infected adults Mean age: 39.1 years	—	Convenience sample	HIV clinics, AIDS service organizations, social service agencies

Measure	Reported Demographic Associations with Low Health Literacy	Prevalence of Literacy Levels

		South Florida
		English Spanish
		  Inadequate: 17.3% Inadequate: 34.3%
		  Marginal: 11.6% Marginal: 20.3%
		  Adequate: 71.1% Adequate: 45.4%
		
		Tampa, FL
		English Spanish
		  Inadequate: 16.6% Inadequate: 60.0%
		  Marginal: 10.2% Marginal: 16.0%
		  Adequate: 73.2% Adequate: 24.0%

TOFHLA (abbreviated version)	Lower education level Health literacy levels were not significantly associated with age, race, marital status, employment status, and poverty status	9.6% scored less than 80% on the TOFHLA
TOFHLA	Fewer years of education Ethnic/minority status Health literacy level was not related to age, income level, gender, or sexual orientation	TOFHLA Scores: 0%–20%: 2% 21%–40%: 2% 41%–60%: 3% 61%–80%: 11% 81%–90%: 23% 91%–100%: 59%
TOFHLA		41% scored below 85% on the TOFHLA

Continued

TABLE 3-2 Continued

Citation	Population	Participation Rate	Study Design	Setting
Kaufman et al., 2001	N = 61 First-time mothers aged 18 years or older who had an infant between 2 and 12 months	—	Convenience sample	Public health clinic, Albuquerque, NM
Li et al., 2000	N = 55 (REALM scores available on 39) Women with early-stage breast cancer	71% 39 patients participated in REALM testing out of 55 identified by retrospective chart review	Convenience sample	Clinic in the rural south
Lindau et al., 2002	N = 529 English-speaking patients older than 18 years Median age: 27	91%	Prospective Cohort	Ambulatory Obstetrics and Gynecology clinic and a women's HIV clinic
Montalto and Spiegler, 2001	N = 70 Female: Mean age: 45 Male: Mean age: 55	38.%		Rural community health center
Schillinger et al., 2002	N = 408 English- and Spanish-speaking type-2 diabetes patients older than 30 years (San Francisco General Diabetic Patients with Low Health Literacy Study)	91%	Cross-sectional	Two primary care clinics, public hospital, San Francisco, CA

Measure	Reported Demographic Associations with Low Health Literacy	Prevalence of Literacy Levels	
REALM	—	3rd and below: 0% 4th–6th: 0% 7th–8th: 36% 9th and above: 64%	
REALM	—	3rd and below: 0% 4th–6th: 12.8% 7th–8th: 12.8% 9th and above: 74.4%	
REALM	Non-white participant Those with no or public health insurance	6th and below: nearly 10% 7th–8th: 33% 9th and above: 61%	
TOFHLA		Inadequate: 2.86% Marginal: 11.43% Adequate: 85.71%	
S-TOFHLA	Older age Female gender Non-white Spanish-speakers Lower education level Medicare coverage Longer time with diabetes	English Inadequate: 27.7% Marginal: 12.7% Adequate: 59.6%	Spanish Inadequate: 56.8% Marginal: 14.2% Adequate: 29.9%

Continued

TABLE 3-2 Continued

Citation	Population	Participation Rate	Study Design	Setting
Shea et al., 2003. Published abstract	N = 2494 (Health literacy and patient satisfaction study)	—	Cohort	Urban community-based practices
Weiss et al., 1994	N = 402 Medicaid enrollees, 21.6% Male, 78.4% Female 45.8% Hispanic 42.8% Caucasian 5.5% African American Mean age: 49.0	75%	Cohort	University Family Care, a health care organization in Tucson, AZ
Williams et al., 1998a	N = 483 273 from emergency department (ED) 210 from asthma clinic (AC) ED Mean age: 37 AC Mean age: 47	ED = 79% AC = 90%	Cohort	ED and AC at urban public hospital, Atlanta, GA
Williams et al., 1998b	N = 516 Patients with hypertension (n = 402) and patients with diabetes (n = 114)	94% (LA) 86% (Atlanta)	Cohort	General medical clinics of two urban public hospitals (Atlanta and Los Angeles)

Measure	Reported Demographic Associations with Low Health Literacy	Prevalence of Literacy Levels
S-TOFHLA	—	Inadequate: 25% Marginal: 11% Adequate: 65%
Instrument for the Diagnosis of Reading/ Instrumento Para Diagnosticar Lecturas (IDL)	Spanish-speaking	0: 8.7% 1st: 4.7% 2nd: 5.1% 3rd: 5.6% 4th: 4.2% 5th: 5.2% 6th: 13.7% 7th: 14.2% 8th and above: 38.6%
REALM	Older age	3rd and below: 13% 4th–6th: 27% 7th–8th: 33% 9th and above: 27%
TOFHLA	Older age Spanish-speaking	Diabetes patients* Inadequate: 44% Marginal: 11% Adequate: 45% Hypertension patients* Inadequate: 49% Marginal: 12% Adequate: 39% *results include both Spanish- and English-speaking individuals

Continued

TABLE 3-2 Continued

Citation	Population	Participation Rate	Study Design	Setting
Williams et al., 1995	N = 2,659 Patients presenting for acute care, 1892 English speakers, 767 Spanish speakers (Literacy in Health Care study)	77.% Atlanta, 84% Los Angeles	Cohort	Two urban public hospitals in Atlanta and Los Angeles

REALM: 4 levels: (1st–3rd, 4th–6th, 7th–8th, 9th and above).
TOFHLA: Inadequate health literacy (score 0–59), marginal health literacy (score 60–74), adequate health literacy (score 75–100).

Gazmararian et al., 1999b; Schillinger et al., 2002; Williams et al., 1995, 1998a, b). Limited literacy and health literacy as measured by these studies in older adults is an important problem. Older individuals generate high health-care costs (Berk and Monheit, 2001). High health-care costs, in turn, are associated with limited literacy (see below for a detailed discussion). While older individuals have some of the highest rates of limited health literacy scores and limited functional literacy scores, they also have some of the most demanding health-care needs. Limited health literacy in older adults may contribute to a situation in which those most in need of health care may be those least able to access and benefit from the care.

Studies with current health literacy measures have reported that demographic associations with limited health literacy include racial or ethnic minority status (Arnold et al., 2001; Beers et al., 2003; Bennett et al., 1998; Gazmararian et al., 1999b; Kalichman et al., 2000; Lindau et al., 2002; Schillinger et al., 2002), fewer years of schooling or lower education level (Beers et al., 2003; Benson and Forman, 2002; Gazmararian et al., 1999a, b; Kalichman et al., 2000; Schillinger et al., 2002), and being a Spanish-speaker (tested in Spanish; Weiss et al., 1994). Notably, these demographic groups identified by several assessments conducted in different settings are the same demographic groups identified by the NALS, discussed earlier. However, none of these studies have involved a sufficiently large random sample of adults that would allow us to extrapolate these findings to other populations.

Measure	Reported Demographic Associations with Low Health Literacy	Prevalence of Literacy Levels	
TOFHLA	Age 60 years or above Spanish-speaking	Los Angeles	
		English	Spanish
		Inadequate: 12.5%	Inadequate: 41.9%
		Marginal: 9.5%	Marginal: 19.8%
		Adequate: 78%	Adequate: 38.3%
		Atlanta	
		Inadequate: 34.7%	
		Marginal: 12.7%	
		Adequate: 52.6%	

S-TOFHLA: Inadequate health literacy (score 0–53), marginal health literacy (score 54–66), adequate health literacy (67–100).
IDL: Grade level scores from 0 to 8, 0 indicating failure at grade level 1, 8 indicating reading comprehension at or above the 8th grade level.

THE ASSOCIATIONS OF LIMITED HEALTH LITERACY

Research study findings linking the presence of limited health literacy as currently measured to poor health are accumulating, although the causal relationship between health literacy and health is unknown. This research can be thought of as addressing two types of costs associated with limited health literacy: economic costs to society and the health-care system, and costs in terms of the human burden of disease. This section will review both peer-reviewed and new evidence of the association of limited health literacy as measured by the REALM or TOFHLA with health outcomes, health-related knowledge and behaviors, and economic costs. The personal costs of limited health literacy also bear consideration. Many adults overestimate their knowledge and understanding of health information, including instructions for their own care (Davis et al., 1996; Doak et al., 1996). Others may be all too aware of their difficulty understanding health information. Limited health literacy may also take a psychological toll; one study found that those with limited health literacy as measured by the S-TOFHLA reported a sense of shame about their skill level (Parikh et al., 1996).

Finding 3-2 On the basis of limited studies, public testimony, and committee members' experience the committee concludes that the shame and stigma associated with limited literacy skills are major barriers to improving health literacy.

Associations with Health Knowledge, Behavior, and Outcomes

Individuals with inadequate health literacy as currently measured report less knowledge about their medical conditions and treatment, worse health status, less understanding and use of preventive services, and a higher rate of hospitalization than those with marginal or adequate health literacy (for review, see Parker et al., 2003). Table 3-3 displays a sampling of studies that provide evidence of health-related associations with health literacy as measured by currently available assessments of print literacy in the health context. These studies were identified using the same methodology as described in the previous section.

A number of researchers examined relationships between patients' scores on the REALM or TOFHLA, knowledge of illnesses, and chronic condition management. Studies included in Table 3-3 demonstrate that hypertension, diabetes, asthma, and HIV/AIDS patients with lower scores have less knowledge of their chronic illness and its management than those with higher scores (Kalichman et al., 2000; Schillinger et al., 2002; Williams et al., 1998a, b). Examination of health literacy scores and health-care management found that patients with limited health literacy as determined by current measures have a decreased ability to share in decision making about prostate cancer treatment (Kim et al., 2001), lower adherence to anticoagulation therapy (Lasater, 2003; Win and Schillinger, 2003), and worse glycemic control (Arnold et al., 2001; Kalichman and Rompa, 2000; Schillinger et al., 2002; Williams et al., 1998a, b).

As noted in Table 3-3, several studies have demonstrated a relationship between hospitalization rates and limited health literacy as measured by the TOFHLA or REALM (e.g., Baker et al., 1997, 2002a). For example, Gordon and colleagues (2002) demonstrated that although rheumatoid arthritis patients of differing literacy levels had similar levels of rheumatoid arthritis-related dysfunction, those scoring lower on the REALM had significantly more hospital visits in the previous 12 months than age- and sex-matched controls with higher scores. Arozullah and colleagues (2002) investigated the relationships between health literacy level, the preventability of hospital admissions, and the causes of preventable hospital admissions. Patients scoring at or below the third-grade level on the REALM had an increased risk (odds ratio (OR) = 8.5) of preventable admission as compared to those scoring at the ninth-grade level and above, while patients with fourth- to eighth-grade literacy had an OR for preventability of 2.5. Furthermore, preventable admissions among patients with literacy levels at or below sixth grade were more likely than preventable admissions among those with above sixth-grade literacy to be related to system-level factors such as the availability of outpatient diagnostic care.

Health literacy level has also been linked to self-reported health status. Baker and colleagues found that among both individuals at a public hospital (1997) and in a Medicare managed care health plan (2002a), those with inadequate health literacy as determined by the TOFHLA were significantly more likely than patients with adequate health literacy scores to report their health as poor.

Health literacy levels may influence health status by affecting care-seeking behavior. A study by Bennett and colleagues (1998) indicated that individuals with lower health literacy scores on the REALM may enter the health-care system when they are sicker than those with higher health literacy scores; among men with prostate cancer, those scoring lower on the REALM were more likely to be initially diagnosed at a more advanced stage of disease than those with higher health literacy. However, this difference was not statistically significant after adjustments for race, age, and location or care. Several studies have showed that individuals with lower health literacy scores are less likely than those with higher health literacy scores to make use of preventive health-care services. Scott and colleagues (2002) found that, among Medicare managed care enrollees, those with inadequate health literacy, as measured by the S-TOFHLA, used preventive health services (including influenza and pneumococcal vaccinations, mammogram, and Pap smear) less than enrollees with higher health literacy. Similarly, Fortenberry and colleagues (2001) administered the REALM test to 1,035 people in four sites across the country, and found that higher REALM scores were independently associated with gonorrhea testing in the previous year. In contrast, Moon and colleagues (1998) found no relationship between parental literacy levels, as measured by the REALM, and use of preventive health services for pediatric patients.

Finding 3-3   Adults with limited health literacy, as measured by reading and numeracy skills, have less knowledge of disease management and of health-promoting behaviors, report poorer health status, and are less likely to use preventive services.

While research in developing countries rarely examines health literacy, a number of studies have examined the association between literacy or reading levels and health outcomes. A Bolivian study found that children of individuals participating in health, literacy, or small business financing programs offered through an international non-governmental organization were at less risk of becoming malnourished than children from comparison communities (Gonzales et al., 1999). A World Bank study of the association between maternal educational attainment and child health in Morocco found that the mother's health knowledge was associated with improved child health and nutrition (Glewwe, 1999). In contrast, a 10-year study of factors influencing infant and child health in Pakistan showed notable improvements in indicators of health, including a 69 percent increase in vacci-

TABLE 3-3 Health-Related Associations of Health Literacy Skills

Citation	Population	Participation Rate	Study Design	Setting
Arnold et al., 2001	N = 600 Pregnant women 296 African American 303 Caucasian Mean age: 23	96%	Convenience sample	Obstetric clinics, Louisiana
Baker et al., 2002b	N = 2,787 Medicare enrollees 354 African American 2,343 Caucasian Mean age: 73	37% 2,787 of 7,471 selected enrollees	Cohort	Prudential Medicare managed care (4 sites)
Baker et al., 2002a	N = 3,260 Medicare enrollees 2,956 English speakers 304 Spanish speakers	44% 3,260 of 7,471 selected enrollees	Prospective cohort	Prudential Medicare managed care (4 sites)
Baker et al., 1998	N = 979 (Literacy in Health Care Study)	—	Prospective cohort	Large public hospital emergency department; Atlanta

Data Collection Method	Health-Related Outcome Associations
REALM Structured interview Urine cotinine levels Self-report of smoking practices	Participants scoring lower on the REALM had less knowledge about the effects of smoking and less concern about the health effects of smoking on their baby than those with higher scores. REALM scores were not related to smoking practices even when race, age, and living with a smoker were controlled.
S-TOFHLA Mini-Mental State Examination (MMSE) Self-report	Health literacy was linearly related to the total MMSE score across the entire range of S-TOFHLA scores.
S-TOFHLA Structured interview MMSE Geriatric Depression Scale Short Form-12 Health Survey (SF-12), a measure of self-rated physical and mental health Managed care organization claims	Participants with inadequate and marginal health literacy reported worse health status. They were also significantly more likely to have been hospitalized than those with adequate health literacy. This relationship remained after adjusting for demographics, income, schooling, cognitive function, and social support. Spanish-speaking individuals at all literacy levels had a lower risk of admission than English speakers.
TOFHLA Structured interview Grady Memorial Hospital information system	Patients with inadequate literacy were significantly more likely to be hospitalized one or more times than those with marginal or adequate literacy. This association remained after adjusting for age, gender, race, self-reported health, socioeconomic status, and health insurance.

Continued

TABLE 3-3 Continued

Citation	Population	Participation Rate	Study Design	Setting
Baker et al., 1997	N = 2,659 979 Atlanta Los Angeles 913 English speakers 767 Spanish speakers (Literacy in Health Care Study)	81%	Prospective cohort	Two large public hospitals: Atlanta and Los Angeles
Bennett et al., 1998	N = 212 Low-income men 109 African American 103 Caucasian Mean age: 70.8	96%	Convenience sample	Prostate clinics in Shreveport, LA and Chicago, IL
Fortenberry et al., 2001	N = 1,035 Mean age: 26	78%	Convenience sample	Clinics, community-based organizations, and by street intercept (4 states: CO, IN, NY, and AL)

Data Collection Method	Health-Related Outcome Associations
TOFHLA Interview	Participants with inadequate health literacy were significantly more likely than participants with adequate health literacy to report poor health. This association remained after controlling for age, gender, race, and socioeconomic indicators. No relationship existed between literacy level and ambulatory care use after adjusting for age, health status, and economic indicators. At one of the study sites (Atlanta, GA), patients with inadequate literacy were more likely to have been hospitalized in the year preceding the study, and this relationship remained after controlling for age, gender, race, socioeconomic indicators, and self-reported health.
REALM Medical record review Pathology reports	Participants with literacy levels below the sixth grade were significantly more likely to present with Stage D cancer than those with higher literacy levels.
REALM Structured interview	After adjustment for missing REALM data, a REALM score of ninth grade or higher was independently associated with gonorrhea testing in the previous year. (Other independent predictors of testing were past suspicion of gonorrhea, self-inspection for gonorrhea, self-efficacy for care seeking, and younger age). Participants scoring lower on the REALM rated themselves more likely to acquire gonorrhea in the next 12 months than those with higher REALM scores.

Continued

TABLE 3-3 Continued

Citation	Population	Participation Rate	Study Design	Setting
Gazmararian et al., 1999a	N = 406 Women enrolled in health plan Age distribution: 19–24: 144 25–29: 86 30: 175	19% 2,197 identified for study: 1,061 not located.	Cohort	Medicaid managed care, Memphis, Tennessee
Gazmararian et al., 2000	N = 3,260 New Medicare enrollees 2,956 English speakers 304 Spanish speakers 76% Caucasian	44%	Cohort	Prudential Medicare managed care (4 sites)
Gordon et al., 2002	N = 123 Patients with rheumatoid arthritis Median age: 56 years Range: 19–77 years	96.8%	Cross-sectional	Arthritis clinic

Data Collection Method	Health-Related Outcome Associations
S-TOFHLA Interview	Higher rates of low health literacy were observed among participants who had ever used an intrauterine device, douching, rhythm, or levonorgestrel implants as methods of birth control than women who had used other methods of birth control. Compared with women with good reading skills, women with low reading skills were 2.2 times (95% confidence interval [CI] 1.1, 4.4) more likely to want to know more about birth control methods and 4.4 times (95% CI 2.2, 9.0) more likely to have incorrect knowledge about when they were most likely to get pregnant. These relationships were significant after controlling for age, race, and marital status. There was no relationship between health literacy levels and either pregnancy intendedness or current use of contraception.
S-TOFHLA Geriatric Depression Scale Interview	Participants with inadequate health literacy skills were significantly more likely to report depressive symptoms than those with adequate health literacy skills. However, this association was no longer significant after controlling for health status.
REALM Interview Case record review Health Assessment Questionnaire Hospital Anxiety and Depression Scale Carstairs Index of social deprivation	REALM scores not related to disease duration, numbers of joint replacements, or number of previous disease-modifying antirheumatic drugs. "Illiterate" patients had three times as many hospital visits as controls in the previous 12 months.

Continued

TABLE 3-3 Continued

Citation	Population	Participation Rate	Study Design	Setting
Guerra and Shea, 2003. Published Abstract	N = 1,301 Patients over 18 years of age insured by Medicaid or Medicare Mean age: 42.2 (Health Literacy and Patient Satisfaction Study)	49%	Convenience sample	Four community- and one university-based primary care practice
Kalichman et al., 2000a	N = 228 HIV-positive adults Mean age: 40		Convenience sample	HIV clinics, AIDS service organizations, social service agencies

Data Collection Method	Health-Related Outcome Associations
TOFHLA Charlson Comorbidity Index SF-12 Questionnaire	Inadequate health literacy was significantly associated with greater comorbidity burden, and this association remained after adjusting for confounders. Inadequate functional health literacy was not related to health status after adjusting for confounders.
TOFHLA Questionnaire or interview	Participants with lower health literacy were significantly less likely than those with higher health literacy: to report an undetectable HIV viral load, to indicate that they understand the meaning of viral load and CD4 cell counts, to state that their doctors ask their opinions about treatment, and to state that their doctors explain things to them so they understand. Participants with lower health literacy were significantly more likely than those with higher health literacy: to visit a doctor at least once per month, to believe that HIV medications reduce HIV-transmission risk, to believe that it is safe to have sex if an HIV+ person has an undetectable viral load, to state that new HIV treatments make it easier to relax about unsafe sex, and to state that they practice more unsafe sex because of new treatments. Health literacy level was not related to CD4 cell counts, amount of time since learning of HIV status, number of HIV-related symptoms, having diagnosed AIDS-related conditions, use of anti-HIV therapies, and some measures of treatment optimism.

Continued

TABLE 3-3 Continued

Citation	Population	Participation Rate	Study Design	Setting
Kalichman and Rompa, 2000	N = 339 HIV-positive adults Mean age: 40	—	Convenience sample	HIV clinics, AIDS service organizations, social service agencies
Kalichman et al., 1999	N = 182 HIV-positive adults Mean age: 39.1	—	Convenience sample	HIV clinics, AIDS service organizations, social service agencies
Kaufman et al., 2001	N = 61 First-time mothers aged 18 years or older who spoke English as their first language and had an infant between 2 and 12 months	—	Convenience sample	Public health clinic

Data Collection Method	Health-Related Outcome Associations
Reading comprehension section of TOFHLA (lower literacy defined as scoring at or below 80%, higher literacy as scoring above 80%) Questionnaire or interview	HIV-infected participants with lower health literacy had lower CD4 cell counts, higher viral loads, were less likely to be taking antiretroviral medications, reported a greater number of hospitalizations, and reported poorer health than those with higher health literacy. After adjusting for years of formal education, lower health literacy was associated with poorer knowledge of one's HIV-related health status, poorer AIDS-related disease and treatment knowledge, and more negative health-care perceptions and experiences.
Adapted reading comprehension section of TOFHLA (lower literacy defined as scoring 85% or below, higher literacy as scoring above 85%) Interview Questionnaire/survey	Participants with fewer years of education and lower health literacy were significantly more likely to be non-adherent in the past 2 days than those with higher health literacy, and this association remained after controlling for age, ethnicity, income, HIV symptoms, substance abuse, social support, emotional distress, and attitudes toward primary care providers. Persons of low literacy were more likely to miss treatment doses because of confusion, depression, and desire to cleanse their body than were participants with higher health literacy.
REALM (higher health literacy defined as high school level or above, and lower health literacy as seventh-eighth-grade level) Survey	Participants with higher health literacy were significantly more likely than those with lower health literacy to initiate and sustain breastfeeding during the first 2 months.

Continued

TABLE 3-3 Continued

Citation	Population	Participation Rate	Study Design	Setting
Lindau et al., 2002	N = 529 English-speaking patients older than 18 years Median age: 27 58% African-American 18% Hispanic	91%	Prospective cohort	Ambulatory OBGYN clinic and a women's HIV clinic
Moon et al., 1998	N = 543 Parents accompanying children to clinic Mean age: 32	85.8%	Prospective cohort	Pediatric acute care clinic
Parikh et al., 1996	N = 202 Patients from Literacy in Health Care Study Mean age: 41 92% African American	65%	Cohort	Emergency department and walk-in clinic, Atlanta, GA

Data Collection Method	Health-Related Outcome Associations
REALM Interview Chart review Physician survey	Health literacy level was the only factor independently associated with knowledge related to cervical cancer screening. This association remained after controlling for education, employment, ethnicity, insurance, and age. Participants with inadequate and marginal health literacy were significantly more likely than those with adequate health literacy to: state that they would seek care for an illness in an emergency department or acute care facility (11% vs. 3%); not seek medical care if informed of an abnormal Pap test (30% vs. 19%).
REALM Interview	REALM score significantly correlated with parental perception of how sick the child was. No relationship between REALM score and use of preventive services, comprehension of diagnosis, medication name and instructions, or ability to obtain and administer prescribed medicines.
TOFHLA Survey Interview	67.4% of participants with inadequate or marginal health literacy stated that they had trouble reading and understanding what they read. 39.7% of these participants acknowledged they have shame about their reading difficulty. Of the participants who had low functional health literacy and admitted having trouble reading, 67.2% had never told their spouses, and 53.4% had never told their children of their difficulties reading. Nineteen percent had never disclosed their difficulty reading to anyone.

Continued

TABLE 3-3 Continued

Citation	Population	Participation Rate	Study Design	Setting
Schillinger et al., 2003	N = 74 English-speaking patients with diabetes mellitus and low functional health literacy Mean age: 64 85% non-white (San Francisco General Diabetic Patients with Low Health Literacy Study)	71%	Cohort	2 primary care clinics, public hospital, San Francisco, CA
Schillinger et al., 2002	N = 408 English- and Spanish-speaking type-2 diabetes patients older than 30 years (San Francisco General Diabetic Patients with Low Health Literacy Study)	91%	Cross-sectional	Two primary care clinics, public hospital, San Francisco, CA
Scott et al., 2002	N = 2,722 New Medicare enrollees between 65 and 80 years old Mean age: 71	36%	Cohort	Prudential Medicare managed care (4 sites) Cleveland, Houston, Tampa, or South Florida

Data Collection Method	Health-Related Outcome Associations
S-TOFHLA Audiotaped patient-physician interaction	After a multivariate logistic regression, 2 variables were independently associated with good glycemic control among a group of diabetes patients with low health literacy: higher health literacy levels, and physicians' use of an interactive communication strategy.

S-TOFHLA
Diabetes care profile social support
  scale
Short form of the Center for
  Epidemiologic Studies Depression
  Scale
Interview
Hospital database
	After adjusting for patients' sociodemographic characteristics, depressive symptoms, social support, treatment regimen, and years with diabetes, three variables were independently associated with HbA1c level: health literacy level, insurance status, and treatment regimen.
	Patients with inadequate health literacy were less likely than those with adequate health literacy to achieve tight glycemic control and were more likely to have to report having retinopathy.

S-TOFHLA Interview	Inadequate health literacy was independently associated with lower use of preventive health services including receiving the influenza and pneumococcal vaccinations, mammogram, or a Pap smear. This association remained significant after adjusting for demographics, years of school completed, income, number of physician visits, and health status.

Continued

TABLE 3-3 Continued

Citation	Population	Participation Rate	Study Design	Setting
Shea et al., 2003 Published Abstract	N = 2,494 62% Hispanic 78% female 50% younger than 40 (Health Literacy and Patient Satisfaction Study)	—	Cohort	Urban community-based practices
Weiss et al., 1994	N = 402 Adult Medicaid enrollees 78.% Female 46% Hispanic 43% Caucasian Mean age: 49	75%	Cohort	University Family Care, a health-care organization Tucson, AZ
Williams et al., 1998a	N = 483 273 from emergency department Mean age: 37 210 from asthma clinic Mean age: 47	90%	Cohort	Emergency department and asthma clinic at urban public hospital, Atlanta, GA
Williams et al., 1998b	N = 516 402 patients with hypertension and 114 patients with diabetes	94% (Los Angeles) 86% (Atlanta)	Cohort	Two urban public hospitals in Los Angeles and Atlanta

Data Collection Method	Health-Related Outcome Associations
S-TOFHLA Interview Consumer Assessment of Health Plans Survey (CAHPS) in 3 different formats: written, with supporting illustrations, and an automated telephone survey	Health literacy level was a significant predictor of reported satisfaction in all subscale and overall satisfaction scores, and this relationship remained when controlling for demographic factors and the type of CAHPS instrument given.
Instrument for the Diagnosis of Reading University Famili Care Records	There was no significant relationship between literacy and health-care costs.
REALM Interview Observation of Metered dose inhaler (MDI) technique	Reading level was the strongest predictor of asthma knowledge score in a multivariate analysis. Poor MDI technique was found in 89% of patients reading at less than the third-grade level compared with 48% of patients reading at the high school level. Reading level was the strongest predictor of MDI technique in multivariate regression analyses.
TOFHLA (in either English or Spanish) Interview	Participants with inadequate or marginal functional health literacy and either hypertension or diabetes had significantly less knowledge of their disease than those with adequate functional health literacy. There were no significant relationships between health literacy and measures of outcome (blood pressure, or HbA1c level).

nation rates, although the numbers of literate women did not change and there was a 12 percent increase in the number of literate men. This study also suggests that health behaviors may improve as a result of changes in health-care delivery without improvements in individual literacy (Northrop-Clewes et al., 1998).

Financial Associations of Low Health Literacy

The limited information available suggests that limited health literacy may be associated with increased consumer, health provider, and the health-care system costs. Weiss and colleagues (1994) initially found no association between literacy skills, as measured by grade-equivalent reading level, and total 1-year health-care charges in 402 randomly selected Arizona Medicaid enrollees. The relationship between costs incurred and reading level as assessed by the IDL in the 72 patients in the original sample who were not seeking prenatal care was reanalyzed since 330 patients in this study were receiving prenatal care that had a fixed cost. The health-care costs of the remaining 72 patients showed greater variation. Consistent with REALM scoring, which categorizes the lowest reading group as third grade and under, the authors divided the sample at grade 3. Patients with a reading level at or below third grade had mean Medicaid charges of $10,688, while patients who read above the third-grade level had mean charges of $2,891 (p = 0.025) (Weiss and Palmer, 2004).

Friedland (1998) presented an analysis of the association of literacy and health-care utilization using data from the Health Care Financing Administration,[6] the NALS, and the Survey of Income and Program Participation. This estimate was derived from predicted levels of functional literacy and estimates of health-care use. Differences in health-care spending were estimated by comparing health-care utilization by people with a lower probability of having functional literacy skills to health-care utilization by people those with a higher probability of having functional literacy skills. Friedland suggested that the additional health-care resource attributable to inadequate health literacy (NALS Level 1) in 1996 was $29 billion if inadequate health literacy was equivalent to inadequate literacy, and would have grown to $69 billion if even half of the marginally literate (NALS Level 2) were also considered not health literate (Friedland, 1998). This estimate has been cited elsewhere and, while illustrating the depth of the problem of limited health literacy, does not directly address the issue of cost.[7]

---

[6]HCFA, now the Centers for Medicare & Medicaid Services.

[7]The committee thanks Robert Friedland, Ph.D., for his contributions to this section of the report.

Associations of patient literacy with health-care utilization were examined by Baker and colleagues (1998, 2002a). Two analyses showed that limited literacy patients have higher rates of hospitalization that may be associated with greater resource use. Of 979 patients seen in the emergency department of Grady Memorial Hospital (Atlanta) in 1994–1995, logistic regression showed that those with inadequate health literacy, as measured by the TOFHLA, were more likely to be hospitalized (31.5 percent) than patients with adequate health literacy (14.9 percent). The OR after adjusting for confounding variables was 1.69. The adjusted relative risk increased to 3.15 among patients with inadequate literacy who had been hospitalized in the previous year (Baker et al., 1998). More recently, Baker and colleagues (2002a) studied a prospective cohort of 3,260 Medicare managed care enrollees. Of the 29 percent of these patients hospitalized over a 2-year period, the risk of admission was inversely related to health literacy as measured by the S-TOFHLA. The adjusted relative risk of admission was 1.29 for those with inadequate literacy and 1.21 for those with marginal literacy; however, it should be noted that education was not controlled for in this study.

> *Jose, a Bolivian man in his early 30s, stayed after class one night so I could help him understand a hospital bill. He had been having bad headaches for some time. Thinking it was his only option for care, he had gone to the emergency department to get treatment. There he was told the headaches would clear up if he got glasses. He was charged $300 for this diagnosis (Singleton, 2002).*

For the purpose of this Institute of Medicine report, the committee commissioned an examination of the expenditure data collected in association with the Baker et al. (2002a) study from David Howard, a health economist at Emory University.[8] Using econometric regression techniques, Howard found that predicted inpatient spending for persons with inadequate health literacy, as measured by the S-TOFHLA, was $993 higher than that of persons with adequate health literacy. This difference fell to $450 after controlling for health status. It is not clear whether this control is appropriate as there may be a bidirectional relationship between literacy and health status. Emergency care costs incurred by individuals with inad-

---

[8]The information in this section is drawn from the background paper "The Relationship Between Health Literacy and Medical Costs," commissioned by the committee from David H. Howard, Ph.D. The committee appreciates his contribution. The full text of the paper can be found in Appendix B of this report.

Finding 3-1   About 90 million adults, an estimate based on the 1992 NALS, have literacy skills that test below high school level (NALS Level 1 and 2). Of these, about 40–44 million (NALS Level 1) have difficulty finding information in unfamiliar or complex texts such as newspaper articles, editorials, medicine labels, forms, or charts. Because the medical and public health literature indicates that health materials are complex and often far above high school level, the committee notes that approximately 90 million adults may lack the needed literacy skills to effectively use the U.S. health system. The majority of these adults are native-born English speakers. Literacy levels are lower among the elderly, those who have lower educational levels, those who are poor, minority populations, and groups with limited English proficiency such as recent immigrants.

Finding 3-2   On the basis of limited studies, public testimony, and committee members' experience, the committee concludes that the shame and stigma associated with limited literacy skills are major barriers to improving health literacy.

equate health literacy scores were higher than in patients with adequate literacy, while pharmacy expenses were similar in both groups and outpatient expenditures were lower. Although this Medicare managed care sample is not representative of the U.S. population as a whole, the results are consistent with previous reports that limited-literacy individuals make greater use of services designed to treat complications of disease and fewer services designed to prevent complications (Baker et al., 1998, 2002; Gordon et al., 2002; Scott et al., 2002).

These data suggest that patients with limited literacy may interact with a complex health-care system in ways that interfere with ideal utilization patterns and therefore could be more expensive. However, since the causal relationships between literacy and health-care utilization and cost have not been discovered, it is not possible to establish a valid cost figure for the impact of limited health literacy. If the magnitudes suggested by Howard and Friedland approach the actual costs, they clearly underscore the importance of addressing this risk factor from a financial perspective, in addition to health outcome implications. More research is needed to expand these limited results and move to a clearer estimation of these effects.

Finding 3-4   Two recent studies demonstrate a higher rate of hospitalization and use of emergency services among patients with limited literacy. This higher utilization has been associated with higher health-care costs.

Finding 3-3 Adults with limited health literacy, as measured by reading and numeracy skills, have less knowledge of disease management and of health-promoting behaviors, report poorer health status, and are less likely to use preventive services.

Finding 3-4 Two recent studies demonstrate a higher rate of hospitalization and use of emergency services among patients with limited literacy. This higher utilization has been associated with higher health-care costs.

Recommendation 3-1 Given the compelling evidence noted above, funding for health-literacy research is urgently needed. The Department of Health and Human Services, especially the National Institutes of Health, the Agency for Healthcare Research and Quality, the Health Resources and Services Administrations, and the Centers for Disease Control and Prevention; the Department of Defense; the Veterans Administration; and other public and private funding agencies should support multidisciplinary research on the extent, associations, and consequences of limited health literacy, including studies on health service utilization and expenditures.

REFERENCES

Arnold CL, Davis TC, Berkel HJ, Jackson RH, Nandy I, London S. 2001. Smoking status, reading level, and knowledge of tobacco effects among low-income pregnant women. *Preventive Medicine.* 32(4): 313–320.

Arozullah AM, Lee SY, Khan T, Kurup S. 2002. Low health literacy increases the risk of preventable hospital admission. Abstract presented at the Midwest Regional Meeting of the Society of General Internal Medicine. September 26–28, 2002: Chicago, IL.

Baker DW, Parker RM, Williams MV, Clark WS, Nurss J. 1997. The relationship of patient reading ability to self-reported health and use of health services. *American Journal of Public Health.* 87(6): 1027–1030.

Baker DW, Parker RM, Williams MV, Clark WS. 1998. Health literacy and the risk of hospital admission. *Journal of General Internal Medicine.* 13(12): 791–798.

Baker DW, Williams MV, Parker RM, Gazmararian JA, Nurss J. 1999. Development of a brief test to measure functional health literacy. *Patient Education and Counseling.* 38: 33–42.

Baker DW, Gazmararian JA, Williams MV, Scott T, Parker RM, Green D, Ren J, Peel J. 2002a. Functional health literacy and the risk of hospital admission among Medicare managed care enrollees. *American Journal of Public Health.* 92(8): 1278–1283.

Baker DW, Gazmararian JA, Sudano J, Patterson M, Parker RM, Williams DW. 2002b. Health literacy and performance on the Mini-Mental State Examination. *Aging and Mental Health.* 6(1): 22–29.

Balsa AI, McGuire TG. 2001. Statistical discrimination in health care. *Journal of Health Economics.* 20(6): 881–907.

Beers BB, McDonald VJ, Quistberg DA, Ravenell KL, Asch DA, Shea JA. 2003. Disparities in health literacy between African American and non-African American primary care patients. Abstract. *Journal of General Internal Medicine.* 18(Supplement 1): 169.

Bennett CL, Ferreira MR, Davis TC, Kaplan J, Weinberger M, Kuzel T, Seday MA, Sartor O. 1998. Relation between literacy, race, and stage of presentation among low-income patients with prostate cancer. *Journal of Clinical Oncology.* 16(9): 3101–3104.

Benson JG, Forman WB. 2002. Comprehension of written health care information in an affluent geriatric retirement community: Use of the test of functional health literacy. *Gerontology.* 48(2): 93–97.

Berk ML, Monheit AC. 2001. The concentration of health care expenditures, revisited. *Health Affairs.* 20(2): 9–18.

Comings JP, Reder S, Sum A. 2001. Building a Level Playing Field: The Need to Expand and Improve the National and State Adult Education and Literacy Systems. NCSALL Report. Cambridge, MA: National Center for the Study of Adult Learning and Literacy.

Davis TC, Long SW, Jackson RH, Mayeaux EJ, George RB, Murphy PW, Crouch MA. 1993. Rapid estimate of adult literacy in medicine: A shortened screening instrument. *Family Medicine.* 25(6): 391–395.

Davis TC, Mayeaux EJ, Fredrickson D, Bocchini JA Jr, Jackson RH, Murphy PW. 1994. Reading ability of parents compared with reading level of pediatric patient education materials. *Pediatrics.* 93(3): 460–468.

Davis TC, Arnold C, Berkel HJ, Nandy I, Jackson RH, Glass J. 1996. Knowledge and attitude on screening mammography among low-literate, low-income women. *Cancer.* 78(9): 1912–1920.

Doak CC, Doak LG, Root J. 1996. *Teaching Patients with Low Literacy Skills.* 2nd edition. New York: Lippincott.

Fortenberry JD, McFarlane MM, Hennessy M, Bull SS, Grimley DM, St Lawrence J, Stoner BP, VanDevanter N. 2001. Relation of health literacy to gonorrhoea related care. *Sexually Transmitted Infections.* 77(3): 206–211.

Friedland R. 1998. New estimates of the high costs of inadequate health literacy. In: *Proceedings of Pfizer Conference "Promoting Health Literacy: A Call to Action."* October 7–8, 1998, Washington, DC: Pfizer, Inc. Pp. 6–10.

Gazmararian JA, Parker RM, Baker DW. 1999a. Reading skills and family planning knowledge and practices in a low-income managed-care population. *Obstetrics & Gynecology.* 93(2): 239–244.

Gazmararian JA, Baker DW, Williams MV, Parker RM, Scott T, Greemn DCFSN, Ren J, Koplan JP. 1999b. Health literacy among Medicare enrollees in a managed care organization. *Journal of the American Medical Association.* 281(6): 545–551.

Gazmararian J, Baker D, Parker R, Blazer DG. 2000. A multivariate analysis of factors associated with depression: Evaluating the role of health literacy as a potential contributor. *Archives of Internal Medicine.* 160(21): 3307–3314.

Glewwe P. 1999. Why does mother's schooling raise child health in developing countries? Evidence from Morocco. *Journal of Human Resources.* 34(1): 124–159.

Gonzales F, Dearden K, Jimenez W. 1999. Do multi-sectoral development programmes affect health? A Bolivian case study. *Health Policy & Planning.* 14(4): 400–408.

Gordon MM, Hampson R, Capell HA, Madhok R. 2002. Illiteracy in rheumatoid arthritis patients as determined by the Rapid Estimate of Adult Literacy in Medicine (REALM) score. *Rheumatology.* 41(7): 750–754.

Greenberg E, Macias RF, Rhodes D, Chan T. 2001. *English Literacy and Language Minorities in the United States.* NCES 2001-464. Washington, DC: National Center for Education Statistics. U.S. Department of Education. [Online]. Available: http://www.nces.ed.gov/pubs2002/2002382.pdf [accessed: June 5, 2003].

Greenberg, J. 2001. *An Updated Overview of Medical and Public Health Literature Addressing Literacy Issues: An Annotated Bibliography of Articles Published in 2000.* [Online]. Available: http://www. hsph.harvard.edu/healthliteracy/literature/lit_2000.html [accessed: October, 2003].

Guerra CE, Shea JA. 2003. Functional health literacy, comorbidity and health status. Abstract. *Journal of General Internal Medicine*. 18(Supplement 1): 174.

Haigler KO. 1994. *Literacy Behind Prison Walls. Profiles of the Prison Population from the National Adult Literacy Survey*. Washington, DC: U.S. Government Printing Office. [Online]. Available: http://www.nces.ed.gov/pubs2002/2002382.pdf [accessed: June 5, 2003].

Hegerfeld M. 1999. *Reading, Writing, and the American Soldier: A Study of Literacy in the American Armed Forces*. Fort Wayne, IN: Department of Education, Indiana University–Purdue University at Fort Wayne.

Kalichman SC, Rompa D. 2000. Functional health literacy is associated with health status and health-related knowledge in people living with HIV-AIDS. *Journal of Acquired Immune Deficiency Syndromes and Human Retrovirology*. 25(4): 337–344.

Kalichman SC, Benotsch E, Suarez T, Catz S, Miller J, Rompa D. 2000. Health literacy and health-related knowledge among persons living with HIV/AIDS. *American Journal of Preventive Medicine*. 18(4): 325–331.

Kalichman SCP, Ramachandran BB, Catz SP. 1999. Adherence to combination antiretroviral therapies in HIV patients of low health literacy. *Journal of General Internal Medicine*. 14(5): 267–273.

Kaufman H, Skipper B, Small L, Terry T, McGrew M. 2001. Effect of literacy on breast-feeding outcomes. *Southern Medical Journal*. 94(3): 293–296.

Kim SP, Knight SJ, Tomori C, Colella KM, Schoor RA, Shih L, Kuzel TM, Nadler RB, Bennett CL. 2001. Health literacy and shared decision making for prostate cancer patients with low socioeconomic status. *Cancer Investigation*. 19(7): 684–691.

Kirsch IS. 2001. *The International Adult Literacy Survey (IALS): Understanding What Was Measured*. Princeton, NJ: Educational Testing Service.

Kirsch IS, Jungeblut A, Jenkins L, Kolstad A. 1993. *Adult Literacy in America: A First Look at the Results of the National Adult Literacy Survey (NALS)*. Washington, DC: National Center for Education Statistics, U.S. Department of Education.

Lasater L. 2003. Patient literacy, adherence, and anticoagulation therapy outcomes: A preliminary report. Abstract. *Journal of General Internal Medicine*. 18(Supplement 1): 179.

Li BDL, Brown WA, Ampil FL, Burton GV, Yu H, McDonald JC. 2000. Patient compliance is critical for equivalent clinical outcomes for breast cancer treated by breast-conservation therapy. *Annals of Surgery*. 231(6): 883–889.

Lindau ST, Tomori C, Lyons T, Langseth L, Bennett CL, Garcia P. 2002. The association of health literacy with cervical cancer prevention knowledge and health behaviors in a multiethnic cohort of women. *American Journal of Obstetrics & Gynecology*. 186(5): 938–943.

Mayer GG. 2003. Confessions of a health illiterate. *Healthcare Advances*. 5(2): 2.

Montalto NJ, Spiegler GE. 2001. Functional health literacy in adults in a rural community health center. *West Virginia Medical Journal*. 97(2): 111–114.

Moon RY, Cheng TL, Patel KM, Baumhaft K, Scheidt PC. 1998. Parental literacy level and understanding of medical information. *Pediatrics*. 102(2): e25.

Morse L. 2002. *Improving Health Literacy: An Educational Response to a Public Health Problem*. Presentation given at a workshop of the Institute of Medicine Committee on Health Literacy. December 11, 2002, Washington, DC.

Northrop-Clewes CA, Ahmad N, Paracha PI, Thurnham DI. 1998. Impact of health service provision on mothers and infants in a rural village in North West Frontier Province, Pakistan. *Public Health Nutrition*. 1(1): 51–59.

Organization for Economic Co-operation and Development and Statistics Canada. 2000. *Literacy in the Information Age: Final Report of the International Adult Literacy Survey*. Statistics Canada Catalogue no. 89-571-XPE. Paris: Organization for Economic Co-operation and Development and Ottawa: Minister of Industry.

Parikh NS, Parker RM, Nurss JR, Baker DW, Williams MV. 1996. Shame and health literacy: The unspoken connection. *Patient Education and Counseling.* 27(1): 33–39.

Parker RM, Baker DW, Williams MV, Nurss JR. 1995. The Test of Functional Health Literacy in Adults: A new instrument for measuring patients' literacy skills. *Journal of General Internal Medicine.* 10(10): 537–541.

Parker RM, Ratzan SC, Lurie N. 2003. Health literacy: A policy challenge for advancing high-quality health care. *Health Affairs.* 22(4): 147.

Profiles of State Programs. 1990. *Profiles of State Programs: Adult Education for the Homeless.* Washington, DC: Division of Adult Literacy and Education, U.S. Department of Education.

Rudd R, Moeykens BA, Colton TC. 2000a. Health and literacy. A review of medical and public health literature. In: *Annual Review of Adult Learning and Literacy.* Comings J, Garners B, Smith C, Editors. New York: Jossey-Bass.

Rudd RE, Colton T, Schacht R. 2000b. *An Overview of Medical and Public Health Literature Addressing Literacy Issues: An Annotated Bibliography.* Report #14. Cambridge, MA: National Center for the Study of Adult Learning and Literacy.

Rudd RE, Kirsch I, Yamamoto K. 2003. Literacy in health contexts: A re-analysis of the NALS. In: *Clear Health Communications: Issues and Solutions, Session 4182.1.* Washington, DC: American Public Health Association Annual Conference.

Schillinger D, Grumbach K, Piette J, Wang F, Osmond D, Daher C, Palacios J, Sullivan GaD, Bindman AB. 2002. Association of health literacy with diabetes outcomes. *Journal of the American Medical Association.* 288(4): 475–482.

Schillinger D, Piette J, Grumbach K, Wang F, Wilson C, Daher C, Leong-Grotz K, Castro C, Bindman AB. 2003. Closing the loop: Physician communication with diabetic patients who have low health literacy. *Archives of Internal Medicine.* 163(1): 83–90.

Scott TL, Gazmararian JA, Williams MV, Baker DW. 2002. Health literacy and preventive health care use among Medicare enrollees in a managed care organization. *Medical Care.* 40(5): 395–404.

Shea JA, Guerra C, Weiner J, Aguirre A, Schaffer M, Asch DA. 2003. Health literacy and patient satisfaction. *Journal of General Internal Medicine.* 18(Supplement 1): 187–188.

Shinagawa S, Foong HL. 2003. *Health literacy challenges for Asian Americans and Native Hawaiians and other Pacific Islanders.* Supplement to oral testimony presented at a workshop of the Institute of Medicine Committee on Health Literacy. February 13, 2003, Irvine, CA.

Singleton K. 2002. ESOL Teachers: Helpers in health care. *Focus on Basics: Connecting Research Practice.* 5(C): 26–30.

Sum A, Kirsch IS, Taggart R. 2002. The twin challenges of mediocrity and inequality: Literacy in the U.S. from an international perspective. In: *Policy Information Report.* Princeton, NJ: Educational Testing Service.

U.S. Census Bureau. 2002. *Race and Hispanic or Latino Origin by Age and Sex for the United States: 2000 (PHC-T-8).* Washington, DC: U.S. Census Bureau. [Online]. Available: http://www.census.gov/population/www/cen2000/phc-t08.html [accessed: December 9, 2003].

U.S. Department of Education. 2001. *English Literacy and Language Minorities in the United States.* Greenberg E, Macias RF, Rhodes D, Chan T, Editors. NCES 2001-464. Washington, DC: National Center for Health Statistics.

Weiss BD. 1999. How common is low literacy? In: *20 Common Problems in Primary Care.* Weiss BD, Editor. New York: McGraw-Hill. Pp. 468–481.

Weiss BD, Palmer R. 2004. Relationship between health care costs and very low literacy skills in a medically needy and indigent Medicaid population. *Journal of the American Board of Family Practice.* 17(1): 44–47.

Weiss BD, Blanchard JS, McGee DL, Hart G, Warren B, Burgoon M, Smith KJ. 1994. Illiteracy among Medicaid recipients and its relationship to health care costs. *Journal of Health Care for the Poor & Underserved.* 5(2): 99–111.

Williams MV, Parker RM, Baker DW, Parikh NS, Pitkin K, Coates WC, Nurss JR. 1995. Inadequate functional health literacy among patients at two public hospitals. *Journal of the American Medical Association.* 274(21): 1677–1682.

Williams MV, Baker DW, Honig EG, Lee TM, Nowlan A. 1998a. Inadequate literacy is a barrier to asthma knowledge and self-care. *Chest.* 114(4): 1008–1015.

Williams MV, Baker DW, Parker RM, Nurss JR. 1998b. Relationship of functional health literacy to patients' knowledge of their chronic disease. A study of patients with hypertension and diabetes. *Archives of Internal Medicine.* 158(2): 166–172.

Win K, Schillinger D. 2003. Understanding of warfarin therapy and stroke among ethnically diverse anticoagulation patients at a public hospital. Abstract. *Journal of General Internal Medicine.* 18(Supplement 1): 278.

Young BA. 2002. *Public High School Dropouts and Completers from the Common Core of Data: School Years 1998–99 and 1999–2000.* NCES 2002-382. Washington, DC: National Center for Education Statistics. U.S. Department of Education. Office of Educational Research and Improvement. [Online]. Available: http://www.nces.ed.gov/pubs2002/2002382.pdf [accessed: June 5, 2003].

Zobel E, Rowe K, Gomez-Mandic C. 2003. *An Updated Overview of Medical and Public Health Literature Addressing Literacy Issues: An Annotated Bibliography of Articles Published in 2002.* [Online]. Available: http://www.hsph.harvard.edu/health literacy/literature/lit_2002.html [accessed: October, 2003].

4

Culture and Society

Escorted by his teenage granddaughter, an elderly old Navajo grandfather was taken to the internal medicine clinic for an infection in his right leg. The granddaughter was fluent in English but had very limited Navajo speaking skills. Speaking in English, the doctor informed the man that the infection in his leg would get worse if he did not take his medication as prescribed. The granddaughter could not translate the scientific concept of infection into Navajo language. The doctor asked one of the nurses for help, and although the she tried as much as she could, she also was unsuccessful. The old man, becoming frustrated, just agreed that he understood everything that he had been told. He told the nurse he wanted to have a traditional ceremony performed for him within a couple of days, and for her to tell the doctor. The nurse translated this to the doctor, who restated the importance of taking the medicines. The grandfather insisted he understood, but in fact because he felt that he did not understand the physician's explanation, he decided to go to a traditional medicine man instead. The medicine man helped him the best he could, but the grandfather's leg had to be amputated, which the doctor ascribed to noncompliance.

Our understanding of health literacy gains greater depth and meaning in the context of culture. This is especially important given the ethnic and linguistic diversity of the U.S. population. In addition to 211,460,626 Americans of European decent, the 2000 U.S. Census identified 69,961,280 people from 19 other ethnic and cultural groups living in America (U.S. Census Bureau, 2000). Many of these diverse American populations have differing systems of belief about health and illness. Cultural health beliefs affect how people think and feel about their health and health problems, when and from whom they seek health care, and how they respond to recommendations for lifestyle change, health-care interventions, and treatment adherence.

Cultures also differ in their styles of communication, in the meaning of words and gestures, and even in what can be discussed regarding the body, health, and illness. Health literacy requires communication and mutual understanding between patients and their families and health-care providers and staff. Culture and health literacy both influence the content and outcomes of health-care encounters.

A definition of health literacy that does not recognize the potential effect of cultural differences on the communication and understanding of health information would miss much of the deeper meaning and purpose of literacy for people (Nutbeam, 2000). Culture provides a context through which meaning is gained from information, and provides the purpose by which people come to understand their health status and comprehend options for diagnoses and treatments. A conceptual understanding of the interconnections between culture and literacy through the idea of cultural literacy can provide insights into the deeper meanings of how diverse populations in the United States come to know, comprehend, and make informed decisions based on valid data regarding their health.

This intersection between culture and literacy is recognized in the U.S. Department of Health and Human Services (HHS) National Standards for Culturally and Linguistically Appropriate Services (CLAS) in Health Care. The standard states that "health care organizations must make available easily understood patient-related materials . . . in the languages of commonly encountered groups . . ." (HHS, 2001: 11). The standard goes on to state explicitly that in addition to being culturally responsive, these materials need also be responsive to the literacy levels of patients and consumers. Issues of culture, language, and learning are interrelated, and to be effective, health education must be conducted in both culturally and linguistically appropriate formats to address the increasingly diverse multicultural and multilingual population (AMA Ad Hoc Committee on Health Literacy, 1999).

Cultural, social, and family influences shape attitudes and beliefs and therefore influence health literacy. Social determinants of health are well documented regarding the conditions over which the individual has little or no control but that affect his or her ability to participate fully in a health-literate society. Native language, socioeconomic status, gender, race, and ethnicity along with mass culture as represented by news publishing, advertising, marketing, and the plethora of health information sources available through electronic channels are also integral to the social–cultural landscape of health literacy.

Traditional and mass culture and society provide a lens through which individuals perceive the mix of opportunities and underlying values and assumptions inherent in the health system. Society influences individuals and collectivities such as families, communities, and professional groups. Social factors work through social networks as well as through government programs, legislation, and private-sector markets. They are reflected in and shaped by the media. They are manifested through access to agency and organizational programs. A wide variety of social factors produce and diffuse information or misinformation, shape bias, develop and support health-promoting or -degrading environments, and provide normative pressures. These influence the actions of individuals, collectivities, and the specialized groups of public health and care providers and therefore suggest critical intervention points.

TRADITIONAL CULTURE

Culture is the shared ideas, meanings, and values acquired by individuals as members of society. It is socially learned, not genetically transmitted, and often influences us unconsciously. Human beings learn through social means—through interactions with others as well as through the products of culture such as books and television (IOM, 2002). Reliance on tools and symbolic resources, notably language, is a hallmark of culture. Language is central to social life and mediates the acquisition of much cultural knowledge. Language "provides the most complex system of the classification of experience" and is "the most flexible and most powerful tool developed by humans" (Duranti, 1997: 49 and 47). Differences in languages and underlying concepts may lead to problems with health-related communication. For example, translating the word "chemotherapy" into the Navajo language might require pages of text. Since the Navajo language has no word or concept for chemotherapy, the translation must start with the idea of cancer, and include what the person might experience as a result of chemotherapy. This is further complicated by the fact that many Navajos believe that if you say something will happen, it will[1] (Billie, 2003).

Beyond the differences of language, culture gives significance to health information and messages. Perceptions and definitions of health and illness, preferences, language and cultural barriers, care process barriers, and stereotypes are all strongly influenced by culture and can have a great impact

---

[1]The committee thanks Alvin Billie for his contributions to this section of the report.

on health literacy and health outcomes. Differing cultural and educational backgrounds among patients and providers, as well as among those who create health information and those who use it, contribute to problems with health literacy. The relationship between culture, patient–provider interaction, and quality of care has been reviewed by Cooper and Roter (2003). Early work showed that European-American cultural groups used language differently in discussing symptoms such as pain (Zborowski, 1952; Zola, 1966). These linguistic differences were associated with differences in diagnoses, irrespective of symptomology. African-American patients frequently experience shorter physician–patient interactions and less patient-centered visits than Caucasian patients (Cooper and Roter, 2003; Cooper-Patrick et al., 1999).

It is crucial to note that culture is not static for individuals or for societies. This dynamic principle of culture is referred to as "cultural processes" when groups are discussed, and "lived experiences" in the case of individuals. Individuals are shaped by their life experiences and are exposed to multiple cultures. Their behavior may reflect an amalgam of this *"experiential identity"* (IOM, 2002). For example, the experiential identity of immigrants includes their experience with the health systems from their country of origin as well as their immigrant experience. This experiential identity will incorporate new experiences with the American health system. Development of adequate health literacy may be hindered by limited English skills or outcomes of poorly understood health experiences.

Today's families and communities consist of people with multiple cultural backgrounds and experiences, who cannot be put into rigid "boxes" by using racial and ethnic labels that are often resented and are misleading. Individuals, families, and communities have belief systems, religious and cultural values, and group identity that serve as powerful filters through which information is received and processed. These concepts of cultural processes and lived identities replace more traditional concepts such as "acculturation" and present measurement challenges to researchers and health service providers.

Culture, cultural processes, and cross-cultural interventions have been discussed in-depth in several Institute of Medicine (IOM) reports (IOM, 2002, 2003a) which suggest that ways of learning, beliefs about health and illness, and patterns of communications contribute to health literacy through their effect on communication, comprehension, understanding, and decision-making. Socioeconomic status was found to affect health in the IOM report *Promoting Health: Intervention Strategies from Social and Behavioral Research* (IOM, 2000). Behavioral and social factors influence a person's susceptibility to disease, especially among individuals of lower socioeconomic status. The 2000 IOM report identified increased prevalence of disease among socio-economically underserved groups and outlined "the need to balance clinical approach to disease with recognized social and class determinants" (IOM, 2000). Social and behavioral interventions were further investigated in *Speaking of Health* (IOM, 2002), which recognized the link between behavior and disease.

In the following section, we examine the relationships between cultural processes and health literacy for indications of how to make Americans more literate about health and illness through health systems that are more responsive to patient needs, preferences, and perspectives.

Cultural Competence

The skills and knowledge of cultural competence provide a trajectory towards the interpersonal skills for effective patient care that can be realized only when comprehension, understanding, and meaning are inherent in the process. Cultural competence has been variously defined by different organizations.[2] *Speaking of Health* (IOM, 2002) notes the following dimensions:

- *Cultural awareness:* A deliberate, cognitive process in which health-care providers become appreciative and sensitive to values, beliefs, lifestyles, practices, and problem-solving strategies of clients' cultures.
- *Cultural knowledge:* The process of seeking and obtaining a sound educational foundation concerning worldviews of various cultures; goal is to understand clients' world views, or the way individuals or groups of people view the universe to form values about their lives and the world around them.
- *Cultural skill:* The ability to collect relevant cultural data regarding clients' health histories and presenting problems, as well as accurately perform culturally sensitive physical histories.
- *Cultural encounter:* A process that encourages health-care providers to engage directly in cross-cultural interactions with clients from culturally diverse backgrounds (IOM, 2002).

Among these four dimensions of cultural competency, common themes emerge: ways of thinking, understanding world views, cultural data, and cross-cultural interactions.

---

[2]For example, the HHS CLAS standards define cultural competence as "the capacity to function effectively as an individual and as an organization within the context of cultural beliefs, behaviors, and needs presented by consumers and their communities" and the National Medical Association defines cultural competence as "the application of cultural knowledge, behaviors, clinical and interpersonal skills that enhances a provider's effectiveness in patient care."

Cultural competence becomes important to health literacy at the point where language and culture interfere with or support effective communication. While health literacy efforts are not limited to cross-cultural situations, and cultural competence efforts are broader than health literacy, initiatives in both these areas would benefit from coordination with each other. Cultural competency is sometimes approached through recommendations for culturally and socially sensitive communication. These approaches must take into consideration the dynamic and ever-changing nature of culture. As culture is constantly being influenced by lived experiences, so must health literacy approaches that are coordinated with cultural competence be responsive to cultural change. In meeting the health needs of diverse peoples, cultural competency is essential for the development of health literacy.

Language

An ob-gyn resident tells of working with an inner city, Hispanic population. Alone on service late one night, she struggled to communicate with a couple who spoke only Spanish in order to learn the pregnant woman's due date. Grasping at a word familiar from popular music, she said "navidad, navidad" over and over again to the puzzled couple. Finally, she located another resident who spoke Spanish and helped her ask the couple about the "fecha" (date) the baby was expected. They all had a good laugh over her puzzling repetition of the Spanish word for "Christmas."

An important component of cultural competence is linguistic competence. Many individuals receiving care from the U.S. health-care system have limited English proficiency (LEP). For individuals whose native language is not English, issues of health literacy are compounded by issues of language and the specialized vocabulary used, both in written and spoken form, to convey health information. The 2000 census indicates that the foreign-born population in the United States is 31 million. More than 300 different languages are spoken in the United States, and 47 million citizens and non-citizens speak a language other than English at home (an increase from 31.8 million in 1990). English is not the primary language spoken in the homes of 41 percent of Hispanics, 34 percent of Koreans, 29 percent of Vietnamese, and 20 percent of Chinese (Collins et al., 2002). Eleven million individuals indicate that they speak English not well or not at all (U.S. Census Bureau, 2000). Some of these individuals live in isolation from English, that is, without personal or social resources to understand English.

The profound effect of primary language on health is widely recognized. It provided the impetus for an Executive Order on improving access to services for persons with LEP[3] and a subsequent report to Congress. The effect of primary language on health remains a central concern of the federal Office of Minority Health Center for Linguistic and Cultural Competence in Health Care, established in 1995 to address the health needs of populations who speak limited English

Individuals with LEP have widely varying levels of literacy and health literacy in their primary language. When LEP individuals are health literate in their primary language, the key is providing language assistance either in the form of care in their primary language or interpreter services and translated materials. When LEP individuals are not health literate in their own language, additional efforts are needed ensure adequate communication. Some languages do not have a written form or individuals may not be able to read, and so translation services are of no use in such cases. These individuals may be unfamiliar with medical terminology in their primary language and, therefore, linguistically competent services alone will be insufficient to ensure adequate communication. Alternatively, individuals may be health literate in their own culture, but not in Western medicine's health system and style of health care.

Cultural Languages

Cultural context gets transformed into cultural language that influences three critical determinants of health literacy: comprehension, understanding, and decision-making. Different cultural groups mobilize creative forces to formulate unique cultural languages that must be considered in culturally competent approaches for implementing interventions to promote health literacy. Two examples of these innovative cultural languages can be found in the language of Aboriginal people and in the dreams of Native American cultures.

In contrast to Westernized people whose language use is dominated by nouns, Aboriginal people use a language dominated by verbs in deference to their worldly vision of all existence as energy or spirit that is in constant transformation (Ross, 1996: 116). A consequence is that there is attention to the "relationship between things" and less focus on the "characteristic of things" (in a noun-driven language such as English). This feature of using "fluidity of verb-phrases" is functional in healing relationships. Thus, a re-thinking and re-framing of the standard inquiries that drive health assess-

---

[3]Executive Order No. 13166. Benefit-Cost Report of Executive Order No. 13166: Improving Access to Services for Persons with Limited English Proficiency. August 2000.

ments via predominant use of nouns, adjectives, and pronouns is necessary when working with Aboriginal people during health and illness encounters.

In Native American cultures, dreams function as a cultural language to communicate realities in everyday life and deal with health and illness. The significance of this for health care is demonstrated by Lincoln (2003) with respect to the Navajo Indians in Arizona: "Diagnosticians are called upon to cure sickness caused by dreams or to prevent sickness predicted by dreams." (Lincoln, 2003). For Native American peoples, therefore, dreams are part of the cultural lexicon that informs health literacy.

> The Hmong language has no word for cancer, or even the concept of the disease. "We're going to put a fire in you," is how one inexperienced interpreter tried to explain radiation treatment to the patient, who as a result, refused treatment (Morse, 2003).

Language and Meaning in the Context of Health

Frequently, words or their underlying concepts have little or no meaning, or a different meaning, for a person from another culture. This is true both of specific terminology as well as the essential meaning of health and illness to different people. For example, instructing a patient to take a teaspoon of medicine assumes that the patient owns a teaspoon that holds 5 cc of liquid, and identifies it as such. Promoting health literacy requires an awareness and understanding of these differences in meaning and providing what is needed to increase the probability of treatment adherence (for example, a teaspoon with which to measure the medicine, or pre-measured quantities of medicine).

As noted, recent IOM reports (IOM, 2002, 2003a) urge a broad, more realistic perspective of culture as fluid processes and lived experiences, in which communications, relationships, and meaning are central themes relevant to health literacy. Conceptual definitions and proposed relationships between culture and health literacy as human experiences have yet to be developed. In-depth theoretical concepts to guide scientific inquiries could arise from conceptual frameworks on the interface between cultural processes, literacy, and health literacy. These frameworks must distinguish between linguistic and cultural processes, both of which are rooted in the concept of meaning. For example, research on epilepsy found that both neurologists and patients use the word "trauma," but neurologists most often mean "a physical blow," while patients and families most often understand the word to imply "psychological damage." This confusion is exacerbated in Latino patients and families since trauma has the same two meanings in Spanish, but cultural views of illness more often focus on the psychological meaning (Long et al., 1992). While specific meaning of the word trauma may differ between individuals and groups, people will act upon the meaning they understand.

> *A 45-year-old Hispanic immigrant, Mr. G., undergoes a job health screening and is told that his blood pressure is very high and he will not be allowed to continue work until his blood pressure is controlled. He goes to the local public hospital and is given a prescription for a Beta-blocker and a diuretic. The doctor prescribes two medications known to be effective and simple for adherence because they each are supposed to be taken once a day.*
>
> *Mr. G. presents to the emergency department one week later with dizziness. His blood pressure is very low, and Mr. G. says he has been taking the medicine just like it says to take it on the bottle. The puzzling case is discussed by multiple practitioners until one that speaks Spanish asks Mr. G. how many pills he took each day. "22," Mr. G. replies. The provider explains to his colleagues that "once" means "11" in Spanish.*

Similarly, work on dissonances between medical staff and pregnant women of Mexican origin in Los Angeles revealed that there is no Spanish word for the English word "labor." Medical Spanish uses a construct that translates labor as "the work of childbirth," but women use the Spanish word for pain ("dolor"). More important than the words themselves, there may be large differences in concept for the process of labor between women and providers. The women described childbirth as "pain and the baby is born." Clinicians, who probably think of childbirth as a longer process with physiological stages, could not understand the women's panic when they were told that it was too soon to be admitted to the hospital (Scrimshaw and Souza, 1982). Communication goes beyond words to encompass the meaning behind the words, a meaning that is affected by culture, knowledge, and experience.

It is also important to consider signage in health-care settings and written materials as well as verbal communications. Recently, a clinic in Guatemala was observed to have the label "Estomocologia" (which translates as "Stomachology"). This may make more sense to people there than "gastro-enterology." There is a tremendous challenge in finding clear and acceptable signage for hospitals and clinics. One project, Hablamos Juntos, funded for ten health-care settings by the Robert Wood Johnson Foundation is currently working on signage, literature, and interpreter qualifications and training.

Anthropologists Good and Good (1981) write about meaning-centered clinical practice, and note that groups vary in

- the specificity of their medical complaints
- their style of communication around medical complaints
- the nature of their anxiety about the meaning of symptoms
- their focus on organ systems
- their response to therapeutic strategies

Therefore, human illness has meaning, in both the biological sense and as a human experience. As a result, clinical practice is inherently interpretive and practitioners must elicit patients' requests, elicit and decode patients' use of language, diagnose disease and illness, and develop plans for managing problems. This includes the need to elicit explanatory modes of patients and families, analyze conflict with the biomedical model, and negotiate alternatives (Good and Good, 1981).

Patient Perspectives and Language

Patients' varied perspectives, values, beliefs, and behaviors regarding health and illness are consistently cited as integral to quality care in several IOM reports (IOM, 2001, 2003a). Because culture is the tapestry of shared ideas, meanings, and values that underlie of human behaviors, references to "patient perspectives" in health care necessitate an understanding of cultural processes that can be harnessed to promote health literacy. Thinking styles influence information processing, and what a person attends to and retains in memory operates within a context that is frequently culturally determined. A classic example is the many different words for describing "snow" in Inuit languages, since qualities of snow are essential to many aspects of life in these cultures. Other cultural groups have two, one, or no words for "snow," depending on whether snow is a central fact of daily life. Similar examples can be identified in health contexts. People with diverse cultural experiences may differ on how a fever is defined or described, how pain is expressed, and how body parts are identified, such as whether there is a word for "hand" but no words for "fingers," or whether there is a different name for each finger. Thus, to be health literate in America means having the cognitive capacity to comprehend the Western biomedical perspective. For a clinician, it means working with patients whose perspectives are shaped by diverse cultural contexts. Cultural processes and lived experiences contribute to widely different and unpredictable ways people understand concepts and spoken words. Culturally responsive communication is an active process by which we discover how the other person decoded or understood the stated messages. Being culturally responsive means discovering differences in frames of reference—the world views, priorities, values, and understanding each speaker brings to the encounter—on an individual basis. It requires the use of skills to seek feedback and to verify the conclusions or assumptions we come to as we communicate with another person. Being culturally responsive also means developing skills to ensure that our communication is being received as intended. Learning to develop communication and interpersonal skills to obtain feedback and verify successful communication is critical to working competently with others, and contributes to addressing the problem of health literacy.

Family relations can be a motivating factor in behavior change. The Latino value of *familialismo* and its influence on health-care interventions and behavioral change in individual Hispanic patients is well documented. Perez-Stable found that the social importance of cigarette smoking was greater for Latinos than for Caucasians. Latinos were also more concerned about the effects of smoking on interpersonal relationships. As a result, they felt more certain that quitting smoking would improve family relationships and provide a better example for their children (Perez-Stable, 1994). Sabogal and colleagues (1987) note that "to motivate a parent to alter a high-fat diet or increase the level of physical activity to prevent a future heart attack, . . . appeal[s] to his or her sense of duty to the children. The extended family network can similarly be used to persuade patient with or at risk for cardiovascular disease to adhere to prescribed or recommended medication, diet and exercise regimens."

The contributions of culture and language to health literacy are rich and complex. Potential approaches to issues of culture, language, and health literacy are discussed in the latter section of this chapter.

Finding 4-1   Culture gives meaning to health communication. Health literacy must be understood and addressed in the context of culture and language.

Measures Can Dissociate Culture, Meaning, and Health Literacy

The interface among individuals, cultural processes, layers of cultural experience, families, communities, health systems, and health-care providers is extremely complex. That complexity affects health literacy for people at every level of education and access to care. The challenge is to develop tools for measuring the health literacy effect of that complexity in order to assess and improve health literacy in the United States from both patient and provider perspectives. While strong evidence suggests an association between cultural diversity and health and illness (e.g., IOM, 2003a), the relationships between diversity and health literacy have yet to be fully delineated and investigated. This must begin with meaningful measures of culture, meaning, and health literacy. These new measures should function to improve the validity of current approaches and provide new knowledge about the impact of health literacy on health outcomes in diverse populations.

MASS CULTURE

Mass culture refers to the institutions, organizations, and individuals that produce and disseminate health messages to Americans. The quantity, quality, and lack of quality control over these messages have exploded in the past 10 years. Hundreds of health organizations across the country from hospitals to advocacy groups to major government agencies like HHS, the Centers for Disease Control and Prevention (CDC), the National Library of Medicine, and the National Institutes of Health (NIH), have created elaborate "user-friendly" information sources. These are often electronically accessible 24 hours a day to provide Americans with up-to-date health information on the care and prevention of disease. But the information sources available to Americans do not stop there. Major advocacy groups such as AARP and The American Cancer Society, plus many others, also offer detailed information on health care and disease prevention. These approaches to providing and accessing information are in their infancy, and must be evaluated and then modified for maximum effectiveness. When consumer needs are at the core of information provision, whether via print, digital media, or intrapersonal communication, the information can be more accessible. With appropriate attention to the information needs of health-care consumers, new technologies can offer all segments of society greater access to health information.

In the private sector, the marketing of pharmaceutical drugs—both over-the-counter and prescription—is now a part of every American's television viewing. The cost of pharmaceuticals promotions rose to $19.1 billion in 2001 (Medvantx, 2003). The industry drug packaging and consumer education programs are another powerful source of health information. Radio programs provide regular advice on both modern and herbal medicines. Products of all kinds make health claims as part of their marketing programs. Indeed, health has become a major consumer motivator along with sex and price promotions in American marketing.

The news media has also taken health information seriously. Dozens of major news outlets have health reporters who are increasingly skilled in interpreting health studies. The *Journal of the American Medical Association* is widely quoted and referenced in news articles in both print and broadcast media. Finally, the Internet has provided an opportunity for any individual to make health claims about any product or procedure with little or no scientific basis. In sum, the American public is now faced with a

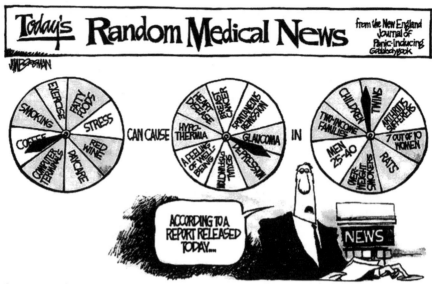

© Reprinted with special permission of King Features Syndicate.

plethora of health information and the arduous task of finding, selecting, reading, understanding, judging, and following the advice presented by multiple sources.

How People Obtain and Use Health Information

How do people obtain and use health information? There is no single reliable answer to this question. While data on health information alone is not available, responses of the National Adult Literacy Survey (NALS) participants indicated over half of individuals at each literacy skill level as measured by the NALS obtain information about current events, public affairs, and government from family and friends, newspapers and magazines, and radio and television (Kirsch et al., 1993). Between 62 and 69 percent of adults at all NALS literacy skill levels reported obtaining information from family and friends. Between 94 and 97 percent of adults at all NALS skill levels reported using radio or television to obtain information. Individuals in the lower literacy levels were less likely to use print media as an information source than were adults in the higher levels. While 69.5 percent of the respondents with NALS Level 1 literacy skills reported getting information from newspapers or magazines, 85.5 percent of adults with literacy skills at NALS Level 2 skills and 90 percent of those with literacy skills at or above NALS Level 3 reported obtaining information from newspapers or magazines.

BOX 4-1
Sources of Health Information Reported in a Gallup Poll

Proportion who reported getting a great deal or moderate amount of healthand medical information from the following sources:

Proportion who reported a great deal or moderate amount of trust and confidence inthe following sources of health and medical information:

Doctor	70%	Doctors	93%
TV	64%	Nurses	83%
Books	56%	Books	82%
Newspapers	52%	Newspapers	64%
Magazines	51%	Magazines	62%
Nurse	49%	Internet	62%
Internet	37%	TV	59%

SOURCE: Gallup Organization (2002).

The National Cancer Institute is presently conducting the Health Information National Trends Survey (HINTS), one of the nation's first national surveys of health information sources.[4] HINTS is designed to provide data regarding pattern of information use and opportunities to inform Americans about cancer; however, survey data is not yet available. In a Gallup Organization poll of 1,004 adults nationwide, several sources of information were cited as "a great deal" or "moderate" sources of health information (Gallup Organization, 2002). These sources are shown in Box 4-1. Confidence levels remain highest about information obtained from doctors and nurses, but confidence levels (great deal or moderate confidence) from other sources are also fairly high.

A September 2001 survey called *Sex Matters* looked at women's knowledge of sex differences in health (Benenson Strategy Group, 2001). Findings from this survey, based on telephone interviews of 962 women, indicate that 44 percent of adult women who said they have a doctor they see regularly for basic health care indicated that their doctor is the major source of information. However, when provided with specific information, only 19 percent said they had heard it from a doctor or nurse, as shown in Box 4-2.

[4]For more information, please see http://dccps.nci.nih.gov/hcirb/hints.html.

BOX 4-2
Selected Findings from Sex Matters

Which of the following would you say you use most often as a source of information about health for you:	Have you ever heard this information before: In addition to the typical chest pain associated with a heart attack, women may suffer from subtle symptoms such as indigestion, abdominal or mid-back pain, nausea or vomiting?	To the best of your recollection, where did you hear this information? (asked only of the 55% who said they had heard it)
Doctor 44%	Yes 55%	Newspaper/TV 25%
Magazines 15%	No 44%	Magazines 22%
Newspapers/TV 14%	Don't know 1%	Doctor 17%
Friends/family 14%		Friends/family 15%
Internet 7%		Don't know 10%
Nurses 4%		Medical text 7%
Don't know 2%		Nurses 2%
		Internet 1%

SOURCE: Benenson Strategy Group (2001).

To understand the full impact of health literacy on America's health system, we need to understand a wide array of information sources, information needs, information contexts, and communication complexity.

Complexity of Materials

Many materials developed to provide health information fail to take into account the needs of the audiences for these materials. Rudd and colleagues (2000) reviewed studies of patient information materials, and found that disparities between the readability of education materials and patient reading level occurred in ambulatory care settings (Cooley et al., 1995; Davis et al., 1990), substance abuse treatment centers (Davis et al., 1993), and pediatric care settings (Davis et al., 1994). Similar findings are reported for patients with diabetes (Hosey et al., 1990), arthritis (Hill, 1997), and lupus (Hearth-Holmes et al., 1997). These studies found that the reading levels of groups of patients with these chronic diseases fell between grade levels 6 and 10, while the readability of the materials designed for them fell between grade levels 7 and 13.

Rudd and colleagues (2000) also showed that several studies examined patient education materials designed for specific ethnic groups. A substantial number of studies report on both readability and comprehension assessments of these documents, deeming most of them inappropriate (Austin et al., 1995; Delp and Jones, 1996; Jolly et al., 1993, 1995; Logan et al., 1996; Powers, 1988; Spandorfer et al., 1995; Williams et al., 1996). Hosey and colleagues (1990) used the Wide Range Achievement Test to measure the reading ability of a group of American Indian diabetic patients and found that although many patients scored at a reading grade level of 5, the diabetes education materials scored at a mean reading grade level of 10. Guidry, Fagan, and Walker (1998) note that less than half of the cancer education materials specifically targeting African Americans reflected the culture of African Americans and that few were written at a reading grade level for those with low literacy skills.

Finding 4-2   More than 300 studies indicate that health-related materials far exceed the average reading ability of U.S. adults.

Popular Sources of Health Information

News Media. The news media is a large part of America's health information revolution. More than a dozen exclusively health-related magazines are easily available at grocery stores and major bookstore chains every month in America. Magazines aimed at women, men, children, parents, and mothers are also widely available and carry numerous articles on a wide variety of health issues. Several of America's largest newspapers, reaching millions of people each day, carry health sections dedicated to health news. These health sections are read by people at all literacy levels. Three quarters of newspaper readers with NALS Level 1 literacy skills reported reading the home, fashion, health, or reviews sections, while 85 percent of newspaper readers with NALS Level 5 skills read these sections (health data alone was not available) (Kirsch et al., 1993). The major broadcast and cable networks have health journalists and health reporting. There are multiple cable channels dedicated to health topics and other channels dedicated to women's issues such as Oxygen, that cover health as a major focus. Some of broadcast TV's most popular shows—Oprah and more recently a spin-off called Dr. Phil, regularly carry health information and advice. Health news, such as SARS, heart disease, obesity, antibiotic resistance, and smallpox vaccination has been a centerpiece in newspaper headlines dozens of times in 2002–2003 alone.

Advertising and Marketing. Advertising is also a prominent source of health information. Scott-Levin, a drug market research firm in Newtown, Pennsylvania, reports that while all visits to physician's offices rose 2 percent in the first nine months of 1998, visits for specific causes related to advertised products and services increased much more dramatically during this time. For example, visits for smoking cessation rose 263 percent, visits for impotence increased 113 percent, visits for hair loss rose 30 percent, and visits for high cholesterol rose by 19 percent (Maguire, 1999).

Commercial and social marketing of health information, products, and services is now a multi-billion-dollar industry. According to the Institute for Policy Innovation, direct-to-consumer advertising of prescription drugs alone increased to $1.8 billion in 1999 (Matthews, 2001). These expenditures are not unique. They represent a small portion of the dollars aimed at providing health information to consumers and motivating specific health behaviors. The United States invested some $1,080,000,000 in its recent 6-year National Youth Anti-Drug Media Campaign (Eddy, 2003). The importance of these expenditures goes beyond the dollar amount. These expenditures are guided by an understanding of consumers and their desires. These are not "information" campaigns, but rather targeted marketing efforts designed to influence what people do by offering new products, new services, lower barriers, and new motivations for changing their behavior—to stop smoking, to avoid fast food, to get a mammogram or to delay getting a mammogram. These expenditures are guided by years of market research studies and experience that have shown what kind of language works, what pictures appeal, and what messages compel people to act (Wilke, 1994). Despite this investment of talent and resources, some programs fail. The most recent evaluation of the Office of National Drug Control Policy's National Youth Anti-Drug Media Campaign program states: "There is little evidence of direct favorable Campaign effects on youth. There is no statistically significant decline in marijuana use to date, and some evidence for an increase in use from 2000 to 2001" (Hornick et al., 2002).

One characteristic of the commercial and social marketing sector is that the information is not provided objectively. The authors of these messages, whether antismoking advocates or the cigarette industry, carefully select facts, stories, and images that fall far short of full information for an intelligent decision (Mazur, 2003: 6–11). This assault on the public may have trained segments of the American public to be skeptical; to expect short sound bites of information and to avoid equivocation in information. As Mazur concludes:

> Although we may talk about shared decision making in medical care and the provider–patient relationship, the original goal of the decision scientist, to provide a full discussion of risks and benefits among a full set of alternatives, may or may not be attainable. And it is far from clear whether patients actually want to participate in such a fully shared decision-making environment (Mazur, 2003: 177).

Family and Friends. The lay network, informal communications among family members and friends, is another source of information about health for many individuals. Health information is often shared through personal experiences recounted by others. Personal stories also come from ethnic media programming and print media coverage. These personal stories may have the power to influence health behavior. This may be particularly true for individuals with limited literacy skills. Friedell and colleagues (1997) found that many individuals with limited literacy more often obtained information about cancer from family and others who have had experiences with a late-stage diagnosis rather than from reading about the disease.

The Internet. The Internet is estimated to reach 70 million Americans with health information. As America's attention moves from the treatment of disease to wellness, the number of health sites has mushroomed. Information about Internet use among adolescents and young adults indicates that most have used the Internet to access health information. A recent survey of 15- to 24-year-olds found that 90 percent of this population has been online (Rideout, 2001). Of this 90 percent, 75 percent used the Internet at least once to find health information. Searches of the Internet for health information exceed searches for sport scores or online purchases and participation in chat rooms (Rideout, 2001).

Questions have been raised regarding whether the Internet is a reliable and understandable information source that appeals to and is accessible by diverse users (e.g., Goldstein and Flory, 1997; IOM, 2002; Sikorski and Peters, 1997). Socioeconomic status and level of education are strongly associated with the likelihood that a consumer will obtain health information from the Internet. Limited literacy in English and disparities in computer access decrease the likelihood that the information will be available to and understood by all health consumers (Houston and Allison, 2002). In addition, the majority of health-related sites on the Internet are English-language-only sites (Kalichman et al., 2001) which also serves to limit access. The Children's Partership conducted an analysis of online content for low-income and underserved Americans and estimate that 44 million adults face literacy barriers in their use of the Internet (Lazarus and Mora, 2000). Of the 1,000 web sites assessed, only 10 were accessible for adults with limited literacy skills. Furthermore, only 20 had content in languages other than in English that provided "practical information for a more productive life in the United States."

Because there is little regulation or oversight of the information posted on the Internet, many consumers and health-care professionals are concerned about the reliability of posted information (Houston and Allison, 2002; Murray et al., 2003). In fact, *Healthy People 2010* includes as an objective increasing the proportion of web sites with health-related information that allow the user to evaluate the quality of that information (HHS, 2000). A meta-analysis of empirical studies of consumer health information on the Internet by Eysenbach et al. (2002) found that 70 percent of the studies analyzed concluded that quality was a problem.

The Internet also can influence the ways health professionals and patients interact. Consumers who use the Internet to look up health-related information may take action based on that information, including bringing the information to their health-care provider. In a telephone survey of 521 people who had used the Internet to search for health information, those in poor or failing health were more likely than those in good or excellent health to talk to their physician about health information they had found online (Houston and Allison, 2002). Murray et al. (2003) reported findings from a telephone survey of a nationally representative sample of 3,209 people. They found that 50 percent of people who had found information relevant to their own health took that information to their physician. Among those who took information to the physician, 83 percent said they felt more in control as a result, 78 percent said they felt more confident as a result, and 6 percent reported negative feelings such as embarrassment as a result. Murray and colleagues further reported that those taking information from the Internet to their physician may experience a change in patient/physician relationship depending primarily on the communication skills of the physician. For example, if the patient perceived that the physician "acted challenged" by the information the relationship was more likely to be damaged.

Finding 4-3 Competing sources of health information (including the national media, the Internet, product marketing, health education, and consumer protection) intensify the need for improved health literacy.

Finding 4-4 Health literacy efforts have not yet fully benefited from research findings in social and commercial marketing.

OPPORTUNITIES TO IMPROVE HEALTH LITERACY

Evidence-Based Approaches[5]

Within the health sciences there is emerging literature on the effectiveness of community-based interventions with culturally diverse groups and increasing cultural competency by health providers (IOM, 2002). The out-

---

[5]The committee would like to thank the Agency for Healthcare Research and Quality for their assistance with this segment of the report.

comes of a number of community-based approaches have been published, and a sample of these are shown in Table 4-1. These approaches, while small in number, are an important contribution to current and future approaches to health literacy, particularly to the degree that they provide evidence of their effectiveness. As noted earlier in this chapter, this collection of approaches is not intended to be an exhaustive review of the work in the field. Studies described in this table represent a sample of the English-language peer-reviewed health literature that investigate the effect of an intervention in a community-based setting. Many studies in this table reflect the contribution of the Agency for Healthcare Research and Quality (AHRQ) research program, which is discussed in more detail in Chapter 6. Additional studies were identified by searching the Medline, PsycInfo, ERIC,[6] Sociological Abstracts, and CINAHL[7] databases, and through testimony to the committee by experts in the field.

Four studies evaluated patient knowledge (Bill-Harvey et al., 1989; Busselman and Holcomb, 1994; Fitzgibbon et al., 1996; Raymond et al., 2002), and of these, only one (Bill-Harvey et al., 1989) showed positive changes in both understanding and health behavior. Three other programs (Fouad et al., 1997; Hartman et al., 1997; Lillington et al., 1995) showed an improved health outcome as a result of the program, but failed to provide evidence of increased understanding. Other evidence-based studies are continually being identified and evaluated by the CDC's Task Force on Guidelines for Community Preventative Services.

Promising Approaches

In addition to these published studies, many unpublished activities are being carried out in the community to improve health literacy. Anecdotal evidence suggests that the limited budgets of these programs, combined with their emphasis on intervention, result in funding being used for the approach itself to the exclusion of formal evaluation of the program outcome. Examples of these approaches are presented below.

Community Opportunities

Community organizations provide an opportunity to address issues of health literacy directly. An example of this is a set of programs to address the needs of the Navajo community. Older Navajos are particularly vulnerable to complications of medical conditions exacerbated by a mismatch in

---

[6]Education Resources Information Center.
[7]Cumulative Index to Nursing and Allied Health Literature.

TABLE 4-1 Examples of Published Studies of Community-Based
Interventions

Citation	Setting	Study Design	Population
Bill-Harvey et al., 1989	Senior centers and community centers for the elderly, Hartford, CT	Uncontrolled trial	n = 76 (100 enrolled, 76 completed program)
Busselman and Holcomb, 1994	WIC voucher distribution sites in 7 urban and rural communities, Kansas	Randomized trial	n = 32 Controls = 31 Participants were receiving WIC vouchers Controls met all WIC criteria except for income Controls had significantly higher reading levels as measured by the WRAT-R than the WIC group (p < 0.001)
Elkind et al., 2002	Three county region of Eastern Washington	Pre-test, post-test	n = 301 185 farmworkers 115 community members Hispanic farmworkers and their families living in eastern Washington
Fitzgibbon et al., 1996	Literacy training program in a Hispanic neighborhood, Chicago, IL	Randomized controlled trial	n = 38 families (mother and at least one child between 7–12 years). Low-income Hispanics

Intervention	Outcome
10-Hour osteoarthritis education program designed for older low-income adults with osteoarthritis. Course taught by indigenous community leaders.	Pre-/post-test outcomes showed significant increase in knowledge on both verbal and picture story tests ($p < 0.001$ for both), significant increase in scores on exercise scale ($p < 0.001$), improvement in attitude toward one's illness, and increase in use of adaptive equipment. No significant improvement in functioning.
Simplified dietary guidelines. Control group received the unmodified tenth grade reading level version of the introduction to dietary guildines, while the WIC group received a simplified seventh grade reading level version.	Differences in comprehension of the seventh and tenth grade materials were not significant.
Four one-act Spanish language plays intended to provide education about health and safety issues for farmworkers.	Participants showed significantly greater knowledge about information from the plays ($p < 0.01$). Participants reported enjoying the plays, remembering the story lines, and were willing to see additional plays if available.
Intervention families participated in a 12-week-long culture-specific dietary intervention intended to reduce cancer risk through the adoption of a low-fat, high-fiber diet. Control families received standard pamphlet on nutrition and health behaviors and no classes.	No significant differences between intervention and control groups, before and after intervention in mothers' fat intake, saturated fat intake, fiber intake, exercise level, or nutrition knowledge; or in children's dietary intake or nutrition knowledge.

Continued

TABLE 4-1 Continued

Citation	Setting	Study Design	Population
Fouad et al., 1997	City of Birmingham, AL	Volunteer participants matched with non-participant controls	n = 81 completed program (130 enrolled, program offered to 600) 81 controls City employees with high blood pressure (BP)
Hartman et al., 1997	Expanded Food and Nutrition Education Program (EFNEP), Twin Cities Metropolitan Area, MN	Randomized controlled trial, randomized by instructor (not participant)	n = 134 participants 70 controls
Kumanyika et al., 1999	Community based Recruitment from supermarkets in Washington, D.C. in primarily African-American neighborhoods	Randomized trial	n = 330 Adults with a history of hypertension or an abnormal total cholesterol level, aged 40–70.
Lillington et al., 1995	4 WIC sites in south and central Los Angeles	Randomized controlled trial	n = 768, 555 at follow-up Pregnant WIC participants who were current smokers or recent ex-smokers

Intervention	Outcome
Educational program designed to reduce risk factors for cardiovascular disease among low-literacy, unskilled workers. Participants attended health education sessions over the course of 1 year on different topics; weight and BP assessed at each session, goals set, culturally appropriate examples used, monetary incentives offered. Participants and controls received materials such as newletters and tipsheets.	Participants showed significant decrease in mean BP (p = 0.03) No significant change in BP of controls.
Nutrition education program. Participants received low-fat nutrition education curriculum. Controls received regular EFNEP materials that focus on food budgeting, safety, and healthy eating.	Mixed model regression analyses showed significant effects for the intervention program related to changes in eating pattern scales and scales related to attitudes of low-fat eating.
Nutrition counseling. Self-help (control) group received food cards and nutrition guide. Full instruction (intervention) group received these materials, video and audiotape series, and a series of 4 monthly classes.	Decreases in total cholesterol and systolic blood pressure observed at 12 months, but there was no significant difference between the control and intervention groups. Outcomes did not differ by literacy scores.
Culturally appropriate low-literacy smoking cessation intervention materials for low-income African-American and Hispanic women. Intervention group received 15-minute, one-on-one interviews, self-help guide, reinforcement cards, and participated in incentive contest. Controls received usual care; included written material on quitting smoking in pregnancy	Twice as many smokers in intervention group reported quitting smoking at 9 months gestation compared to control group (p < 0.01). Differences remained at 6 weeks postpartum. Although no significant differences were observed for relapse during pregnancy among ex-smokers at 6 weeks postpartum, a significantly higher proportion of intervention ex-smokers were still abstinent (79%), compared to control ex-smokers (62%) (p < 0.01).

Continued

TABLE 4-1 Continued

Citation	Setting	Study Design	Population
Raymond et al., 2002	Malls and family planning clinics in eight U.S. cities: Denver, Los Angeles, Chicago, San Antonio, Philadelphia, Phoenix, Miami, Washington, D.C.	Before-after comparison	n = 656 Females, aged 12–50, without a health-care or marketing background, and able to read English well enough to read an over-the-counter label

the health literacy skills of health consumers and care providers. The Gathering Place[8] provides health and literacy programs for Navajo adults and children in their homes and community centers. Bilingual, trained community members provide services that include information on health, safety, mental, and physical wellness, and preventive measures. A "Shima Yazhi" lay health program offers information and support for new baby care, parenting, and health concerns, in locations convenient to the client.

The Gathering Place also represents a collaborative program, as it offers workshops to child care providers throughout Eastern Agency of the reservation using videos, bilingual oral presentations, and hands-on formats.

> *We need to provide opportunities for health professionals to experience the native culture by providing workshops, presentations, or hands-on experience in selected ceremonies. We also need to provide exposure to community members with more formal workshops in health literacy related issues. Some topics may be "what steps need to be taken when visiting with doctors," and "talking about prescriptions and how they are supposed to work."*
>
> Alvin Bille
> The Gathering Place

---

[8]The Gathering Place is located in Thoreau, New Mexico. For more information, see http://www.navajo-coop.com.

Intervention	Outcome
Prototype product packaging and insert for emergency contraceptive pill. Participants were shown the package and then answered questions about the product. Results reported by literacy level as measured by the REALM.	85% of participants showed understanding of at least 7 of 11 communication objectives. Participants with lower literacy significantly less likely than those with higher literacy to understand almost all of the communication objectives, but 8 of the 11 objectives were understood by more than 80% of those with lower literacy.

Asian Health Services[9] takes advantage of community opportunities to provide health education through one-on-one and community outreach at nail salons, bars, sewing factories, massage parlors, beauty schools, and community events (Asian Health Services, 2003). The program provides group education to women thorough Northern California community centers, area businesses, and clinics. These programs offer information on women's health needs such as breast cancer and pap smears, as well as information about health insurance for women and their children. The "Health is Strength" Project run by Asian Health Services provides Korean adults and children with health education materials (brochure, resource list, workshops) in the Korean language. Distributed in churches and other community venues, these materials are designed to improve knowledge and remove barriers to health literacy. Additionally, bilingual (English and Korean) health counselors work within community social structures, primarily churches attended by Koreans, to organize activities, serve as liasons between the Korean and medical communities, provide social support, follow up, and improve health knowledge.

Community centers, homes, and businesses provide the opportunity for the Centro Latino de Salud, Educación y Cultura to serve Missouri-area Hispanic adults and children through a program called Attaining Cultural Competency and Enriching Health Service Solutions. This program provides information and help in accessing needed educational and health resources, a program for new and expectant mothers, interpreter and translation services, and health referrals (Centro Latino, 2003).

---

[9]Asian Health Services is based in Oakland, California. For more information, see http://www.ahschc.org.

Nongovernmental Organizations

Nongovernmental organizations provide an opportunity for informed and effective advocates to have a role in shaping health literacy programs, policies, and interventions. For example, The Institute for Healthcare Advancement has developed a set of books to assist consumers in deciding what health issues can be dealt with at home (and how to best deal with them) and what health issues should initiate a call to a health-care provider. Most of these books, part of a series entitled *What to Do for Health*, are available in English or Spanish; two are also available in Vietnamese. An evaluation of one of the books carried out by Molina Healthcare found that individuals and families who received the books visited the emergency department 6.7 percent less after receiving the books (Institute for Healthcare Advancement, 2003).

Another example is provided by the Managed Care Consumer Assistance Program (MCCAP). The MCCAP works to educate consumers about the concepts of managed care and rights as consumers, and provide assistance with dispute resolution procedures. MCCAP holds consumer education workshops in the appropriate languages and provides one-on-one counseling to consumers needing information or assistance with managed care. Services are provided to low-income, multilingual, and multicultural communities, through a network of 25 community-based organizations. These community-based organizations include neighborhood centers, ethnic organizations, and social service agencies (MCCAP, 2003).

Collaborative Programs

Collaborations between government and community programs offer an opportunity to develop interventions appropriate to the needs of the audience. An example of a collaborative approach is a set of materials on sex education developed though a collaboration between the Program for Appropriate Technology in Health, Austin/Travis County Health Department, the Washington, DC, Center for Youth Services, Delaware (Maryland) Delmarva Rural Ministries, the Tlingit and Haida Indian Tribes Central Council, and the Children's Theatre of Juneau. Entitled "Plain Talk," these materials were developed to educate and inform English-speaking and non-English-speaking low-literate youth in response to a nationwide needs assessment survey of 2,500 U.S. organizations that showed that teens especially need materials on AIDS, other STDs, and condom use (Program for Appropriate Technology in Health, 2003).

Programs between for-profit or nonprofit agencies and community organizations provide an opportunity to develop appropriate interventions, and to reach the intended audience. This type of collaboration can effec-

BOX 4-3
Excerpt from the Introduction to "Language Access: Helping Non-English Speakers Navigate Health and Human Services"

Public and private organizations have begun to address language barriers to ensure effective communication between service providers and patients, particularly in health care. The language gap can lead to delays in or denial of service, unnecessary tests, more costly or invasive treatment of disease, mistakes in prescribing and using medication, and deterrence in patient compliance with treatment. Language barriers are a contributing factor in health care disparities among racial and ethnic minorities and in a lack of health insurance among immigrants and minorities. In a series of federal guidances since 2000, federal agencies have reminded recipients of federal funds of their obligation under civil rights law to provide meaningful access to their services for limited-English proficient individuals. The Office for Civil Rights in the U.S. Department of Health and Human Services (HHS) states that language assistance should result in accurate and effective communication between provider and client, at no cost to the client. Within the health and human services field, affected organizations include state and local health and welfare agencies, hospitals and clinics, managed care organizations, nursing homes, mental health centers, senior citizen centers, Head Start programs and contractors. In three federal programs, federal agencies have approved reimbursement for language services to applicants and recipients who are limited English proficient. HHS, in a November 1999 brief, approved the use of federal Temporary Assistance for Needy Families (TANF) and state Maintenance-of-Effort (MOE) funds to provide language services. In a 2000 letter to state Medicaid directors, the Centers for Medicaid & Medicare Services confirmed that federal matching funds for the State Children's Health Insurance Program (SCHIP) and Medicaid are available for state expenditures on interpretation and translation. At least nine states—Hawaii, Idaho, Maine, Massachusetts, Minnesota, Montana, New Hampshire, Utah and Washington—have obtained federal matching funds for these services. Recently, other states have enacted legislation requiring interpreters in emergency departments and hospitals (Massachusetts and Rhode Island, respectively); a health-care interpreters council (Oregon); and an office to address racial and ethnic disparities in health care, including language and cultural competency (New Jersey).

SOURCE: Morse (2003).

tively create coalitions of existing providers by partnering a for-profit or nonprofit organization with specific ethnic and geographically focused community providers. As an example, the Alzheimer's Association of Los Angeles has developed a model to build the dementia care capability of existing community providers such as hospitals, public health clinics, adult day care centers, and community-based social service agencies. Using focus groups and community input, the Alzheimer's Association identified churches as a visible and trusted source of health information for the Los Angeles area

African-American community. The organization then developed a set of education and outreach projects which involved collaboration with clergy, social service health-care providers, and constituent representatives (Alzheimer's Association of Los Angeles, 2001).

Approaches to Increasing Language Access

In 2003, the National Conference of State Legislatures' Children's Policy Initiative issued a report titled "Language Access: Helping Non-English Speakers Navigate Health and Human Services" (Morse, 2003). This report highlights the importance of language to quality of care and access to care, and reviews the array of promising approaches to improving language access that are currently being carried out on the federal and state levels. An excerpt from this report is presented in Box 4-3.

These studies and programs, both published and unpublished, offer a variety of possible approaches and indicate both the need for effective programs and for outcomes measures of program effectiveness. While little evidence supports the use of any given approach, research into the value of existing and innovative approaches on health behaviors and the effect of participatory action and empowerment strategies can provide further direction for future approaches to address health literacy.

Finding 4-1 Culture gives meaning to health communication. Health literacy must be understood and addressed in the context of culture and language.

Finding 4-2 More than 300 studies indicate that health-related materials far exceed the average reading ability of U.S. adults.

Finding 4-3 Competing sources of health information (including the national media, the Internet, product marketing, health education, and consumer protection) intensify the need for improved health literacy.

Finding 4-4 Health literacy efforts have not yet fully benefited from research findings in social and commercial marketing.

Recommendation 4-1 Federal agencies responsible for addressing disparities should support the development of conceptual frameworks on the intersection of culture and health literacy to direct in-depth theoretical explorations and formulate the conceptual underpinnings that can guide interventions.

4-1.a NIH should convene a consensus conference, including stakeholders, to develop methodology for the incorporation of health literacy improvement into approaches to health disparities.

4-1.b The Office of Minority Health and AHRQ should develop measures of the relationships between culture, language, cultural competency, and health literacy to be used in studies of the relationship between health literacy and health outcomes.

Recommendation 4-2 AHRQ, the CDC, Indian Health Service, Health Resources and Services Administration, and Substance Abuse and Mental Health Services Administration should develop and test approaches to improve health communication that foster healing relationships across culturally diverse populations. This includes investigations that explore the effect of existing and innovative communication approaches on health behaviors, and studies that examine the impact of participatory action and empowerment research strategies for effective penetration of health information at the community level.

REFERENCES

Alzheimer's Association of Los Angeles. 2001. *Faith-Centered Partnerships: A Model for Reaching the African-American Community.* [Online]. Available: http://www.alzla.org/resources/faithcentered/index.html [accessed: December, 2003].

AMA Ad Hoc Committee on Health Literacy. 1999. Health literacy: Report of the Council on Scientific Affairs. Ad Hoc Committee on Health Literacy for the Council on Scientific Affairs, American Medical Association. *Journal of the American Medical Association.* 281(6): 552–557.

Asian Health Services. 2003. *Asian Health Services Home Page.* [Online]. Available: http://www.ahschc.org/ [accessed: October 20, 2003].

Austin PE, Matlack R 2nd, Dunn KA, Kesler C, Brown CK. 1995. Discharge instructions: Do illustrations help our patients understand them? *Annals of Emergency Medicine.* 25(3): 317–320.

Benenson Strategy Group. 2001. Sex Matters Survey. Available from: Roper Center for Public Opinion Research In: *Public Opinion Online.* Storrs, CT: The Roper Center for Public Opinion Research.

Bill-Harvey D, Rippey R, Abeles M, Donald MJ, Downing D, Ingenito F, Pfeiffer CA. 1989. Outcome of an osteoarthritis education program for low-literacy patients taught by indigenous instructors. *Patient Education and Counseling.* 13(2): 133–142.

Billie A. 2003. *Health and Literacy: A Native American Point of View.* Presentation given at a workshop of the Institute of Medicine Committee on Health Literacy. February 13, 2003, Irvine, CA.

Busselman KM, Holcomb CA. 1994. Reading skill and comprehension of the dietary guidelines by WIC participants. *Journal of the American Dietetic Association.* 94(6): 622–625.

Centro Latino. 2003. *Centro Latino de Salud, Educación, y Cultura Home Page.* [Online]. Available: http://centrolatino.missouri.org [accessed: October 20, 2003].

Collins KS, Hughes DL, Doty MM, Ives BL, Edwards JN, Tenney K. 2002. *Diverse Communities, Common Concerns: Assessing Health Care Quality for Minority Americans.* New York: The Commonwealth Fund.

Cooley ME, Moriarty H, Berger MS, Selm-Orr D, Coyle B, Short T. 1995. Patient literacy and the readability of written cancer educational materials. *Oncology Nursing Forum.* 22(9): 1345–1351.

Cooper LA, Roter DL. 2003. Patient-provider communication: The effect of race and ethnicity on process and outcomes in health care. In: *Unequal Treatment: Confronting Racial and Ethnic Disparities in Health Care.* Smedley BD, Stith AY, Nelson AR, Editors. Washington, DC: The National Academies Press. Pp. 336–354.

Cooper-Patrick L, Gallo JJ, Gonzales JJ, Vu HT, Powe NR, Nelson C, Ford DE. 1999. Race, gender, and partnership in the patient-physician relationship. *Journal of the American Medical Association.* 282(6): 583–589.

Davis TC, Crouch MA, Wills G, Miller S, Abdehou DM. 1990. The gap between patient reading comprehension and the readability of patient education materials. *Journal of Family Practice.* 31(5): 533–538.

Davis TC, Jackson RH, George RB, Long SW, Talley D, Murphy PW, Mayeaux EJ, Truong T. 1993. Reading ability in patients in substance misuse treatment centers. *International Journal of the Addictions.* 28(6): 571–582.

Davis TC, Mayeaux EJ, Fredrickson D, Bocchini JA Jr, Jackson RH, Murphy PW. 1994. Reading ability of parents compared with reading level of pediatric patient education materials. *Pediatrics.* 93(3): 460–468.

Delp C, Jones J. 1996. Communicating information to patients: The use of cartoon illustrations to improve comprehension of instructions. *Academic Emergency Medicine.* 3(3): 264–270.

Duranti A. 1997. *Linguistic Anthropology.* Cambridge: Cambridge University Press.

Eddy M. 2003. *War on Drugs: The National Youth Anti-Drug Media Campaign.* Congressional Research Service, The Library of Congress.

Elkind PD, Pitts K, Ybarra SL. 2002. Theater as a mechanism for increasing farm health and safety knowledge. *American Journal of Industrial Medicine.* (Supplement 2): 28–35.

Eysenbach G, Powell J, Kuss O, Sa ER. 2002. Empirical studies assessing the quality of health information for consumers on the world-wide web: A systematic review. *Journal of the American Medical Association.* 287(20): 2691–2700.

Fitzgibbon ML, Stolley MR, Avellone ME, Sugerman S, Chavez N. 1996. Involving parents in cancer risk reduction: A program for Hispanic American families. *Health Psychology*. 15(6): 413–422.

Fouad MN, Kiefe CI, Bartolucci AA, Burst NM, Ulene V, Harvey MR. 1997. A hypertension control program tailored to unskilled and minority workers. *Ethnicity and Disease*. 7(3): 191–199.

Friedell GH, Linville LH, Rubio A, Wagner WD, Tucker TC. 1997. What providers should know about community cancer control. *Cancer Practice*. 5(6): 367–374.

Gallup Organization. 2002. Gallup Poll. Roper Center for Public Opinion Research. In: *Public Opinion Online*. Storrs, CT: The Roper Center for Public Opinion Research.

Goldstein D, Flory J. 1997. Health care commerce on the net: The revolution begins. *Medical Interface*. 10(8): 56–58.

Good BJ, Good MJD. 1981. The meaning of symptoms: A cultural hermeneutic model for clinical practice. In: *The Relevance of Social Science for Medicine*. Eisenberg L, Kleinman A, Editors. Dordecht, Holland: Reidel. Pp. 165–196.

Guidry JJ, Fagan P, Walker V. 1998. Cultural sensitivity and readability of breast and prostate printed cancer education materials targeting African Americans. *Journal of the National Medical Association*. 90(3): 165–169.

Hartman TJ, McCarthy PR, Park RJ, Schuster E, Kushi LH. 1997. Results of a community-based low-literacy nutrition education program. *Journal of Community Health*. 22(5): 325–341.

Hearth-Holmes M, Murphy PW, Davis TC, Nandy I, Elder CG, Broadwell LH, Wolf RE. 1997. Literacy in patients with a chronic disease: Systemic lupus erythematosus and the reading level of patient education materials. *Journal of Rheumatology*. 24(12): 2335–2339.

HHS (U.S. Department of Health and Human Services). 2000. *Healthy People 2010: Understanding and Improving Health*. Washington, DC: U.S. Department of Health and Human Services. [Online]. Available: http://www.health.gov/healthypeople [accessed: January 15, 2003].

HHS. 2001. *National Standards for Culturally and Linguistically Appropriate Services in Health Care. Executive Summary*. Washington, DC: U.S. DHHS Office of Minority Health.

Hill J. 1997. A practical guide to patient education and information giving. *Baillieres Clinical Rheumatology*. 11(1): 109–127.

Hornick R, Maklan D, Cadell D, Barmada CH, Jacobsen L, Prado A, Romantan A, Orwin R, Sridharan S, Zanutto E, Baskin R, Chu A, Morin C, Taylor K, Steele D. 2002. *Evaluation of the National Youth Anti-Drug Campaign: Fifth Semi-annual Report of Findings. Delivered to: The National Institute on Drug Abuse*. WESTAT Corporation and Annenberg School for Communication.

Hosey GM, Freeman WL, Stracqualursi F, Gohdes D. 1990. Designing and evaluating diabetes education material for American Indians. *Diabetes Educator*. 16(5): 407–414.

Houston TK, Allison JJ. 2002. Users of Internet health information: Differences by health status. *Journal of Medical Internet Research*. 4(2): E7.

Institute for Healthcare Advancement. 2003. *Health Literacy: An Overview and Research-Supported Solutions*. [Online]. Available: http://www.iha4health.org/pdf/research_brochures.pdf [accessed: December 9, 2003].

IOM (Institute of Medicine). 2000. *Promoting Health: Intervention Strategies from Social and Behavioral Research*. Smedley BD, Syme SL, Editors. Washington, DC: National Academy Press.

IOM. 2001. *Crossing the Quality Chasm: A New Health System for the 21st Century*. Washington, DC: National Academy Press.

IOM. 2002. *Speaking of Health: Assessing Health Communication Strategies for Diverse Populations*. Washington, DC: The National Academies Press.

IOM. 2003a. *Unequal Treatment: Confronting Racial and Ethnic Disparities in Health Care*. Smedley BD, Stith AY, Nelson AR, Editors. Washington, DC: The National Academies Press.

IOM. 2003b. *Priority Areas for National Action: Transforming Healthcare Quality*. Adams K, Corrigan JM, Editors. Washington, DC: The National Academies Press.

Jolly BT, Scott JL, Feied CF, Sanford SM. 1993. Functional illiteracy among emergency department patients: A preliminary study. *Annals of Emergency Medicine*. 22(3): 573–578.

Jolly BT, Scott JL, Sanford SM. 1995. Simplification of emergency department discharge instructions improves patient comprehension. *Annals of Emergency Medicine*. 26(4): 443–446.

Kalichman SC, Benotsch E, Weinhardt L. 2001. Quality of health information on the Internet. *Journal of the American Medical Association*. 286(17): 2092–2093; author reply 2094–2095.

Kirsch IS, Jungeblut A, Jenkins L, Kolstad A. 1993. *Adult Literacy in America: A First Look at the Results of the National Adult Literacy Survey (NALS)*. Washington, DC: National Center for Education Statistics, U.S. Department of Education.

Kumanyika SK, Adams-Campbell L, Van Horn B, Ten Have TR, Treu JA, Askov E, Williams J, Achterberg C, Zaghloul S, Monsegu D, Bright M, Stoy DB, Malone-Jackson M, Mooney D, Deiling S, Caulfield J. 1999. Outcomes of a cardiovascular nutrition counseling program in African-Americans with elevated blood pressure or cholesterol level. *Journal of the American Dietetic Association*. 99(11): 1380–1391.

Lazarus W, Mora F. 2000. *Online Content for Low-income and Underserved Americans: The Digital Divide's New Frontier. A Strategic Audit of Activities and Opportunities*. Santa Monica, CA: The Children's Partnership.

Lillington L, Royce J, Novak D, Ruvalcaba M, Chlebowski R. 1995. Evaluation of a smoking cessation program for pregnant minority women. *Cancer Practice*. 3(3): 157–163.

Lincoln JS. 2003. *The Dream in Native American and Other Primitive Cultures*. New York: Dover Publications.

Logan PD, Schwab RA, Salomone JA 3rd, Watson WA. 1996. Patient understanding of emergency department discharge instructions. *Southern Medical Journal*. 89(8): 770–774.

Long A, Scrimshaw SC, Hernandez N. 1992. Transcultural epilepsy services. In: *Rapid Assessment Procedures: Qualitative Methodologies for Planning and Evaluation of Health Related Programmes*. Scrimshaw NS, Gleason GR, Editors. Boston, MA: International Nutrition Foundation for Developing Countries. Pp. 205–214.

Maguire P. 1999. How direct-to-consumer advertising is putting the squeeze on physicians. *ACP-ASIM Observer*. March.

Matthews M Jr. 2001. Who's Afraid of Pharmaceutical Advertising? A Response to a Changing Health System. Policy Report 155. Lewisville, TX: Institute for Policy Innovation.

Mazur DJ. 2003. *The New Medical Conversation: Media, Patients, Doctors and the Ethics of Scientific Communication*. New York: Rowman and Littlefield.

MCCAP. 2003. *Who We Are. How Does MCCAP Work?* [Online]. Available: http://www. mccapny.org/about.htm [accessed: December, 2003].

Medvantx. 2003. *How Can Medvantx Help You Manage Escalating Drug Costs?* [Online]. Available: http://www.medvantx.com/ [accessed: October, 2003].

Morse A. 2003. *Language Access: Helping Non-English Speakers Navigate Health and Human Services*. National Conference of State Legislature's Children's Policy Initiative.

Murray E, Lo B, Pollack L, Donelan K, Catania J, White M, Zapert K, Turner R. 2003. The impact of health information on the internet on the physician-patient relationship: Patient perceptions. *Archives of Internal Medicine*. 163(14): 1727–1734.

Nutbeam D. 2000. Health literacy as a public health goal: A challenge for contemporary health education and communication strategies into the 21st century. *Health Promotion International*. 15(3): 259–267.

Perez-Stable EJ. 1994. *Cardiovascular Disease in Latino Health in the US: A Growing Challenge*. Washington, DC: American Public Health Association.

Powers RD. 1988. Emergency department patient literacy and the readability of patient-directed materials. *Annals of Emergency Medicine*. 17(2): 124–126.

Program for Appropriate Technology in Health. 2003. *Plain Talk: Teaching Low-Literate Youth in the United States about HIV, AIDS, and STDs*. [Online]. Available: http://www.path.org/about/f_plain_talk.htm [accessed: December, 2003].

Raymond EG, Dalebout SM, Camp SI. 2002. Comprehension of a prototype over-the-counter label for an emergency contraceptive pill product. *Obstetrics and Gynecology*. 100(2): 342–349.

Rideout V. 2001. *Generation Rx.com. How Young People Use the Internet for Health Information*. Menlo Park, CA: Henry J. Kaiser Family Foundation. [Online]. Available: http://www.kff.org/content/2001/20011211a/GenerationRx.pdf [accessed: February 3, 2003].

Ross R. 1996. *Returning to the Teachings: Exploring Aboriginal Justice*. Toronto: Penguin Books.

Rudd R, Moeykens BA, Colton TC. 2000. Health and literacy. A review of medical and public health literature. In: *Annual Review of Adult Learning and Literacy*. Comings J, Garners B, Smith C, Editors. New York: Jossey-Bass.

Sabogal F, Marin G, Otero-Fabogal R, Marin BV, Perez-Stable EF. 1987. Hispanic familialismo and acculturation: What changes and what doesn't? *Hispanic Journal Behavioral Sciences*. 9: 397–412.

Scrimshaw SC, Souza R. 1982. Recognizing active labor. A test of a decision-making guide for pregnant women. *Social Science and Medicine*. 16(16): 1473–1482.

Sikorski R, Peters R. 1997. Allergy and immunology on the Internet. *Journal of the American Medical Association*. 278(22): 2029–2030.

Spandorfer JM, Karras DJ, Hughes LA, Caputo C. 1995. Comprehension of discharge instructions by patients in an urban emergency department. *Annals of Emergency Medicine*. 25(1): 71–74.

U.S. Census Bureau. 2000. *United States Census 2000. Profile of General Demographic Characteristics*. Washington, D.C.: U.S. Census Bureau.

U.S. Census Bureau. 2003. *American Fact Finder*. [Online]. Available: http://factfinder.census.gov [accessed: December, 2003].

Wilke WL. 1994. *Consumer Behavior*. 4th edition. New York: Wiley.

Williams DM, Counselman FL, Caggiano CD. 1996. Emergency department discharge instructions and patient literacy: A problem of disparity. *American Journal of Emergency Medicine*. 14(1): 19–22.

Zborowski M. 1952. Cultural components in response to pain. *Journal of Social Issues*. 8(4): 16–30.

Zola IK. 1966. Culture and symptoms: An analysis of patients' presenting complaints. *American Sociological Review*. 31(5): 615–630.

5

Educational Systems

"People are hearing about overweight and obesity. So they're trying to figure out how much food they should eat. How much is too much? They're asking about calories, carbohydrates, vitamins, and fiber. They're asking about salt, sugar, and portion sizes.

. . . As young medical students, you and I learned more about the pathophysiology of disease than we learned about answering these questions for our future patients."

Vice Admiral Richard H. Carmona, M.D., M.P.H., F.A.C.S.
United States Surgeon General
American Medical Association House of Delegates Meeting
June 14, 2003

Overall, the U.S. educational systems offer a primary point of inter vention to improve the quality of literacy and health literacy. The educational systems discussed in this chapter are the K-12 system, the adult education system, and education for health professionals. Public educational systems in the United States are influenced by national policy and funding, but remain under the jurisdiction of and are funded by states and localities.

THE K-12 AND UNIVERSITY EDUCATION SYSTEMS

Elementary, middle school, high school, and university education provide an opportunity to promote health literacy, to reduce health-risk behaviors, and to prepare children to navigate the health-care system. Effective health education programs should begin in early childhood and continually build on previous knowledge (NRC, 1999). Achieving health literacy in students is hindered by a lack of continuity in health education programs across the many age groups.

K-12 Education

Health Education Programs

The School Health Policies and Programs Study 2000, conducted by the Centers for Disease Control and Prevention (CDC), indicated that most elementary, middle, and high schools require health education classes as a part of the curriculum (Kann et al., 2001). The majority of these states (75 percent) use the National Health Education Standards (NHES) as a framework to develop these programs (Kann et al., 2001). Box 5-1 displays the NHES and some background about these standards. Some states have made significant progress in establishing guidelines in accordance with the NHES.

A lack of consistent, cross-grade health curriculums may reduce student health literacy. Although most elementary, middle, and high schools require students to take health education, classes in different grades tend not to build upon previous grades. The absence of a coordinated health education program across grade levels may impede student learning. Kann et al. (2001) report an increase in the percentage of elementary schools that require health education from 33 percent in kindergarten to 44 percent in grade 5. However, only 27 percent of schools require health education in grade 6, 20 percent in grade 8, 10 percent in grade 9, and 2 percent in grade 12.

Teacher education may affect teacher effectiveness in implementing health and health literacy curriculums. National and international strategies developed to help schools implement effective policies and programs (e.g., Kolbe et al., 1997, 2001) are complicated by the fact that few health education teachers majored in health education (Collins et al., 1995; Hausman and Ruzek, 1995; Kann et al., 2001; Patterson et al., 1996; Ubbes et al., 1999). Only 10 percent of health education classes or courses have a teacher who majored in health education, or in health and physical education combined (Kann et al., 2001). Peterson and colleagues (2001) suggest that inadequate attention to teacher health literacy has impeded student health literacy. Many teachers feel that they are not prepared to teach specific health topics (Peterson et al., 2001). For example, a sample of 156

BOX 5-1
The National Health Education Standards

In 1995, the Joint Committee on National Health Standards published the *National Health Education Standards* (NHES) subtitled *Achieving Health Literacy* (Joint Committee on National Health Education Standards, 1995). The standards describe the knowledge and skills essential for health literacy and detail what students should know and be able to do in health education by the end of grades 4, 8, and 11. The standards describe a health-literate person as a critical thinker and problem solver, a responsible, productive citizen, a self-directed learner, and an effective communicator.

The National Health Education Standards:

1. Students will comprehend concepts related to health promotion and disease prevention.
2. Students will demonstrate the ability to access valid health information and health-promoting products and services.
3. Students will demonstrate the ability to practice health-enhancing behaviors and reduce health risks.
4. Students will analyze the influence of culture, media, technology, and other factors on health.
5. Students will demonstrate the ability to use interpersonal communication skills to enhance health.
6. Students will demonstrate the ability to use goal-setting and decision-making skills to enhance health.
7. Students will demonstrate the ability to advocate for personal, family, and community health.

The NHES identified obstacles that continue to impede health education programs, including:

- Lack of appreciation for the relationship between health status and success in academic and work performance,
- Low levels of commitment by school board members and administrators,
- Inadequately prepared teachers,
- Insufficient funding for resources and staff development,
- Overcrowded curricula with little or no time for health education (Pateman, 2002; Thackeray et al., 2002),
- Unconnected and seemingly irrelevant health instruction,
- Lack of recognition of the contribution made by health education to the achievement of the academic goals of schools,
- Failure to adequately document student performance in achievement of health literacy.

elementary school staff from five schools in Philadelphia felt only "somewhat prepared" to teach health education (Hausman and Ruzek, 1995). These findings highlight the importance of professional development for teachers who provide classroom health education to young students.

Many teachers are also required by state guidelines to include specific topics and standards within their curriculums, often in response to state-mandated tests. Even within good health education curricula, teachers cannot address all topics and issues at a single grade level. Although health education may be included within the required curriculum, it might not be included within state-mandated tests and therefore these topics will receive less attention in the classroom (Pateman et al., 1999). A call to strengthen school health education by health education with state assessment requirements was made soon after the NHES were published (Collins et al., 1995), but a low level of grant support for health literacy assessment persists.

A national health promotion and disease prevention report recommends that the United States increase the proportion of middle, junior, and senior high schools that provide health education to prevent health problems in areas such as unintentional injuries; violence; suicide; tobacco use and addiction; alcohol and other drug use; unintended pregnancy; HIV/ AIDS and STD infection; unhealthy dietary patterns; inadequate physical activity; and environmental health (HHS, 2000).

The World Health Organization (1996) has described several barriers that may impede the implementation of school health programs at local, state, national, and international levels. First, education, health, and political leaders, as well as the public at large, often do not possess accurate knowledge of modern school health programs and their potential impact on health. Second, many believe the most important function of schools to be the improvement of language, mathematical, and scientific skills. Third, some may not support modern school health programs because some elements of some programs may be controversial (e.g., school programs to educate about, and prevent, HIV infection, other prevalent STDs, and unintended pregnancy). Fourth, modern school health programs require effective collaboration, especially among separate education and health agencies.

Unfortunately, among 38 states that participated in the School Health Education Profiles Study, the percentage of schools that required a health education course decreased between 1996 and 2000, as did the percentage of schools that taught about dietary behaviors and nutrition, and about how HIV is transmitted. During the year 2000, only 27 percent of schools required health education in grade 6, a number that fell to 2 percent in grade 12 (Storch et al., 2003). A similar pattern is observed in Canadian schools. In 1999, over 70 percent of Canadian school districts reported that health education was mandatory in grades 3 through 5, but only 20 percent reported that it was mandatory in grade 12 (McCall et al., 1999). When children are at an age when health risk behaviors increase (Smith, 1999), American schools require little education about health (Grunbaum et al., 2002). Unless health education is considered part of basic education, the quantity and quality of health education in U.S. elementary and secondary schools are likely to deteriorate further.

A report from an Institute of Medicine Committee on Comprehensive School Health Programs in Grades K-12 (IOM, 1997) recommended that the United States improve its school health programs. A report from the World Health Organization (1997) made similar recommendations for all nations to take similar measures. Recent surveys show that school administrators, parents, students, and the public at large all want elementary and secondary schools to implement more comprehensive school health programs (The Gallup Organization, 1994; Marzano et al., 1998).

Health professionals, such as school nurses, food service directors, health teachers, physical education teachers, and school psychologists, are already working in many elementary and secondary schools (Marx et al., 1998). Many state education and health departments also employ staff to help schools implement school health programs, as do many national nongovernmental education and health organizations (CCSSO, 2003). These programs provide a potential target for further intervention.

Science Education

Science education provides a clear opportunity for implementation of health literacy education programs and content. An example of this association is the Curriculum Linking Science Education and Health Literacy program. This project transformed inner-city children's, teachers', and parents' or care givers' experiences with food into an inquiry-based science program. Guidelines for science education include content standards for personal and community health (American Association for the Advancement of Science, 1993; NRC, 1996).

Science teachers have indicated that scientist participation can strengthen science education. A survey called "The Bayer Facts of Science Education V," conducted by Bayer Corporation and the National Science Teachers Association (1999), indicated that 98 percent of the science teachers believe that direct student–scientist interaction within classroom was important. These findings suggest an opportunity for science and health-care professionals to participate in school science and health education programs to improve the health literacy of pre-college students. In fact, more than half of 107 elementary school teachers at 31 schools reported wanting classroom visits by health professionals (Thackeray et al., 2002).

Literacy Education

The subject of literacy instruction and achievement in schools, particularly reading, is more conspicuous in the political and mainstream arenas than is health education. While health education holds promise in promoting full health literacy insofar as it leads to the acquisition of the necessary health-related knowledge, the issue of basic literacy is equally essential to full health literacy. As detailed in previous chapters, much of the research on health literacy documents the difficulties with printed health texts experienced by adults who are low in overall literacy skill.

Two influential reports have been issued by the National Research Council (NRC, 1998) and the National Institute of Child Health and Human Development (National Reading Panel, 2000) addressing the failure of schools to produce adults who are sufficiently literate to participate in an increasingly information-driven and competitive economy. These reports, along with a collection of Congressional mandates, helped lead to the *No Child Left Behind* legislation,[1] which is driving major instructional change designed to improve the levels of achievement in the schools. The major strategy of *No Child Left Behind* is to hold all schools accountable for ensuring that students achieve certain standards in subjects that comprise basic education, including language, science, and mathematics. It is too soon to report any results of these changes, but increasing numbers of schools and school districts are attending to the issues raised by the national concern with literacy achievement.

College and University Health Education

Nearly two-thirds of the 27 million 18- to 24-year-olds in the United States become college undergraduates (U.S. Department of Education, 2001). Unfortunately, relatively few of the nation's 2- and 4-year colleges and universities currently require or provide education about health (Keeling, 2001; Patrick et al., 1992). In a summary from a symposium on health and higher education, the Association of American Colleges and Universities suggested that these institutions are well situated to address issues critical to health literacy, ". . . to discover the causes and cures for diseases and to explain how people can be engaged, individually and collectively, in the improvement of their own lives and the lives of others" (Burns, 1999). But a summary from their 2001 symposium noted that: ". . . as a nation, we have not made the health of college students a priority; we lack a strong commitment to addressing health on campus, a coordinated strategy to

---

[1]*No Child Left Behind Act of 2002.* P.L. 107-110.

improve health among students, and—most important—a focus on the capacity of students themselves to contribute to solving health problems" (Association of American Colleges and Universities, 2002).

One of the National Health Objectives calls for the United States by the year 2010 to "increase to 25 percent the proportion of college and university students who receive information from their institution on each of the six priority health-risk behavior areas (injuries, tobacco use, alcohol and illicit drug use, sexual behaviors that cause unintended pregnancies and sexually transmitted diseases, dietary patterns that cause disease, and inadequate physical activity)" (HHS, 2000). In 1995, only 6 percent of 18- to 24-year-old undergraduates in the United States received information about all six topics (Douglas et al., 1997), despite the fact that these college students were substantially more likely to engage in most of these health risk behaviors than high school students (Kann et al., 1996). Neither standards nor instruments to assess their attainment have been developed to support critical health knowledge and skills that undergraduate students could acquire as part of their college education.

Finding 5-1   Significant obstacles and barriers to successful health literacy education exist in K-12 education programs.

Strategies and Opportunities in K-12 and University Systems

Although the difficulties in addressing health literacy in education are considerable, targeted solutions can be developed if the factors that contribute to these difficulties are identified. State and local programs can use the educational system's potential for addressing the issue of health literacy to produce change. St. Leger (2001) proposes that government investment into teacher professional development, research into school health frameworks, and wider dissemination of effective school health programs will improve health literacy. In addition to health education programs, opportunities for health literacy instruction exist that embed health literacy content into basic literacy teaching. In this section, these two types of approaches are described, issues with the assessment of health literacy in educational settings are explored, and examples of ongoing approaches are offered.

Opportunities for Health Education Programs

Many studies have provided evidence that school health programs can improve critical health knowledge, attitudes, and skills among elementary and secondary school students and the evidence suggests that school health programs can improve health behaviors and health outcomes (Kolbe, 2002). The CDC has initiated a project called "Programs-That-Work" to identify effective health education programs that reduce health-risk behaviors (for review, see Collins et al., 2002). These health-risk behaviors are those stressed by the U.S. Department of Health and Human Services *Healthy People 2010* program (2000). Lohrmann and Wooley (1998) have proposed that successful health education curriculums should meet the following criteria:

1. Be research-based and theory-driven.
2. Include information that is accurate and developmentally appropriate.
3. Actively engage students using interactive activities.
4. Allow students to model and practice relevant social skills.
5. Discuss how social or media influences affect behavior.
6. Support health-enhancing behavior.
7. Provide adequate time for students to gain knowledge and skills.
8. Train teachers to effectively convey the material.

Health education programs have the opportunity to provide students with practice in negotiating the health-care system. Specific instruction might include such activities as roleplaying to become familiar with the many different interactions that occur between the health-care provider and the patient (Purtilo and Haddad, 1996). Arguably the most effective means to improve health literacy is to ensure that education about health is a part of the curriculum at all levels of education. Schools and colleges could incorporate health literacy education into a range of exiting programs and services such as health services, health education, food services, physical education, and counseling, psychological, and social services (Kolbe, 1986).

Strategies for Health Literacy Instruction

With the increasing pressure on schools today to include more and more academic content, educators are justifiably reluctant to add one more content area to their already overflowing plates. However, health literacy instruction can be embedded into existing science and health education, and even mathematics and social studies, as well as literacy instruction for children and adults.

There is a sound justification for embedding health literacy instruction into existing literacy instruction for children and adults. Educational research for at least the last few decades has documented the impact of context and content on learning, retention, and transfer. This research has shown that learners retain and apply information best in contexts similar to those in which they learned it (Bereiter, 1997; Mayer and Wittrock, 1996; Perkins, 1992).

Literacy practitioners and scholars have taken these findings and applied them to the vexing problem of why literacy skills learned in school are often not applied to literacy tasks in life. One obvious implication of this research is that reading and writing skills must be learned in the context of texts and literacy purposes that readers will encounter out in the world. Therefore, one needs to teach reading skills in those contexts. Health texts and purposes for reading them make up one of those real-life literacy domains. A survey conducted by Bayer and the National Science Teachers Association (Bayer Corporation and the National Association of Science Teachers, 1999) indicated that 98 percent of science teachers surveyed believe that direct interaction within classroom with health professionals was important. These findings suggest that the participation of health-care professionals in school health education programs would improve the health literacy of pre-college students.

Embedding health literacy instruction can be done with the two types of literacy instruction needed to improve health literacy: basic print literacy instruction and literacy instruction in text types common to the field of health literacy. This latter type of instruction introduces the idea of teaching functional print literacy based on using and understanding real-life text types. Several studies, funded by the National Science Foundation and the Interagency Educational Research Initiative, have examined the outcomes of introducing more expository texts[2] into primary-grade instruction during years typically devoted to basic literacy learning. One study looked at the effect on basic literacy growth of adding non-narrative texts to the typical mix of stories used by first- and second-grade teachers (Duke, 2000). Results indicate that students whose teachers diversified their materials learned as much as those who did not, confirming that this approach was not detrimental to the development of beginning reading skill and writing abilities.

A longitudinal study, termed the TEXT study (Purcell-Gates and Duke, 2000), has shown that children as young as second and third graders can grow in their abilities to read and to write two types of texts often found in the health field: science informational texts and science procedural texts. Since individual unfamiliarity with different text types often used to convey health information is a health literacy challenge, this study is important in that it is the only one to date that addresses the teaching of text types specifically, and, in this case, the teaching of health literacy-significant text types. For this study, second- and third-grade teachers were randomly assigned to one of two conditions: (a) The Authentic Only condition, where teachers had their students reading science informational and science proce-

---

[2]Expository texts are statements or rhetorical discourse intended to give information about or an explanation of difficult material.

dural texts that were constructed similar to those found in the real world for real-world purposes of learning new science information or for actually conducting experimental procedures. They also wrote science informational texts and science procedural texts for real-world purposes of providing readers with information of providing written procedures that allow readers to conduct scientific investigations. (b) The Authentic-plus-Explicit conditions added explicit teaching of language features associated with each text type to the authentic reading and writing just described for condition (a). Examples of language features include (for science informational texts) generic nouns (*whales* rather than *Willy the Whale*) and timeless verbs (*whales eat* rather than *Willy the Whale ate*) and (for science procedural texts) a materials section before the ordered steps that are usually numbered.

Analysis of the TEXT data indicates that the children in both conditions grew significantly in their abilities to read and write these science-related text types. Although no significant differences were found due to explicit teaching of the language features, their reading comprehension and writing ability of these two types of texts were significantly related to how authentic the reading and writing assignments were in each class. All of the students learned the features of these two text types commonly employed in the health field, and those students whose teachers used more 'authentic' texts and purposes for reading and writing them learned them to a greater degree. The fact that this can occur at such an early age implies that one does not need to wait until middle or high school to begin teaching about the different text types so commonly used to convey health information. This study was funded by the National Science Foundation and the Interagency Education Research Initiative.

Several studies funded by the National Science Foundation and the Interagency Educational Research Initiative have examined the outcomes of introducing more expository texts into primary-grade instruction during years typically devoted to basic literacy learning. A study by Duke (2000) looked at the effect on basic literacy growth of adding non-narrative texts to the typical mix of stories used by first- and second-grade teachers. Results are showing that students whose teachers utilized different types of texts in the lessons grew as much as those who did not, confirming that children this young could read and learn from non-narrative texts and that this approach was not detrimental to the development of beginning reading skill and writing abilities.

Assessment of Health Literacy in Educational Settings

It is possible to evaluate basic literacy and functional print literacy, and it is important to be clear when conceptualizing and building valid assessments. Effective recommendations depend on clear, accurate assessments. But much work remains to be done on the specific and targeted issue of health literacy assessment in educational settings.

Educational assessments generally include formative and summative components. Formative assessments are constructed so that test results can directly inform and shape ongoing instruction. They should provide feedback to teachers and to school systems regarding how well the instruction meets the learning needs of their students. The major effort of assessment should be devoted to informed formative assessment.

Summative assessments are a part of instructional contexts, and serve primarily to rate, or grade, the student on how well they learned what was taught. Within the health literacy context, summative assessments can be used to make judgments about individual persons regarding their "level" of health literacy.

Health literacy programs in schools and colleges can be designed to accomplish four distinct, but overlapping and interdependent, types of goals (Kolbe, 2002). First, such programs can be designed to improve health literacy; that is, improve important health knowledge, attitudes, and skills. The Council of Chief State School Officers (which represents the nation's state school superintendents) established a State Collaborative on Assessment and Student Standards (SCASS) to assess student achievement in several context areas. To assess health literacy, SCASS created an Assessment Framework Matrix (Council of Chief State School Officers and State Collaborative on Assessment and Student Standards, 1998) that was used to develop test items within nine content areas[3] and six core concepts and skills[4] that reflect the NHES for elementary, middle, and high school students (Joint Committee on National Health Education Standards, 1995). The major purpose of the SCASS Health Education Assessment Project is to improve health literacy by guiding improvements in school health education planning and delivery (Pateman, 2003).

Examples of Current Approaches

Several state organizations have developed programs to address health literacy education in kindergarten through high school. Many examples of programs are detailed in the *State Official's Guide to Health Literacy*

---

[3]These nine content areas are: alcohol and other drugs, injury prevention, nutrition, physical activity, sexual health, tobacco, mental health, personal and consumer health, and community and environmental health.

[4]These six core concepts and skills are: accessing information, self-management, internal and external influences, interpersonal communication, decision-making/goalsetting, and advocacy.

(Matthews and Sewell, 2002). For example, the state of California has developed a tool to aid health education curriculum development at the local level and to promote collaborations between schools, parents, and the community, called "Health Framework for California's Public Schools, Kindergarten through Grade Twelve" and the State of Alaska produced "Healthy Reading Kits" for grades 2 through 8 (Matthews and Sewell, 2002). The state of New Jersey has implemented core curriculum content standards for comprehensive health and physical education programs which include health literacy. The goal of the standards is to develop citizens who are both health-literate and physically educated. The standards for comprehensive health and physical education emphasize six primary areas (Morse, 2002):

- Behaviors that cause intentional and unintentional injuries
- Drug and alcohol use
- Tobacco use
- Sexual behaviors that lead to sexually transmitted diseases, including HIV infection, and unintended pregnancy
- Inadequate physical activity
- Dietary patterns that cause disease

Federal programs to address health literacy include the "*Media Smart Youth*" program developed by the National Institute of Child Health and Human Development (NICHD), and associated with Centers for Disease Control youth media "VERB" campaign (CDC, 2002). With support from the Academy for Educational Development (Academy for Educational Development, 2002), NICHD has developed this youth health and fitness media literacy campaign, which has the potential to enhance 9- to 13-year-old after-school programs' curriculums in health literacy. Another example of federal activity in health literacy is the Curriculum Linking Science Education and Health Literacy program, funded by the National Center for Research Resources. The goal of this project was to transform the food experiences of inner-city children, teachers and parents, and caregivers into an inquiry-based science program. Barton and colleagues (2001) reported that mothers who spend time engaged in science activities with their children are more likely to have a more personal, dynamic, and inquiry-based view of science; whether this also affects parent's or children's health literacy is unclear.

The private sector has also developed approaches which may improve health literacy in youth. Inflexxion® Incorporated has developed "*Special Report*" (Inflexicon, 2001), a curriculum-based tobacco education program for middle and junior high school students, supported by the National Cancer Institute small business innovative research program. The short program includes an interactive game, animation, and audio; a section on media literacy helps students analyze tobacco advertisements; and a skill-building module includes video of situations in which actors are presented with tobacco and peer stories from older youths who have used or avoided tobacco. The effectiveness of this program is being examined in a controlled clinical trial of 270 children from 12 schools throughout the Massachusetts region representing diverse urban, suburban, and rural populations as well as socioeconomic, racial, and cultural backgrounds. Inflexxion® hopes to distribute this program to schools, community organizations associated with tobacco control, and pediatric practices.

THE ADULT EDUCATION SYSTEM[5]

Individuals were asked to provide information on their use of adult education programs to improve reading, writing, math, or English language skills in the 1992 National Adult Literacy Survey (NALS). Nearly half (46.8 percent) of those who reported using English language instruction took either a basic skills or English language adult education course. In addition, 11.3 percent of high school dropouts and 13.3 percent of high school graduates with NALS Levels 1 or 2 skills reported participation in basic skills classes. This suggests that adult education is an important resource, and may be particularly important to individuals with limited literacy or limited English proficiency.

The Context of the Adult Education System

A major source of support for American adult education programs in literacy is the U.S. adult basic education and literacy (ABEL) system. ABEL, founded through the 1998 Workforce Investment Act,[6] receives $500 million in federal funds and $800 million in state funds annually. ABEL programs provide classes in topics that support health literacy including basic literacy and math skills, English language, and high school equivalence.

ABEL is administered by state agencies, usually education, labor, or employment departments, which in turn fund local service programs. Some ABEL programs also receive local governments or private support. ABEL administration, research, and information activities are carried out by the U.S. Department of Education's Office of Vocational and Adult Education,

---

[5]The committee thanks John Comings, Ed.D., for his contributions to this section of the report.

[6]Workforce Investment Act of 1998. P.L. 105-220, 1998 H.R. 1385, enacted on August 7, 1998, 112 Stat 936. Codified as: Section 504 of the Rehabilitation Act, 29 U.S.C. § 794d.

the National Institute for Literacy, and the National Center for the Study of Adult Learning and Literacy (NCSALL). Thus, ABEL represents a collaborative activity that spans government, private, and volunteer activities at the federal, state, and community levels, which could have a large effect on health literacy.

In fiscal year 1998, the ABEL system provided English language services to approximately 2 million adults, high school equivalence preparation services to 800,000 adults, and basic skills services to 1,300,000 adults (U.S. Department of Education, 1999). Each year, between 3 million and 4 million adults spend some time in an ABEL program. Though the mean hours of participation is only 72, a significant percentage of students drop out within the first 30 hours, and so more than half of the students are receiving at least 100 hours of instruction. Most of these adults are in the primary target population of health literacy programs. ABEL programs are, therefore, an effective venue for health literacy activities. However, the potential demand for these services was much greater and may be affected by the fact that the ABEL system has limited resources for one-time developmental costs that produce curriculum, materials, and teacher training designs. These efforts, and effective adult education programs to improve health literacy, could be made available to more people through a cooperative effort between the health system and the ABEL system to undertake a research and development agenda that would lead to educational programs that served the needs of health literacy and the needs of English language and basic skills instruction.

Strategies and Opportunities in the Adult Education System

Adult education theory maintains that people prefer and want information that is relevant to their current situation, and they tend to learn better when the environment is open and encouraging (or facilitative) rather than narrow and passive (or restrictive) (Knowles, 1980). The complexities of the health-care system today require that information be constructed and delivered with consideration for literacy and culture, and cast within a problem-solving or behavioral context (the "how-to" approach). This how-to approach should be geared to the behavioral information needed to act. While general facts about cancer, nutrition, or care-giving are helpful, unless the health information is cast within a problem-solving context, it is often lost. In many print and oral instructions, the reader does not encounter the behavior information early enough. Most people need to have advice that makes sense to them and is logical from their own perspective (Doak et al., 1996). For example, instructions provided to an elderly man with diabetes on the importance of foot care would be more effective if the information is presented within the context of how to achieve the necessary care.

Green and Kreuter (1999) reported that simple acquisition of knowledge does not necessarily produce change: there may be motivational and informational gaps. In other words, "getting the message out" does not mean that people will act on the information. There is a need for better understanding of how people learn, as well as what factors influence information-seeking and how literacy contributes to health behaviors. Theories of learning and health education principles can offer explanations for health behaviors and actions and can point to promising ways to create meaningful messages (Meade, 2001). Learning theories can aid in recognizing the mechanisms whereby knowledge, attitudes, and behaviors can be potentially modified and adopted (Bandura, 1977; Becker, 1974; Becker et al., 1977; Bigge, 1997; Hochbaum, 1958; Pender, 1996; Rosenstock, 1966). Freire (1973) suggests that knowledge about health issues can be gained through participatory methods. This approach, called problem-solving education, encourages learners to be critical thinkers about health issues: the process encourages ongoing learner participation and input. This perspective of involving consumers in the educational process is consistent with literacy solutions that value the voice of the people.

Incorporating Health Content into Adult Education Programs

Most classes for adults studying for their high school equivalence are narrowly focused on the requirements of the GED test or other certification system. However, health content has always been part of basic skills and English language services. About 10 years ago, a number of professionals in the field became interested in expanding health content in the ABEL curriculum. This interest arose out of a need to find content that was compelling for adults so as to increase their motivation to practice the language, literacy, and math skills learned in class, and health is a topic of high interest to almost all students. Initial efforts focused on specific diseases, such as breast cancer, and traditional school health topics, such as nutrition. Work by NCSALL has expanded this focus to include the issues of access, navigation, prevention, screening, and chronic disease management (Rudd, 2002).

Adult literacy researchers have begun to empirically examine the effects of using authentic (real-life) materials and activities for teaching adults to read and write. For example, Howard-Pitney et al. (1997) tested the effect of dietary intervention for low-literacy, low-income adults and found an increase in nutrition knowledge. A federally funded study, using a nationwide sample of adult literacy classes and students, found that students whose teachers incorporated texts for real-life purposes (like reading newspapers to learn the news rather than underline the verbs) began to read and write more often in their lives and to read and write more complex texts

(Purcell-Gates et al., 2000, 2002)[7] In contrast to these findings, Murphy et al. (1996) reported no significant change in nutrition knowledge or self-reported consumption behaviors.

These findings are beginning to be incorporated into adult literacy teaching. For example, a handbook has been published for teachers who wish to begin to use more real-life texts and literacy activities while still teaching their students the skills of reading and writing (Jacobson et al., 2003). Teachers are encouraged to identify the types of life activities their students engage in that require more advanced reading skills. The domain of health and health maintenance is one obvious topic.

Within this type of instruction, teachers obtain typical health-related texts like prescription labels, consent forms, health history forms, and health-related Internet sites and construct lessons in which students learn not only how to decode and comprehend health-specific words but also what information is being conveyed by different texts and why it is important. The students are taught measurement terms, commonly used abbreviations, how to keep track of vaccinations and medications, and so on. Reports from existing programs for adult health literacy instruction have been positive (Doak et al., 1996). Building on students' present needs and experiences may add to already existing programs to bring more relevancy and meaning to the instruction (Perkins, 1992; Purcell-Gates et al., 2000). Findings from national surveys indicate that both state directors of adult education programs and adult education teachers are interested in and supportive of an integration of literacy skill development and health-related tasks and content (Rudd and Moeykens, 1999; Rudd et al., 1999).

Finding 5-2 Opportunities for measuring literacy skill levels required for health knowledge and skills, and for the implementation of programs to increase learner's skill levels, currently exist in adult education programs and provide promising models for expanding programs. Studies indicate a desire on the part of adult learners and adult education programs to form partnerships with health communities.

EDUCATION FOR HEALTH PROFESSIONALS

There are many demands for time and space in the curricula of health professional schools, including schools of medicine, dentistry, pharmacy, nursing, and public health. Further, continuing education efforts compete with thousands of topics for the attention of busy health-care providers. Regardless, improved education in health literacy is critical to the develop-

---

[7]The reading and writing of more complex texts is associated with higher levels of literacy as defined by the NALS assessment.

ment of competent physicians and other health-care providers who can help to improve health literacy and to limit the negative effects of limited health literacy among patients. Furthermore, research should investigate whether increased health literacy skills in care providers such as medical assistants, home health-care workers, and home health aides could contribute to improved health-care quality and reduced medical errors. Approaches to education for health professionals should include both curricular and continuing education to reach the greatest number of providers at all stages of career development. The approaches described below may provide a starting point for increased integration of health literacy concepts and skills into professional and continuing education programs. Further information on the relationship of health literacy to health-care quality for all categories of providers could help to develop future directions for such integration.

Curricular Approaches

Few official requirements or curricula address health literacy in schools of medicine, public health, nursing, dentistry, or pharmacy. Health literacy issues may be addressed under topics such as patient communication, but they are generally not systematically included in these topics. Plomer and colleagues (2001) reported on the development and implementation phases of a project to improve medical students' communication with limited literacy patients by incorporating literacy content into the medical student curriculum. In this study, the use of standardized patient cases regarding cancer screening was implemented and results revealed that group discussion about literacy was prompted.

There are a few examples of courses or curriculums that should be noted. In 1995, the Harvard School of Public Health initiated an ongoing graduate course for students in public health that focused on health literacy studies, research, theories, and implications (NCSALL, 2001). In addition, the Harvard School of Public Health provides a web site (http://www.hsph. harvard.edu/healthliteracy) about health literacy for researchers and practitioners that includes a video slide show, curriculums, literature reviews, annotated bibliographies, and policy initiatives. Another curricular approach took place at the University of Colorado Medical School in Denver where a course on health literacy for medical students was developed and taught during 2000 as part of a grant. This was a temporary initiative however, and was not made a permanent part of the curriculum.

A more formal approach has been instituted at the University of Virginia School of Medicine (Dalton, 2003). This curriculum includes an introductory lecture for first-year medical students, departments, residents, and external institutions that request a presentation on health literacy. A faculty development handbook is given to all faculty teaching courses in the first and second year, which provides background information and a list of available health literacy materials. Health literacy concepts are also integrated into other courses in the medical school curriculum; for example, patient case studies are presented in the second-year "Clinical Problems" course in which patients experience barriers related to communication misunderstandings and language issues. Also in the second year, the required community preceptorship includes a health literacy component. A fourth-year elective focusing on health literacy issues and including a service component is currently in development and will likely be offered in the spring of 2004. The University of Virginia (UVA) School of Medicine also provides a web interface to help other institutions develop health literacy curricula. It is made up of three main groups of information which can be individually tailored to the needs of an institution: (1) an outline on how UVA established its curriculum, with reference materials that include a faculty development handbook and examples of written cases used at various points of the curriculum; (2) an introductory health literacy lecture, examples of illustrations, and a bibliography and resources list; (3) standardized patient cases that illustrate work with patients with limited literacy, that also show how to work with interpreters for the deaf and for non-English-speaking patients; some of these case studies also integrate cultural competency issues.

Continuing Education Approaches

Most health literacy training for health professionals is done under continuing education umbrellas. Continuing medical education (CME) consists of those educational activities that serve to increase knowledge, skills, and performance of health professionals. They often are intended to update health professionals on new techniques as well as to expose them to new ideas and concepts relevant to their daily practice (ACCME, 2002). The Accreditation Council for Continuing Medical Education (ACCME) reports that over 45,000 directly sponsored CME courses were offered in 2002 to both physician and nonphysician participants (ACCME, 2003).

The Coalition for Allied Health Leadership (CAHL) formed a health literacy team during their 2003 meeting to assess health literacy practices of allied health professionals at the national level. The CAHL team developed a survey to assess further the current level of awareness of the allied health community and to develop materials to help the allied health community better meet their needs. The survey was electronically sent to members of the Health Professions Network and the National Network of Health Career Programs in Two Year Colleges. Approximately one-third of the respondents were unaware of the issues surrounding health literacy, or unaware of its impact on patient care. In addition, the same percentage also reported a lack of any institutional policy within their organization addressing health literacy or no assessment of the effectiveness of existing policies (Brown et al., in press).

The American Medical Association (AMA) has developed several programs in professional continuing education in health literacy since adopting a policy in 1998 that recognized that limited patient literacy affects medical diagnosis and treatment. The AMA and the AMA Foundation have since raised awareness and shared best practices about health literacy. In 2003, the AMA Foundation, American Public Health Association, the National Council on the Aging, and other public health organizations formed the Partnership for Clear Health Communication, a coalition to increase awareness of health literacy and its impact on the nation's health, and introduced a solution-oriented program that includes the "Ask Me 3" program that promotes communication between health-care providers and patients (AMA, 2003b; Ask Me 3, 2003). In conjunction with California Literacy, Inc., and the California Medical Association (CMA), the AMA and AMA Foundation developed the California Statewide Health Initiative that promotes provider–patient communication as a basis for patient understanding (AMA, 2003a). The AMA Foundation, with support from Pfizer, Inc., also links organizations across the country through Health Literacy Coalition, and provides grants to health literacy community service projects.

The AMA Foundation has developed and distributed educational kits to physicians and health-care professionals. This program, *"Health Literacy, Let Your Patients Understand,"* includes a CD-ROM for use by providers in a continuing education curriculum. The 2003 Health Literacy Educational Kit is the Foundation's primary tool for informing physicians, health-care professionals, and patient advocates about health literacy. The 2003 Health Literacy Educational Kit is an expanded version of the kit introduced in 2001. Included are a manual for clinicians, a new video documentary, reprintable information, guidelines for continuing medical education credit, and additional resources for education and involvement. The AMA Foundation provides these kits free to AMA Alliance chapters and state, county, and specialty medical societies that make a formal commitment to launch health literacy educational programs of their own, and to that end provide an extensive "train the trainer" program with a faculty guide to the clinician workshop and guidelines for local implementation planning.

Finding 5-3 Health professionals and staff have limited education, training, continuing education, and practice opportunities to develop skills for improving health literacy.

Finding 5-1 Significant obstacles and barriers to successful health-literacy education exist in K-12 education programs.

Finding 5-2 Opportunities for measuring literacy skill levels required for health knowledge and skills, and for the implementation of programs to increase learner's skill levels, currently exist in adult education programs and provide promising models for expanding programs. Studies indicate a desire on the part of adult learners and adult education programs to form partnerships with health communities.

Finding 5-3 Health professionals and staff have limited education, training, continuing education, and practice opportunities to develop skills for improving health literacy.

Recommendation 5-1 Accreditation requirements for all public and private educational institutions should require the implementation of the NHES.

Recommendation 5-2 Educators should take advantage of the opportunity provided by existing reading, writing, oral language skills, and mathematics curriculums to incorporate health-related tasks, materials, and examples into existing lesson plans.

Recommendation 5-3 HRSA and CDC, in collaboration with the Department of Education, should fund demonstration projects in each state to attain the NHES and to meet basic literacy requirements as they apply to health literacy.

Recommendation 5-4 The Department of Education in association with HHS should convene task forces comprised of appropriate education, health, and public policy experts to delineate specific, feasible, and effective actions relevant agencies could take to improve health literacy through the nation's K-12 schools, 2-year and 4-year colleges and universities, and adult and vocational education.

Recommendation 5-5 The National Science Foundation, the Department of Education, and the NICHD should fund research designed to assess the effectiveness of different models of combining health literacy with basic literacy and instruction. The Interagency Education Research Initiative, a federal partnership of these three agencies, should lead this effort to the fullest extent possible.

Recommendation 5-6 Professional schools and professional continuing education programs in health and related fields, including medicine, dentistry, pharmacy, social work, anthropology, nursing, public health, and journalism, should incorporate health literacy into their curricula and areas of competence.

REFERENCES

Academy for Educational Development. 2002. *AED@work—Media Smart Youth Program.* [Online]. Available: http://www.aed.org/about/atWork/mediasmartyouth.html [accessed: September, 2003].

ACCME (Accreditation Council for Continuing Medical Education). 2002. *Definition of CME.* [Online]. Available: http://www.accme.org/incoming/pol_05_def_cme.pdf [accessed: October, 2003].

ACCME. 2003. *ACCME Annual Report Data 2002.* [Online]. Available: http://www.accme. org/incoming/156_2002_Annual_Report_Data.pdf [accessed: October, 2003].

AMA (American Medical Association). 2003a. *Health Literacy Top Concern of CMA/AMA.* [Online]. Available: http://www.ama-assn.org/ama/pub/article/2403-7454.html [accessed: October, 2003].

AMA. May 1, 2003b. *AMA Foundation Teams Up to Help Fight Low Health Literacy.* [Online]. Available: http://www.ama-assn.org/ama/pub/article/2403-7627.html [accessed: October, 2003].

American Association for the Advancement of Science. 1993. *Benchmarks for Science Literacy.* Washington, DC: American Association for the Advancement of Science.

Ask Me 3. 2003. *Good Guestions for Your Health.* [Online]. Available: http://www.askme3. org/ [accessed: October, 2003].

Association of American Colleges and Universities. 2002. *Summary of the 2001 Summer Symposium of the Program for Health and Higher Education.* College Students As a Challenge and Opportunity for Public Health. Occasional Paper 1. Washington, DC: Association of American Colleges and Universities.

Bandura A. 1977. *Social Learning Theory.* Englewood Cliffs, NJ: Prentice-Hall.

Barton AC, Hindin TJ, Contendo IR, Trudeau M, Yang K, Hagiwara S, Koch PD. 2001. Underprivelaged urban mothers' perspectives on science. *Journal of Research in Science Teaching.* 38(6): 688–711.

Bayer Corporation and the National Association of Science Teachers. 1999. *Nation's Science Teachers Register Concern over U.S. Science Education in New Survey.* [Online]. Available: http://www.bayerus.com/msms/news/pages/factsofscience/survey99.html [accessed: August, 2003].

Becker MH. 1974. *The Health Belief Model and Personal Health Behavior.* Thorofare, NJ: Charles B. Slack.

Becker MH, Maiman LA, Kirscht JP, Haefner DP, Drachman RH. 1977. The Health Belief Model and prediction of dietary compliance: A field experiment. *Journal of Health and Social Behavior.* 18(4): 348–366.

Bereiter C. 1997. Situated cognition and how to overcome it. In: *Situated Cognition: Social, Semiotic and Psychological Perspectives.* Kirschner D, Whitsun JA, Editors. Mahwah, NJ: Erlbaum.

Bigge ML. 1997. *Learning Theories for Teachers.* 5th edition. Reading, MA: Addison-Wesley Educational Publishers.

Brown DR, Ludwig R, Buck GA, Durham D, Shumard T, Graham SS. In press. Health literacy: Universal precautions needed. *Journal of Allied Health.*

Burns W. 1999. *Learning for Our Common Health: How an Academic Focus on HIV/AIDS Will Improve Education and Health.* Washington, DC: Association of American Colleges and Universities.

CCSSO (Council of Chief State School Officers; Society of State Directors of Health, Physical Education, and Recreation; and Association of State and Territorial Health Officials). 2003. *Coordinated School Health Programs Staff: 2002–2003 Directory.* Washington, DC: Council of Chief State School Officers.

CDC (Centers for Disease Control and Prevention). 2002. *Youth Media Campaign: VERB Working Together.* [Online]. Available: http://www.cdc.gov/youthcampaign/working_together/index.htm [accessed: September, 2003].

Collins J, Robin L, Wooley S, Fenley D, Hunt P, Taylor J, Haber D, Kolbe L. 2002. Programs-that-work: CDC's guide to effective programs that reduce health-risk behavior of youth. *Journal of School Health.* 72(3): 93–99.

Collins JL, Small ML, Kann L, Pateman BC, Gold RS, Kolbe LJ. 1995. School health education. *Journal of School Health.* 65(8): 302–311.

Council of Chief State School Officers and State Collaborative on Assessment and Student Standards. 1998. *Assessing Health Literacy: Assessment Framework.* Santa Cruz, CA: Toucan Education.

Dalton, C (University of Virginia Health System). 2003. *Building a Health Literacy Curriculum.* [Online]. Available: http://www.healthsystem.virginia.edu/internet/som-hlc/home.cfm [accessed: December, 2003].

Doak LG, Doak CC, Meade CD. 1996. Strategies to improve cancer education materials. *Oncology Nursing Forum.* 23(8): 1305–1312.

Douglas KA, Collins JL, Warren C, Kann L, Gold R, Clayton S, Ross JG, Kolbe LJ. 1997. Results from the 1995 National College Health Risk Behavior Survey. *Journal of American College Health.* 46(2): 55–66.

Duke NK. 2000. 3.6 minutes a day: The scarcity of informational texts in first grade. *Reading Research Quarterly.* 35: 202–224.

Freire P. 1973. *Education for Critical Consciousness.* New York: Seabury Press.

The Gallup Organization. 1994. *Values and Opinions of Comprehensive School Health Education in U.S. Public Schools: Adolescents, Parents, and School District Administrators.* Atlanta, GA: American Cancer Society.

Green LW, Kreuter MW. 1999. *Health Promotion Planning: An Educational and Ecological Approach.* 3rd edition. Mountain View, CA: Mayfield.

Grunbaum JA, Kann L, Kinchen SA, Williams B, Ross JG, Lowry R, Kolbe L. 2002. Youth risk behavior surveillance—United States, 2001. *Journal of School Health.* 72(8): 313–328.

Hausman AJ, Ruzek SB. 1995. Implementation of comprehensive school health education in elementary schools: Focus on teacher concerns. *Journal of School Health.* 65(3): 81–86.

HHS (U.S. Department of Health and Human Services). 2000. *Healthy People 2010: Understanding and Improving Health.* Washington, DC: U.S. Department of Health and Human Services. [Online]. Available: http://www.health.gov/healthypeople [accessed: January 15, 2003].

Hochbaum GM. 1958. *Public Participation in Medical Screening Programs: A Sociopsychologiocal Study.* Public Health Service Publication No. 572. Washington, DC: Government Printing Office.

Howard-Pitney B, Winkleby MA, Albright CL, Bruce B, Fortmann SP. 1997. The Stanford Nutrition Action Program: A dietary fat intervention for low-literacy adults. *American Journal of Public Health.* 87(12): 1971–1976.

Inflexicon. 2001. *Inflexicon Products: Special Report.* [Online]. Available: http://www.inflexxion.com/inf/products/prod_special.html [accessed: September, 2003].

IOM (Institute of Medicine). 1997. *Schools and Health: Our Nations Investment.* Allensworth D, Lawson E, Nicholson L, Wyche J, Editors. Washington, DC: National Academy Press.

Jacobson E, Degener S, Purcell-Gates V. 2003. *Creating Authentic Materials for the Adult Literacy Classroom: A Handbook for Practitioners.* Cambridge, MA: World Education Inc.

Joint Committee on National Health Education Standards. 1995. *National Health Education Standards: Achieving Health Literacy*. Atlanta, GA: American Cancer Society.

Kann L, Warren CW, Harris WA, Collins JL, Williams BI, Ross JG, Kolbe LJ. 1996. Youth risk behavior surveillance—United States, 1995. *Journal of School Health*. 66(10): 365–377.

Kann L, Brener ND, Allensworth DD. 2001. Health education: Results from the School Health Policies and Programs Study 2000. *Journal of School Health*. 71(7): 266–278.

Keeling R. 2001. *Briefing Paper: College Students As a Challenge and an Opportunity for Public Health*. Washington, DC: Association of American Colleges and Universities.

Knowles MS. 1980. *The Modern Practice of Adult Education: From Pedagogy to Andragogy*. Chicago, IL: Association Press/Follet.

Kolbe L, Jones J, Birdthistle I, Whitman C. 2001. Building the capacity of schools to improve health. In: *Critical Issues in Global Health*. Koop CE, Pearson C, Schwarz M, Editors. San Francisco, CA: Jossey-Bass.

Kolbe LJ. 1986. Increasing the impact of school health promotion programs: Emerging research perspectives. *Health Education*. 17(5): 47–52.

Kolbe LJ. 2002. Education reform and the goals of modern school health programs. *The State Education Standard*. 3(4): 4–11.

Kolbe LJ, Collins J, Cortese P. 1997. Building the capacity of schools to improve the health of the nation. A call for assistance from psychologists. *American Psychologist*. 52(3): 256–265.

Lohrmann DK, Wooley SF. 1998. Comprehensive school health education. In: *A Guide to Coordinated School Health Programs*. Marx E, Wooley SF, Northrop D, Editors. New York: Teachers College Press. Pp. 43–66.

Marx E, Wooley S, Northrup D. 1998. *Health Is Academic: A Guide to Coordinated School Health Programs*. New York: Teachers College Press.

Marzano R, Kendall J, Cicchinelli L. 1998. *What Americans Believe Students Should Know: A Survey of U.S. Adults*. Washington, DC: U.S. Department of Education, Office of Educational Research and Improvement.

Matthews TL, Sewell JC. 2002. *State Official's Guide to Health Literacy*. Lexington, KY: The Council of State Governments.

Mayer RE, Wittrock MC. 1996. Problem-solving transfer. In: *Handbook of Educational Psychology*. Berliner DD, Calfee RC, Editors. New York: Macmillan.

McCall D, Beazley R, Doherty-Poirier M, Lovato C, MacKinnon D, Otis J, Shannon M. 1999. *Schools, Public Health, Sexuality and HIV: A Status Report*. Toronto: Council of Ministers of Education, Canada.

Meade CD. 2001. Community health education. In: *Community Health Nursing: Promoting the Health of Aggregates*. 3rd edition. Nies M, McEwen M, Editors. Philadelphia: W.B. Saunders Co.

Morse L. 2002. *Improving Health Literacy: An Educational Response to a Public Health Problem*. Presentation given at a workshop of the Institute of Medicine Committee on Health Literacy. December 11, 2002, Washington, DC.

Murphy PW, Davis TC, Mayeaux EJ, Sentell T, Arnold C, Rebouche C. 1996. Teaching nutrition education in adult learning centers: Linking literacy, health care, and the community. *Journal of Community Health Nursing*. 13(3): 149–158.

National Reading Panel. 2000. *Teaching Children to Read: An Evidence-Based Assessment of the Scientific Research Literature on Reading and Its Implications for Reading Instruction*. Bethesda, MD: National Institute of Child Health and Human Development.

NCSALL. 2001. *Health Literacy Curricula*. [Online]. Available: http://www.hsph.harvard.edu/healthliteracy/curricula.html [accessed: September 26, 2003].

NRC (National Research Council). 1996. *National Science Education Standards.* Washington, DC: National Academy Press.

NRC. 1998. *Preventing Reading Difficulties in Young Children.* Snow CE, Burns MS, Griffen P, Editors. Washington, DC: National Academy Press.

NRC. 1999. *Designing Mathematics or Science Curriculum Programs. A Guide for Using Mathematics and Science Education Standards.* Washington, DC: National Academy Press.

Pateman B. 2002. A sharper image for school health education: Hawaii's "seven by seven" curriculum focus. *Journal of School Health.* 72(9): 381–384.

Pateman B. 2003. Healthier students, better learners. *Educational Leadership.* 61(4).

Pateman B, Grunbaum JA, Kann L. 1999. Voices from the field—A qualitative analysis of classroom, school, district, and state health education policies and programs. *Journal of School Health.* 69(7): 258–263.

Patrick K, Grace TW, Lovato CY. 1992. Health issues for college students. *Annual Review of Public Health.* 13: 253–268.

Patterson S, Cinelli B, Sankaran G, Brey R, Nye R. 1996. Health instruction responsibilities for elementary classroom teachers in Pennsylvania. *Journal of School Health.* 66(1): 13–17.

Pender NJ. 1996. *Health Promotion in Nursing Practice.* 3rd edition. Stamford, CA: Appleton and Lange.

Perkins DN. 1992. *Smart Schools: From Training Memories to Educating Minds.* New York: Free Press/Macmillan.

Peterson FL, Cooper RJ, Laird JM. 2001. Enhancing teacher health literacy in school health promotion: A vision for the new millennium. *Journal of School Health.* 71(4): 138–144.

Plomer K, Schneider L, Barley G, Cifuentes M, Dignan M. 2001. Improving medical students' communication with limited-literacy patients: Project development and implementation. *Journal of Cancer Education.* 16(2): 68–71.

Purcell-Gates V, Duke NK. 2000. *Explicit Explanation of Genre Within Authentic Literacy Activities in Science: Does it Facilitate Development and Achievement? Grant Proposal funded by NSF/IERI.* Grant Proposal funded by NSF/IERI.

Purcell-Gates V, Degener S, Jacobson E, Soler M. 2000. Affecting Change in Literacy Practices of Adult Learners: Impact of Two Dimensions of Instruction. NCSALL Report No. 17. Boston, MA: National Center for the Study of Adult Learning and Literacy.

Purcell-Gates V, Degener S, Jacobson E, Soler M. 2002. Impact of authentic literacy instruction on adult literacy practices. *Reading Research Quarterly.* 37: 70–92.

Purtilo R, Haddad A. 1996. *Health Professional and Patient Interaction.* 5th edition. Philadelphia, PA: W.B. Saunders Co.

Rosenstock IM. 1966. Why people use health services. *Milbank Memorial Fund Quarterly.* 44(Supplement 3): 94–127.

Rudd RE. 2002. A maturing partnership. *Focus on Basics: Connecting Research and Practice.* 5(3).

Rudd RE, Moeykens BA. 1999. *Adult educators' perceptions of health issues and topics in adult basic education.* NCSALL Report #8. Cambridge, MA: National Center for the Study of Adult Learning and Literacy.

Rudd RE, Zahner L, Banh M. 1999. *Findings from a National Survey of State Directors of Adult Education.* NCSALL Report #9. Cambridge, MA: National Center for the Study of Adult Learning and Literacy.

Smith AM. 1999. *Age of Risk Behavior Debut: Trends and Implications.* Washington, DC: Institute for Youth Development.

St. Leger L. 2001. Schools, health literacy and public health: Possibilities and challenges. *Health Promotion International.* 16(2): 197–205.

Storch P, Grunbaum J, Kann L, Williams B, Kinchen S, Kolbe L. 2003. *School Health Education Profiles: Surveillance for Characteristics of Health Education Among Secondary Schools (Profiles 2000).* Atlanta, GA: Centers for Disease Control and Prevention.

Thackeray R, Neiger BLBH, Hill SC, Barnes MD. 2002. Elementary school teacher's perspectives on health instruction: Implications for health education. *American Journal of Health Education.* 33: 77–82.

Ubbes VA, Cottrell RR, Ausherman JA, Black JM, Wilson P, Gill C, Snider J. 1999. Professional preparation of elementary teachers in Ohio: Status of K-6 health education. *Journal of School Health.* 69(1): 17–21.

U.S. Department of Education, Office of Vocational and Adult Education, Division of Adult Education and Literacy. 1999. *State-Administered Adult Education Program 1998 Enrollment.* [Online]. Available: http://www.ed.gov/offices/OVAE/98enrlbp.html [accessed: December, 2003].

U.S. Department of Education. 2001. *Digest of Education Statistics.* Washington, DC: U.S. Government Printing Office.

WHO (World Health Organization). 1996. *Improving School Health Programs: Barriers and strategies.* Geneva: World Health Organization.

WHO. 1997. *Promoting Health Through Schools: Report of a WHO Expert Committee on Comprehensive School Health Education and Promotion.* Geneva: World Health Organization.

6

Health Systems

Mr. G. is a 64-year-old man with chronic hypertension, diabetes, a high cholesterol level, and gout. He saw his primary care doctor because his left leg was swollen and painful. His doctor diagnosed an early cellulitis and prescribes an antibiotic to be taken for 10 days.

After 4 days, Mr. G. went to the emergency department, unable to walk because of intense pain and swelling of his entire left leg. His blood sugar and blood pressure were both very high, and he was admitted to the hospital to treat his infection and control his blood pressure. During his emergency department treatment and admission, he was examined by, and spoke to, four different doctors.

The fifth doctor to take a history and examine Mr. G discovered that he had taken none of his seven chronic medications, nor the newly prescribed antibiotic given to him when his infection first appeared. Mr. G. explained "You see, I already take 19 pills a day, and when I got another one I got confused about my timing, and I was just so scared I might mess up. My daughter usually helps me with my medicines, but she's been sick and I didn't want to worry her."

THE CONTEXT OF HEALTH SYSTEMS

Navigating the U.S. health-care and public health delivery systems is a complex task with numerous layers of bureaucracy, procedures, and processes. Consequently, an adult's ability or inability to navigate these systems may reflect systemic complexity as well as individual skill levels. Patients, clients, and their family members are typically unfamiliar with these systems and the associated jargon. Even highly educated individuals may find the systems too complicated to understand, especially when people are made more vulnerable by poor health. Official documents, including informed consent forms, social services forms, and public health and medical instructions, as well as health information materials often use jargon and technical language that make them unnecessarily difficult to use (Rudd et al., 2000).

> *When you have medical forms and stuff, I don't think it should be complicated for a person to understand what its saying* (Rudd and DeJong, 2000).

Some of the complexity of the health-care system arises from the nature of health care and public health itself, the mix of public and private financing, and the health information and health-care delivery settings. Unlike many other countries, the United States does not have a single organized national health-care system. Furthermore, the United States has no national health surveillance system, and few common norms exist for basic preventive services such as immunizations. Threats of bioterrorism and new emerging diseases such as SARS continue to complicate the picture of health care.

In the past, health management was primarily the domain of the physician, but greater responsibility for health management has shifted to the patient as health care has evolved and cost pressures on care have increased. This has been called self-management, and was identified in the Institute of Medicine (IOM) *Priority Areas for National Action* report (IOM, 2003b) as one of two cross-cutting issues in improving health-care quality that present the opportunity to improve health across the lifespan, at all stages of health service. In order to make appropriate self-management decisions, health information consumers must locate health information, evaluate the information for credibility and quality, and analyze the risks and benefits, activities that rely on health literacy skills. Consumers must be able to express health concerns clearly by describing symptoms in ways the providers can understand. Both patients and health-care providers must be able to ask pertinent questions and fully understand the available medical information.

Improvement of health literacy was identified by the IOM report as an essential component of self-management that would affect nearly all aspects of health care. The IOM report further noted that system and policy changes to improve self-management would require involvement by most health-care organizations and providers to address all types of health conditions, providing a means to improve health care for all Americans. Figure 6-1 below is a depiction of the "ecology of health service organizations" that form the U.S. health system (Shortell and Kaluzny, 2000). This figure illustrates the complex relationships of organizations and programs that form the basis of the U.S. health-care system that adults are expected to navigate.

The organizations with the most direct impact on patients are in the inner circles and those with a more indirect influence are in the outer circles. Although this complex system could be simplified somewhat by consolidating some of the depicted organizations (such as hospitals and physician groups) into a variety of health networks and health systems, other factors deter such consolidation. For example, tightly integrated managed care systems have failed to grow in response to consumer demands for more choice. Accessing and using the systems effectively is further complicated by the mix of private and public financing mechanisms and interrelationships.

Individuals and families must learn how to interact with employers, supplemental private insurance companies, federal and state government

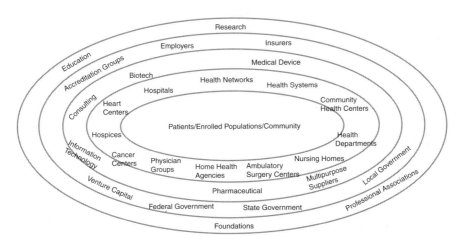

FIGURE 6-1 The concentric ecology of organizations in the health-care sector. SOURCE: Health Care Management: Organization, Design, and Behavior, 4th Edition, by Shortell and Kaluzny. © 2000. Reprinted with permission of Delmar Learning, a division of Thomson Learning: www.thomsonrights.com. Fax 800 730-2215.

programs, and providers who are paid directly, "out-of-pocket." To complicate matters further, individuals seldom interact with only one aspect of the health-care system. They make decisions about the severity of illness, the ease and cost of various treatment options, and move from self-care to seeking advice, from public to private options, and from primary to tertiary care in complex "patterns of resort" (Scrimshaw and Hurtado, 1987). Yet studies indicate that individuals and families lack the information needed for these activities. Chapter 2 provides evidence that health literacy affects the interaction of individuals with components of the health-care system, and may further affect health status and outcomes. Studies suggest that health information is often more difficult to comprehend than other types of information (Root and Stableford, 1999). Extensive research shows that communication of health information through printed material, multimedia, and interpersonal exchange is often not successful (Baker and Wilson, 1996; Berland et al., 2001; Davis et al., 1996; Graber et al., 1999; MacKinnon, 1984; Meade et al., 1989; Meeuwesen et al., 2002; Reid et al., 1995; Roter et al., 2001; Rudd, 2003; Rudd et al., 2000; Smith et al., 1998). Print and interactive materials have been consistently found to be less understandable by their audience than the authors intended (Kerka, 2000; Rudd et al., 2000). Complex materials frequently used by employers, insurance companies, government programs, and providers, such as consent forms and questionnaires, are difficult for many people to use appropriately (Gaba and Grossman, 2003; Hochhauser, 1997; Kaufer et al., 1983; Morales et al., 2001; Osborne and Hochhauser, 1999).

All but the most sophisticated health policy experts have difficulty understanding the many facets of health and health care. Most of us are confused by our hospital and medical bills, the choices we have to make regarding health plans and health coverage, and the often contradictory news accounts about the most effective treatments or preventive strategies. Imagine having to face this complexity if you are one of the 90 million American adults who this committee has found "lack the functional literacy skills in English to use the U.S. health care system."[1]

---

[1]See Finding 3-1: "About 90 million adults, an estimate based on the 1992 National Adult Literacy Survey (NALS), have literacy skills that test below high school level (NALS Levels 1 and 2). Of these, about 40–44 million (NALS Level 1) have difficulty finding information in unfamiliar or complex texts such as newspaper articles, editorials, medicine labels, forms, or charts. Because the medical and public health literature indicates that health materials are complex and often far above high school level, the committee notes that approximately 90 million adults may lack the needed literacy skills to effectively use the U.S. health system. The majority of these adults are native-born English speakers. Literacy levels are lower among the elderly, those who have lower educational levels, those who are poor, minority populations, and groups with limited English proficiency such as recent immigrants."

Finding 6-1 Demands for reading, writing, and numeracy skills are intensified due to health-care systems' complexities, advancements in scientific discoveries, and new technologies. These demands exceed the health literacy skills of most adults in the United States.

Emerging Issues in the Health System Context[2]

In addition to the general complexity of the current system, the committee has identified a number of emerging themes or issues that are important aspects of the health system context with respect to health literacy. These include

- Chronic disease care and self-management
- Patient–provider communication
- Patient safety and health-care quality
- Access to health care and preventive services
- Provider time limitations
- Health expenditures
- Consumer-directed health care

Each of these topics is briefly discussed in the section that follows, with particular attention to the ways in which these issues may function as barriers to those with limited health literacy. Other issues that are currently salient in the health-care context include health disparities and the increasingly complex health information context; these topics are discussed in Chapter 5.

Chronic Disease Care and Self-Management

Chronic disease, and the problem of people having to cope with multiple, comorbid conditions, is a critical issue in health care, particularly as the health-care delivery system becomes more and more complex and patients must become the integrators of their own care. Chronic disease exemplifies the interaction of health literacy and health, as patients' health is often dependent on their ability and willingness to carry out a set of health activities essential to the management and treatment of chronic diseases (IOM, 2002c). The last few decades have seen tremendous advances in the

---

[2]The information in this section is drawn in part from the background paper "Improving Chronic Disease Care for Populations with Limited Health Literacy," commissioned by the committee from Dean Schillinger, M.D. The committee appreciates his contribution. The full text of the paper can be found in Appendix B.

care of chronic conditions, including an array of therapeutic options, risk factor modification for secondary prevention of comorbid conditions, the availability of home monitoring tools, and the growth of disease management programs (Bodenheimer, 1999; McCulloch et al., 2000). Despite these advances, health quality and clinical outcomes of patients with chronic diseases vary significantly across sociodemographic lines (Fiscella et al., 2000; Piette, 1999, 2000; Vinicor et al., 2000).

Care for those with chronic diseases is more difficult for patients, providers, and families when patients cannot understand or remember the given directions, and or when directions that are given are incomplete and unclear (IOM, 2003b). This is also true in other contexts, such as acute care and public health interventions. The collaboration between patients, providers, the system of care, and the community that is required to optimize health outcomes adds a significant layer of complexity to the delivery of health care to individuals with chronic disease. Effective disease management is predicated on systematic, interactive communication between a population of patients with the disease and the providers and health system with whom they interact (Norris et al., 2002a, b; Von Korff et al., 1997), all occurring in the context of a supportive community whose resources are aligned with patients' needs (Wagner, 1995).

Chronic care involves an ongoing process of patient assessments, adjustments to treatment plans, and reassessments to measure change in patient health status. Without timely and reliable information about patients' health status, symptoms, and self-care, the necessary health education, treatments, or behavioral adjustments may come late or not at all, compromising patients' health and increasing the likelihood of poor outcomes. Self-management is essential to successful chronic disease care; patients must remember any self-care instructions they have received from their provider, be able to correctly interpret symptoms or results of self-monitoring, and appropriately problem-solve regarding adjustments to the treatment regimen. Patients also must know when and how to contact the provider should the need arise. A number of studies demonstrate that patients remember and understand as little as half of what they are told by their physicians (Bertakis, 1977; Cole and Bird, 2000; Crane, 1997; Rost and Roter, 1987; Roter, 2000). In addition, because they have knowledge deficits, patients with limited health literacy may be less equipped to overcome such gaps in understanding and memory once they are at home (Williams et al., 1998a, b) and difficulties reading or interpreting instructions (Crane, 1997; Williams et al., 1998b). Cross-sectional studies involving patients with diabetes suggest that traditional self-management education may not eliminate health literacy-related disparities in chronic disease outcomes (Schillinger et al., 2002; Williams et al., 1998b). Focus groups of patients with limited health literacy have identified "health system navigation" (such as knowing whom, for what, and when to call for assistance with a problem) as a particularly daunting aspect of chronic disease management (Baker et al., 1996).

Building on the Chronic Care Model of Wagner et al. (2001), Schillinger has developed a framework that explores ways to improve chronic disease care and is based on health literacy and related research. This framework is discussed in greater detail in Appendix B, but briefly, the model represents the evidence base for chronic disease care and supports the importance of executive leadership and incentives to promote quality, systems to track and monitor patients' progress and support timely provider decision-making (Piette, 2000), patient self-management training (Lorig et al., 1999; Von Korff et al., 1997), and community-oriented care. Since self-management practices and clinical outcomes in chronic disease care appear to vary by patients' level of health literacy (Kalichman and Rompa, 2000; Schillinger et al., 2002; Williams et al., 1998b), the Chronic Care Model, and similar comprehensive, population-based disease management approaches, may offer insights into the ways in which limited health literacy affects chronic disease care and could identify points for potentially successful intervention.

Patient–Provider Communication

To Err Is Human reported that communication failure was the underlying cause of fully 10 percent of adverse drug events (IOM, 2000b). Management of complex drug therapies, especially in elderly patients, is extremely difficult and requires special attention to the ability of the patient to understand and remember the amount and timing of dose, as well as behavioral modifications required by the regimen (e.g., dietary restrictions) (IOM, 2000b). The patient's health literacy level as it affects the communication process is therefore an important consideration in health outcomes.

There is some evidence of a failure of communication with patients with limited health literacy as currently measured. Patients with chronic diseases and limited health literacy have been shown to have poor knowledge of their condition and of its management (Williams et al., 1998a, b), often despite having received standard self-management education. Patients with limited health literacy have greater difficulties accurately reporting their medication regimens and describing the reasons for which their medications were prescribed (Schillinger et al., 2003a; Williams et al., 1995) and more frequently have explanatory models[3] that may interfere with adher-

---

[3]"Explanatory models are the lenses through which cultures perceive and understand illness. They consist of interpretive notions about aspects of illness and treatment including the cause, the timing and mode of onset of the symptoms, the pathophysiological processes involved, the natural history and severity, and the appropriate treatment" (Kleinman, 1980).

ence (Kalichman et al., 1999). Understanding these explanatory models is essential to good communication regarding care (Good and Good, 1981; Kleinman, 1980).

While, by definition, patients with limited health literacy have problems with literacy- and numeracy-related tasks in the health-care setting, a recent study among patients with diabetes demonstrated that these patients also experience difficulties with oral communication (Schillinger et al., 2004). Patients appear to have particular problems with both the decision-making and the explanatory, technical components of dialogue. Furthermore, patients with limited health literacy may be less likely to challenge or ask questions of the provider (Baker et al., 1996; Street, 1991) and may cope by being passive or appearing uninterested (Cooper and Roter, 2003; Roter, 2000; Roter and Hall, 1992; Roter et al., 1997).

Health literacy is one of a number of influences on the communication process. Communication between a health-care provider and patient during outpatient visits may also be hampered by several related factors. These include the relative infrequency and brevity of visits, language barriers, differences between providers' and patients' agendas and communication styles and other cultural barriers, lack of trust between the patient and provider, overriding or competing clinical problems, lack of timeliness of visit in relation to disease-specific problem, and the complexity and variability of patients' reporting of symptoms and trends in their health status.

The complexities that arise from the interplay of cultural processes and variations in health literacy underlie communications and interactions in the health-care system. Typically this balance is part of a healing relationship governed by cultural beliefs and rituals that manifest as a cultural language. Health-care providers need to comprehend this cultural language in order to reduce misunderstanding. Reciprocal to this understanding are the skills of the people among the different cultural groups to understand what health-care providers are communicating regarding their diagnosis, risks, and treatment options.

Diverse cultural groups value distinct processes by which harmony and balance is maintained in the relationships of everyday life. Typically this balance is referred to as healing and along with the dynamics surrounding human relationships, these become "healing relationships" governed by cultural beliefs and rituals that manifest as culturally based language during health and illness. Cultural contexts dominate healing relationships. "Physicians and other health care providers need communication skills . . . to reduce misunderstanding and the risk of incorrect diagnosis and . . . to develop . . . treatment plans that are compatible with the patient's reality" (Molina et al., 1994: 35). Reciprocal to this communication are the skills of the people (individual, families, and communities among different cultural groups) to understand what health-care providers are discussing about diagnoses, risks, and treatment options. In contrast, aboriginal peoples have a vision of healing that informs the "process of healing oneself, relationships with families" and "maintaining balance among their mental, physical, emotional and spiritual dimensions as human beings" (Ross, 1996: 147). In Westernized health care, the concept of healing is typically used during experiences with illness or disruptions in health status. In contrast, some aboriginal cultural languages present healing as an aspect of health and everyday living. "Instead healing is seen as an everyday thing for everyone, something which, like sound nutrition, creates health. In short, the healing perspective must be built into the attitudes and process that shape every aspect of everyday" (Ross, 1996: 147).

In another example, Native Hawaiians comprehend healing through a system for maintaining harmonious relationships and resolving conflicts within the extended family; this system is called Ho'oponopono, which means setting to right. The Ho'oponopono process is a conceptual framework informed by several cultural concepts that become evident as the steps in the cultural ritual. These include problem identification, discussion, seeking forgiveness; release of conflicts and hurts; and the closing phase. Ho'oponopono is especially useful as a mental health intervention (e.g., for alcohol or substance abuse, domestic violence, anger) but also complements interventions for coping with diseases.

> *"Then the ho'ola said Mom should confess to me and before God Jehovah. She did. She asked me to forgive her and I did. I wasn't angry. . . . And later Mom's sickness left her. Of course, she still had diabetes, but the rest—being so confused and miserable—all that left her"* (Shook, 1985: 109).

This broader humanistic perspective of healing is critical to comprehend aboriginal and Native Hawaiian health behaviors and to understand the importance of healing rituals for inclusion in treatment options and caring interventions during health and illness. These culturally based views of health suggest a trajectory for forming healing relationships in that they illuminate a fuller range of human experiences during health and illness. Understanding a greater diversity of healing relationships supports health literacy among different cultural groups. To this end, good health communications are a key pathway to building the continuous healing relationships that have been cited as an important goal for twenty-first century health-care system design (IOM, 2001). Poor communications and relationships translate into unfavorable outcomes, particularly delays in care seeking, refusal, lack of continuity of care, and disparities (IOM, 2003a).

Patient Safety and Health-Care Quality[4]

The IOM report *To Err Is Human* (IOM, 2000b) clarifies the links between miscommunication and medical and health errors and adverse events. Lack of cultural competence and inattention to health literacy can both compromise patient safety through a number of mechanisms. For example, a variety of problems can result if culture and language are not taken into account including

- Failure to get accurate medical histories
- Failure to obtain informed consent
- Poor health knowledge and understanding of health conditions
- Poor treatment adherence
- Medication errors
- Lower utilization of preventive and other health-care services
- Poor patient satisfaction

To the extent that low health literacy may be more prevalent among some racial and ethnic minority groups, these individuals may be at higher risk for adverse events stemming from poor communication. There is a need to understand the independent contributions of cultural competence and health literacy to patient safety, as well as the interactions between cultural competence and health literacy.

Patients' varied perspectives, values, beliefs, and behaviors regarding health and illness are consistently cited as integral to quality care in several IOM reports (2001, 2003a). To protect people from undue harm, eliminate errors and adverse events, prevent unnecessary human suffering, and be more accountable to quality and cost-effective care, cultural processes beckon attention, particularly to erode the culture of blame, reform team-work, and redesign organizational dynamics within health-care systems. A principle of patient safety is to include patients in safety designs and the processes of care (IOM, 2000b). To do so, it is essential to understand cultural nuances of what patient safety means to different people and what beliefs, values, and actions inform people's understanding of safe care come into play.

The communication process plays a central role in this understanding. For example, a recent study in California of pediatric outpatient visits that used Spanish-language interpreters found an average of 31 interpretation errors per pediatric clinic visit (Flores et al., 2003), two-thirds of which had clinical consequences. The errors included errors in the dose and duration

---

[4]The committee thanks Arlene Bierman, M.D., M.S., for her contributions to this section of the report.

of prescribed drugs and missed information on patient allergies. Errors were most common with untrained interpreters. Amoxicillin for an ear infection was translated as one teaspoon three times a day in the ears, rather than by mouth. Steroid ointment for a baby's face was translated as "rub on the body" and twice a day for three or four days was translated as "in four days."

In building a safer health-care system, strategies are needed to include culture and communication, inclusive of patients and families, as an integral component of interventions to reduce medical and health errors and adverse events like these.

The interaction of health literacy, culture, language, and safety is not limited to patient safety. Worker safety is also influenced by health literacy. Workers must employ safeguards against hazardous materials and procedures. They are expected to read warning labels and right-to-know postings and take important precautionary measures. Yet, for some, the information may not accessible. The potential of low literacy and limited English proficiency to affect worker safety has been noted by health and safety educators and unions (Wallerstein, 1992). A recent National Academies workshop on Latino worker safety (NRC, 2003) noted that Spanish-speaking workers are four times more likely to be injured or killed on the job than English-speaking workers. The need to improve and properly translate signage, safety and use instructions, and training procedures is noted in that report (NRC, 2003). Strategies suggested to improve worker safety training include participatory education and popular education approaches (e.g., Wallerstein, 1992). Further research in this area is critical to the development of successful safety programs.

> I prepared all my material, cut all my pieces of Formica, and I opened the can and I didn't really read the label. There was a red label on the can and even if I would have looked at it, I didn't know what it was. I couldn't even read it. Come to find out my lung was poisoned from that material I was using (Rudd and DeJong, 2000).

Crossing the Quality Chasm: A New Health System for the 21st Century (IOM, 2001) proposed that health-care processes are to be redesigned according to 10 rules, 6 of which allude to cultural context and 5 of which relate to health literacy via information and communications. These rules are shown in Box 6-1. Twenty-first century health care will unravel the complexities that arise from the interplay of cultural processes and health literacy. Proposed changes include customizing care based on patient needs and values and accommodating differences in patient preferences and an-

BOX 6-1
Rules for Redesigning Health-Care Processes

1. Care based on continuous healing relationships. Patients should receive care whenever they need it and in many forms, not just face-to-face visits. This rule implies that the health-care system should be responsive at all times (24 hours a day, every day) and that access to care should be provided over the Internet, by telephone, and by other means in addition to face-to-face visits.
2. Customization based on patient needs and values. The system of care should be designed to meet the most common types of needs, but have the capability to respond to individual patient choices and preferences.
3. The patient as the source of control. Patients should be given the necessary information and the opportunity to exercise the degree of control they choose over health-care decisions that affect them. The health system should be able to accommodate differences in patient preferences and encourage shared decision making.
4. Shared knowledge and the free flow of information. Patients should have unfettered access to their own medical information and to clinical knowledge. Clinicians and patients should communicate effectively and share information.
5. Evidence-based decision making. Patients should receive care based on the best available scientific knowledge.
6. Safety as a system property. Patients should be safe from injury caused by the care system.
7. The need for transparency. The health-care system should make available to patients and their families information that allows them to make informed decisions when selecting a health plan, hospital, or clinical practice, or choosing among alternative treatments.
8. Anticipation of needs. The health system should anticipate patient needs, rather than simply reacting to events.
9. Continuous decrease in waste. The health system should not waste resources or patient time.
10. Cooperation among clinicians. Clinicians and institutions should actively collaborate and communicate to ensure an appropriate exchange of information and coordination of care.

SOURCE: IOM (2001).

ticipating patient needs. Customizing (to match individual specifications) and tailoring (to adapt for special needs or purpose) approaches to patient care services are based on the assumption that understanding of people's needs, characteristics, and respect for beliefs and values are operating. Such understanding and respect is rooted in patient-centered care (Gerteis et al., 1993). Customized and tailored information, communication, and education are integral to individualized care (IOM, 2001). To customize and tailor care means that health literacy is subsumed within a cultural context during clinical encounters. This report also recommended that a "patient-centered" approach be implemented to ensure that patients have full understanding of all of their options (IOM, 2001).

Access to Health Care and Preventive Services

Literacy and disparities are two sides common to a health phenomenon rather than two separate problems. Data continue to emerge to support the idea that the different needs of particular individuals and groups who have been historically marginalized or disenfranchised due to their ethnic or racial heritage, or social group identity or membership, continue to be unmet by the health-care system (IOM, 2003a). Inattention to patient preferences, lack of patient-centered care, and insufficient English proficiency (written or verbal) are contextual qualities that fuel health disparities among particular groups and individuals in the United States. In this way, limited health literacy may be a precursor to and condition of health disparities. Interventions to increase communications, improve access to health information, promote the understanding of meaning from facts, and transfer knowledge to actions are likely to reduce the negative impact of low literacy on patients' access and use of health services.

Health services access involves many factors. These include financial ability to use services, lack of appropriate services located where people can reach them, times when services are available, health-care staff's ability to appropriately navigate language and culture with patients, and respectful treatment of patients. Ethnic background and minority status also influence access to care (IOM, 2003a). Across all populations, the individuals most likely to be dissatisfied with seeking care are members of minority groups. These minority groups indicated they felt their race, ethnicity, and ability to pay for services directly affected their level of care (IOM, 2002b). An IOM report found differences in access and in treatment of patients who are poor, African American, Latino, and American Indian, among others (IOM, 2003a). Health literacy is an additional factor that should be considered when examining access to care and use of preventive services. Preliminary research supports such a link. This research is reviewed in Chapter 3. Briefly, individuals with limited health literacy as determined by the available measures are less likely to use preventive services such as mammograms and pap smears (Scott et al., 2002), and may come to the attention of the health-care system at a more advanced stage of disease (Bennett et al., 1998).

A lack of health insurance and lack of access to affordable services may lead people to postpone or not participate in care, particularly preventative care such as screenings, but also including recommended medical tests, treatments, and prescribed medications (Kaiser Commission on Medicaid and the Uninsured, 2003a). Rates of uninsurance in the United States vary by race and ethnicity at 12 percent of Caucasians, 20 percent of Asian Americans, 22 percent of African Americans, more than 25 percent of Native Americans, and more than 33 percent of Hispanics (Kaiser Commission on Medicaid and the Uninsured, 2003b). Uninsured patients are more likely to have poorer health than they would if insured (IOM, 2002a). Many African-American women who are uninsured or underinsured put their families' welfare ahead of their own, especially when financial resources are limited. They seek treatment too late or not at all (IOM, 1999). Further, people who are uninsured or underinsured are more likely to rely on emergency departments for care (IOM, 2002b). An example of this can be seen in asthma. If someone cannot afford the appropriate workup, consultation, and medications to properly control asthma, they (or their children in the case of childhood asthma) will be less likely to prevent attacks that may lead to emergency department use (IOM, 2002b).

The problems created by the financial inability to use services may be exacerbated by health literacy issues, including limited knowledge and information surrounding early symptoms of serious illness and the value of prevention. Preliminary evidence discussed in Chapter 3 suggests that these socioeconomic, cultural, and health literacy factors may be associated with higher costs in the long run, when expensive tertiary care and emergency department services become necessary.

Limited local health resources and services can also impede access to care. Grocery stores and heath services are among the many resources that are limited in low-income and remote areas. Transportation may be a major obstacle; if services are difficult to get to or far away, people may do without, or postpone the use of the service. For some individuals often only limited primary care treatment services are available conveniently. So, for example, women needing mammograms may have to travel to a facility where this can be done, which can be a deterrent to obtaining that service. Limitations on hours of availability can also reduce access. Some clinics operate only or primarily during business hours. This may create problems for many people seeking health services. In particular, low-income patients may have a harder time getting time off from work, or finding child care, in order to seek care or take a family member to get care. Health services that have weekend and evening hours could potentially help prevent the unnecessary use of emergency departments.

Limitations on Provider Time

A major impediment to appropriate communication about health is the limitation on provider time that is often required by HMOs, public clinics, and health-care reimbursement plans. For example, most plans do not reimburse for time spent in instructing patients on how to manage diabetes. It is nearly impossible to deal with literacy, language, and cultural issues within the context of a 10–15-minute patient visit. Ironically, the result of poor communication and abbreviated or no patient education is higher use of emergency services, greater severity of illnesses, failure to follow instructions and use medications properly, and other "errors" which ultimately result in increased health-care costs.

In this regard, Linzer and colleagues (2000) have established that time pressure is related to lower levels of physician career satisfaction, especially in the managed care setting. Federman and others (2001) have demonstrated that failure of physicians to acknowledge patient concerns, provide explanations of care, and spend sufficient time with patients may contribute to patients' decisions to discontinue care at their usual site of care. Discussing these papers in an editorial Warde (2001) states that "it seems that a physicians ability to engage the patient without distraction from other activities is an important determinant in the quality of an encounter with a patient ... true access means being psychologically available to conduct interviews that center on the physical, social, and psychological needs of each patient." She goes on to suggest that "through its effect on the doctor–patient relationship, time pressure may diminish the very outcomes that health plans strive to achieve: high quality of care, access, cost-effective resource utilization, and patient satisfaction" (Warde, 2001). Encounters with limited-literacy patients can only require more time to overcome these barriers.

Health Expenditures

Health expenditures are of concern to decision makers in both the public and private sectors, and particularly to private employers and small businesses. Health spending has increased as a percentage of gross domestic product (GDP) as growth in health expenditures has outpaced growth in the economy as a whole. The Department of Health and Human Services (HHS)[5] projects that the increase in health expenditures will fall to about 7 percent in the 2003–2007 period, and to 6.6 percent during 2008–2011 (Heffler et al., 2002). During this period health spending will continue to

---

[5]National health expenditures and future projections are reported annually by the Office of the Actuary in the Department of Health and Human Services. It reports on total national health expenditures, including all services such as hospitalization, physician and dentist care, pharmaceuticals, nursing homes, home health, and other costs; these also cover all sources of payment such as Medicare, Medicaid, different forms of private insurance and managed care plans, and out-of-pocket payments by individuals.

outpace the overall economy by 2.5 percent per year, resulting in growth from 13.2 percent of GDP in 2000 to 17 percent in 2011. There is no reason to believe that these increases will moderate in the near term, and policy attention from both public and private sectors will continue. This attention has led to a renewed discussion of health-care policy as a national- and state-level issue that has included fundamental questions such as whether health insurance should be tied to employment, the relative roles of the public and private sectors, and whether consumers themselves should assume more responsibility for health-care costs and quality.

The most recent national estimate of expenditures for 2001 is $1.4 trillion or $5,035 per capita, based on a growth rate of 8.7 percent in 2001 (Levit et al., 2003). These expenditures are the highest in the world. The reasons for these high rates are complex. Although greater volume is often cited as the primary reason for higher costs in the United States as compared to other countries, it has been found that prices of services, rather than volume, are responsible for higher costs in the United States. Administrative costs in the private sector are also much higher than in other countries or in Medicare. While some combination of new technology and increased demand has led to increases in both prices and utilization, these vary across the nation. A recent study indicates that variation in expenditures between states is in part due to underlying demographics like age and wage rates, and in part due to the supply of hospitals and physicians (Martin et al., 2002). In addition, states with higher managed care penetration have lower expenditures. This is thought to be attributable to "both lower premium rates charged by HMOs and spillover effects of competition on non HMO premiums" (Martin et al., 2002).

Preliminary evidence on the cost implications of limited health literacy (presented in Chapter 3), while not conclusive, give some idea of the magnitude of impact of health literacy on national medical expenditures. Efforts to improve health literacy, or to limit its detrimental effects, may provide an important contribution to health-care policy addressing rising health expenditures (Heffler et al., 2002; Levit et al., 2002; Martin et al., 2002).

Consumer-Directed Health Care

A major emerging issue in the health system is increased consumer involvement in health-care choices. This movement has evolved primarily from self-insured employers who have developed a series of "consumer-driven" or "consumer-directed" health plans. These plans require consumers to make decisions about how they want to spend their health-care dollars, including how much co-insurance and out-of-pocket expenses to budget, which providers to see, and what services are really necessary

(Edlin, 2002). Consumer-directed health care appears to have developed because of the failure of both regulation and market forces to produce satisfactory cost containment results, and a belief that providing consumers with incentives can produce a more efficient and responsive system. The Foundation for Accountability, with support from the Agency for Healthcare Research and Quality (AHRQ), produced in June 2002 a "how-to guide" called *"Who's in the Driver's Seat? Increasing Consumer Involvement in Health Care"* (FACCT, 2002). This guide describes 48 different strategies currently being tried, which encompass employers implementing disease management programs, purchasing coalitions teaching enrollees about quality, health plans improving doctor–patient communications, consumer organizations relying on members' expertise to develop communication materials, and researchers studying how people acquire and use information to improve their health. More narrowly, much attention is being given to health insurance vehicles which run the gamut from flexible spending accounts, medical savings accounts and defined contribution plans to new Internal Revenue Service-approved "health reimbursement arrangements" (Scandlen, 2003). Several new companies, such as Definity and Lumenos, have formed to market new consumer-driven vehicles (Elswick, 2003). These specific insurance products are still too new to assess their impact and effectiveness and some are skeptical that they will grow dramatically (Elswick, 2003).

In a broader sense, many in both the public and private sectors see increased consumer involvement in coverage and care decisions as a major force to improve the cost and quality issues that other approaches have not been able to achieve. If this is the case, the burden for persons with limited health literacy—who already face the challenges outlined in this report—will surely increase significantly.

Finding 6-2   Health literacy is fundamental to quality care, and relates to three of the six aims of quality improvement described in the IOM Quality Chasm Report: safety, patient-centered care, and equitable treatment. Self-management and health literacy have been identified by IOM as cross-cutting priorities for health-care quality and disease prevention.

Health Law and Health Literacy[6]

Legislatures and courts are beginning to respond to the issues raised by limited health literacy in the context of health care. Current laws require

---

[6]The committee thanks Frank McClellan, J.D., for his contributions to this section of the report. Mr. McClellan summarized and interpreted the law in relation to health literacy for the committee.

health-care providers to furnish translators for patients who do not speak English, and interpreters to patients who have seeing or hearing disabilities.[7] Current laws do not address the problem of patients with limited literacy. We found only a few cases in which literacy itself was pivotal in resolving the tort[8] claim or lawsuit, two of which are discussed briefly below.

Cases in which literacy is pivotal to the tort claim are likely to be more common in the near future. The identification of health literacy as a cross-cutting contributor to health services quality (IOM, 2003b) indicates a need for legislative policies supporting health literacy as a contributor to good health care. These policies would affect the development of common law, which is driven by policy considerations. In this context, these policy considerations are likely to be defined on the basis of what is good health care. Each state has the power to develop its own common law or statutory law, which, in the absence of a single national policy, may contribute to variations between states in the recognition of health literacy as a contributor to good health care.

Two areas of health law and health care that are particularly central to health literacy are the standard of reasonable care and the informed consent process. It is around these areas that policy likely to affect common law could be developed.

The Standard of Reasonable Care

When a patient suffers an injury that was either directly caused by the health care rendered, or which could have been avoided by appropriate health care, the injured patient (or his or her family) may consult an attorney to determine whether the health-care provider is legally responsible for the injury. In making that assessment, the attorney will examine federal and state statutes, administrative regulations, and court decisions to determine what the legal standard is for the particular service provided. The court decisions, referred to as the common law, will in most instances include a reference to the standard of reasonable care. In most circumstances, reasonable care means care rendered in accordance with the standards of the profession. Courts seek to determine what a prudent health-care worker would do in similar circumstances on the evidence of professional standards. Practice standards developed by professional groups provide part of

---

[7]Title VI of the Civil Rights Act, and its implementing regulations. Americans with Disabilities Act.

[8]A wrongful act other than a breach of contract for which relief may be obtained in the form of damages or an injunction.

this evidence; other evidence may be found in federal and state statutes and their implementing regulations, accreditation standards of professional associations, and by-laws of hospitals.

The treating physician or nurse is held liable for an injury only where ordinary care in accordance with the standards of the profession would have avoided the accident, rather than as a guarantor of a good outcome. Therefore, in most instances the professions control the standards by which their members are judged. There are two important qualifications to the profession's control of the standards. First, the provider may be found negligent if he or she has special knowledge indicating that following the ordinary standard in the particular circumstances involved will expose the patient to an unreasonable risk of harm. Second, in rare instances, a court may declare that the whole profession may be found negligent for following a practice that new information or alternatives have shown to be unduly dangerous.

The concept of reasonable care can be applied to considerations of health literacy in the context of health care. The case of *Incollingo* v. *Ewing*[9] provided a court opinion reflecting both the rule that a profession (or a large percentage of it) may be found negligent, and the rule that each physician must use his or her own personal knowledge. This case involved a child who died as a result of suffering aplastic anemia due to the consumption of a wide-spectrum antibiotic (Chloromycetin) prescribed at first by the child's pediatrician for a throat infection and abdominal pains, and then renewed by a second physician after a telephone request by the child's mother.

The doctor who initially prescribed Choloromycetin sought to justify his conduct on the ground that he was aware of the risk that the drug could cause aplastic anemia and therefore made sure not to allow for a renewal of the prescription. In his view, the child first presented to him with a throat infection that he regarded as a major ailment. He argued that even the plaintiff's expert agreed that in prescribing this antibiotic he acted in the same manner as 95 percent of the doctors in Philadelphia where he practiced. The court noted that the drug's package insert warned that the drug should not be prescribed for minor ailments, and the mother produced expert testimony at trial that the child indeed had a minor ailment when the drug was first prescribed. Consequently, the court found that the jury was allowed to find the first doctor negligent for not using his personal knowledge appropriately.

The doctor who renewed the prescription sought to defend his action

---

[9]444 Pa. 263, 282 A.2d 206 91971.

on the ground that most doctors in Philadelphia would have prescribed the same drug for a minor ailment at that time, based on a belief that the drug was effective and posed a very small risk of serious harm. He acknowledged that the package insert warned against such prescriptions of the drug, but contended that the medical community often prescribes the drug because the manufacturer had minimized its risks in communications directly to the prescribing doctors. Rejecting this argument, the court emphasized that medical custom is not always controlling, reflecting the rule that a profession (or a large percentage of it) may be found negligent. The health-care provider must exercise reasonable care, "giving due regard to the advanced state the profession at the time."[10]

A similar view was expressed in *Helling* v. *Carey*[11] (1974), in which the appellate court declared as a matter of law that a prevailing medical custom was negligent. A patient suffered blindness as a result of undiagnosed and untreated glaucoma. The patient had been under the care of the physicians for a number of years, and had never received a test of intraocular pressure. The prevailing custom of ophthalmologists was to perform routine pressure tests for early glaucoma only on patients who were over 40 years of age, because the risk of glaucoma was, in their view, too small in persons under 40 to justify routine pressure tests. The court ruled that the doctors were negligent as a matter of law, notwithstanding the evidence that they followed the custom of their specialty at the time. Noting that a low-risk, inexpensive test could have prevented a serious illness such as blindness in a long-term patient who was experiencing loss of vision, the court declared that reasonable care dictated the performance of the test.

This suggests that if future health literacy research supports the existence of associations between low-risk, inexpensive approaches to limited health literacy and reduced morbidity or mortality, the rule that a profession (or a large percentage of it) may be found negligent could apply to the failure to use health literacy interventions in clinical settings, including programmatic changes in health information provision. Providers could also be responsible when their knowledge indicated that a lack of patient understanding would expose the patient to an unreasonable risk of harm.

The Doctrine of Informed Consent

The doctrine of informed consent, which obligates the physician to inform the patient of the risks, benefits, and alternatives to undergoing or

---

[10]282 A.2d at 216.
[11]83 Wash. 2d 514, 519 P.2d 981.

refusing to undergo the treatment recommended by the physician, has extensive legal and research implications when addressing health literacy.

Informed consent in health care and research. In most cases, consent forms involve the use of structured and technical language to disclose subjects' rights, roles, and responsibilities. They contain complex descriptions of institutional practices, financial and insurance considerations, legal concerns, advanced medical technologies, and potential risk/benefit considerations. Cumulative research over the past two decades and across three continents shows that consent forms for treatment and research are written at a level beyond the skills of most patients involved in research (Criscione et al., 2003; Freda et al., 1998; Goldstein et al., 1996; Gribble, 1999; Grossman et al., 1994; Grundner, 1980; Hammerschmidt and Keane, 1992; Hopper et al., 1995, 1998; Jubelirer, 1991; Lawson and Adamson, 1995; LoVerde et al., 1989; Mader and Playe, 1997; Mathew and McGrath, 2002; McManus and Wheatley, 2003; Meade and Byrd, 1989; Ogloff and Otto, 1991; Ordovas et al., 1999; Osuna et al., 1998; Rivera et al., 1992; Tait et al., 2003; Tarnowski et al., 1990). Examples of consent form text at different reading levels are provided in Table 6-1.

The readability of consent forms is often at a scientific level that contributes to information overload, poor understanding, and misinformed consent (Benson and Forman, 2002; Davis et al., 1994; Hopper et al., 1995; Meade and Howser, 1992; Philipson et al., 1995; Raich et al., 2001; Reicken and Rovich, 1982; Sugarman et al., 1998, 2002). In 2003, Paasch-Orlow et al. (2003) reported results of a cross-sectional study of 114 web sites from U.S. medical schools regarding their Institutional Review Board (IRB) readability standards and informed consent templates. Specific readability standards were found on 61 web sites (54 percent) and were found to range from a fifth-grade reading level to a tenth-grade reading level, while other sites contained descriptive guidelines such as "simple lay language." Results revealed that informed consent text often falls short of the institutions' own readability standards and suggest that federal oversight is associated with better readability. Figure 6-2 shows the difference between the readability of informed consent forms and the readability required by the IRBs.

Furthermore, while patients who sign consent documents often report their understanding of the research or treatment and satisfaction with the consent process, they may not fully understand the consent given (Horng et al., 2002; Pope et al., 2003; Vohra et al., 2003; Williams et al., 2003).

As pointed out in Chapter 1 of this report, all people (not just those with low educational levels) are at risk for low health literacy. The informed consent process brings with it particular challenges that may further impede understanding. This is in part attributable to the inherent complex-

TABLE 6-1 Examples of Informed Consent Text Provided by Institutional Review Boards at U.S. Medical Schools*

Readability Level	Voluntary Participation	No Direct Benefits
4th Grade†	"You don't have to be in this research study. You can agree to be in the study now and change your mind later. Your decision will not affect your regular care. Your doctor's attitude toward you will not change."	"There is no benefit to you from being in the study. Your taking part may help patients in the future."‡
8th Grade†	"Participation in this study is entirely voluntary. You have the right to leave the study at any time. Leaving the study will not result in any penalty or loss of benefits to which you are entitled."	"There is no direct benefit to you from being in this study. However, your participation may help others in the future as a result of knowledge gained from the research."
12th Grade§	"Your participation in this study is strictly voluntary. You have the right to choose not to participate or to withdraw your participation at any point in this study without prejudice to your future health care or other services to which you are otherwise entitled."	"There may be no direct benefit to me, however, information from this study may benefit other patients with similar medical problems in the future."

*All the examples are taken directly from medical-school Web sites unless otherwise noted.
†The readability level is based on the Flesch-Kincaid readability scale.
‡The passage was modified to present key concepts at a fourth-grade reading level.
§The readability level is based on the Fry readability formula.
SOURCE: Excerpted from Table 1 in Paasche-Orlow et al. (2003). Copyright © 2003 Massachusetts Medical Society. All rights reserved. Reprinted with permission.

ity and nature of informed consent information. But, it also relates to the multitude of psychosocial, ethical, and situational factors that may surround the clinical need for informed consent, such as hospitalization, emergency heart surgery, participation in Phase I cancer clinical trial, genetic testing, new vaccine for HIV, use of surgical placebos for Parkinson's disease, or separation of conjoined twins.

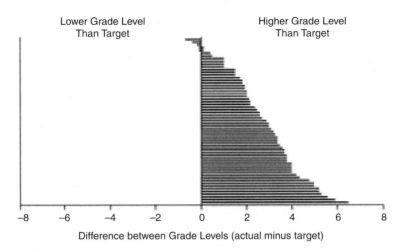

FIGURE 6-2 Difference between actual readability and target readability of informed consent documents. Each bar represents 1 of the 61 institutional review boards that indicated a specific grade-level target as a readability standard.
SOURCE: Paasche-Orlow et al. (2003). Copyright © 2003. Massachusetts Medical Society. All rights reserved.

A signature on a consent form is not adequate evidence that informed consent has been obtained. In providing informed consent, a research participant faces significant challenges, which are not adequately addressed through standard policy procedures (Triantafyllou et al., 2002). In many cases, patients and providers may disagree about the need for and adequacy of consent. Patients tend to see consent as necessary more frequently than providers, hold different views on whether true informed consent was obtained, and may be less than satisfied with the amount of information exchanged (Bray and Yentis, 2002; Cox, 2002; Gardner and Jones, 2002; King, 2001; Mathew and McGrath, 2002; McManus and Wheatley, 2003; Osuna et al., 2001; Schopp et al., 2003). These differences in views and biases in information may not be recognized by the provider or patient (Hewlett, 1996), and affect the patient's right to self-determination[12] and self-decision,[13] that is, the right to make any informed decision. Appelbaum (1997) notes that in communicating with patients, clinicians and researchers often underplay the risks associated with the randomized trials, and the benefits associated with standard care.

---

[12]*Schloendorrf* v. *Society of New York Hospitals*, 211 NY 125;105 NE 92 (1914).
[13]*Canterbury* v. *Spence*, 464 F 2d 772 (1972).

"I was in my early 30s and having problems with my girl parts. I was bulging in the vaginal area and I knew this was not normal. The doctor told me that it would be an easy repair and could be done. The surgery was set up. On the night before surgery, I remember having lots of papers pushed toward me to sign. I signed them because I needed to do this. I had surgery the next day and my recovery went very well. I had a large scar on my lower abdomen. I went for my six-week follow-up visit and was asked by the nurse how I was doing since my hysterectomy. No one had ever used those words before, but I knew what they meant. I had never asked any questions. I made the assumption that all doctors knew exactly what they were doing and had better intelligence than me. I was too humiliated to reveal to the doctor and nurse that I did not know what had been done to me. Communication had broken down and failed me."

"No one knew that I could not read well. Actually, I could read . . . but only one word at a time. By the time I got to the end of a sentence—I had no comprehension of what I had just read. I struggled to read. All that I read I would read three times. I kept books in front of me so others would not find out. I thought that if others found out, that they would think I was stupid. To check on the spelling of a word, I would call the library (that way no one could see me). There are many ways to hide poor reading from others."

Personal story graciously provided by Toni Cordell, Adult Learner and Literacy Advocate, as told to C.D. Meade, September 2003.

Legal precedents. While no case directly addresses health literacy, cases exist in which theories of negligence, informed consent, and literacy have been brought to bear. A case that illustrates the potential issues that must be considered when examining literacy and informed consent is *Hidding* v. *Williams*[14] (1991). The patient underwent a laminectomy that resulted in complete loss of control of his bowel and bladder. Prior to surgery he signed a consent form that stated that a risk of the surgery was "loss of bodily function." Since the patient died prior to trial his wife prosecuted his personal injury claim and offered the only testimony from the patient's view regarding the consent process. She testified that although her husband signed the form, he had only a fifth-grade education and minimal reading skills. She read the consent form for him and did the best she could to explain it. However, she thought "loss of function of bodily organs" meant that he might not be able to get up and walk around right away after the

---

[14]578 so. 2d 1192, La. App.

surgery. She had no idea that it meant he faced a risk of loss of control of his bladder, and thus she did not include that information when she attempted to explain the risks he was confronting. In light of this testimony the judge, sitting without a jury, ruled that informed consent was not obtained. The court explained:

> The physician is required to disclose material risks in such terms as a reasonable doctor would believe a reasonable patient would understand. In order for a reasonable patient to have awareness of a risk he should be told in lay language the nature and severity of the risk and the likelihood of its occurrence. A bland statement as to a risk of 'loss of function of bodily organs' when not accompanied by any estimate of its frequency does not amount to understandable communication of any specific real risk.[15]

The case supports the concept that a written document of a patient's consent is evidence that an informed consent was obtained, but is not conclusive and can be rebutted by other evidence. Thus, while it is important to have documentary evidence of advising a patient of risks, benefits, and alternatives, the existence of that document does not prevent the court from considering whether the information deemed critical to making a meaningful expression of consent to the treatment was conveyed to the patient by a means that was likely to enable patient comprehension. Signed consent documents are treated in this manner in most states. Evidence that the patient could not read or comprehend the form leaves the issue of whether an informed consent was given to evidence regarding the communication process, such as verbal conversations, picture displays, and videos. The same is true with respect to instructions given to the patient or the patient's family as to monitoring physical condition, administering medication, and so forth.

Finding 6-3 The readability levels of informed consent documents (for research and clinical practice) exceed the documented average reading levels of the majority of adults in the United States. This has important ethical and legal implications that have not been fully explored.

Governmental and Agency Roles

Roles of the Federal Government

Many of the federal health agencies have programs and activities for documenting and improving the health literacy of our nation. These agen-

---

[15]578 So. 2d at 1196.

cies can influence the health-care and public health systems to develop and support integrated strategies addressing health literacy and can increase the scientific knowledge base about health literacy by fostering research and collaboration.

In addition, the federal government plays a central role in the production and dissemination of health-related information and the regulation of such information from other sources. The involvement of specific agencies such as the Food and Drug Administration (FDA) and the Centers for Disease Control and Prevention (CDC) in these activities is described below. One widely known regulatory action in this regard is the Health Insurance Portability and Accountability Act of 1996. On April 14, 2003, as mandated by this act and in accordance with the Office of Civil Rights National Standards to Protect the Privacy of Personal Health Information, a notice of privacy practices was disseminated to all consumers entering the health-care system across the country (in hospitals, dental offices, pharmacies, and other health service locations).[16] The law requires that this information be "read and understood" by consumers. Printed information was distributed in a variety of formats and languages to convey how medical information may be used and disclosed including information relating to treatment, payment and health-care operations, business associates, fundraising, research, appointment reminders, treatment alternatives, benefits and services, and persons involved in a patient's care. However, the committee observed that the text disseminated to convey this important information varied widely in its nature, scope, and complexity. It is very likely that the privacy documents were written above the reading level of many Americans. Until formal evaluations are conducted, it remains unknown how well consumers fully understand the federal regulations that must be "read and understood" before care is provided.

We summarize here the activities of those agencies with important roles relating to health literacy in the health system context. This is not an exhaustive list of all federal agencies with related work, but is intended to highlight those that either have ongoing activity in this area or show particular promise to influence the issue. Chapters 4 and 5 highlight some of the health literacy-related activities of federal agencies in the contexts of the educational system and culture and society, including those related to language issues and interpretation in health care.

Office of the Secretary, Office of Disease Prevention and Health Promotion
As the lead agency for the health literacy objective of *Healthy People 2010*

---

[16]Health Insurance Portability and Accountability Act of 1996. http://www.hhs.gov/ocr/hipaa/.

(HHS, 2000), the Office of Disease Prevention and Health Promotion (ODPHP) has been actively working to raise awareness about health literacy, to identify and coordinate health literacy activities across HHS, to convene HHS agencies to work collaboratively on health literacy, and to identify external partners. In 2000, ODPHP established a partnership with the National Center for Education Statistics of the U.S. Department of Education to develop the health literacy measures that are included in the 2003 National Assessment of Adult Literacy. These data represent the first national measures on health literacy, and will be used to assess the *Healthy People 2010* objective. ODPHP has also collaborated with outside organizations on health literacy by including health literacy in its Memoranda of Understanding with several organizations, including the American Medical Association (AMA) and the Academy of General Dentistry.

Centers for Medicare & Medicaid Services (CMS)   Individuals considered at highest risk for limited education and low health literacy are the elderly and those with low incomes. Many are enrolled in the Medicare and Medicaid programs administered by the Centers for Medicare & Medicaid Services (CMS). Medicare is a federally run health insurance plan covering nearly 40 million people in the United States who are 65 years of age and older, disabled, or have permanent kidney failure. Medicaid provides health assistance to certain individuals and families with low incomes or resources, and, in contrast to Medicare, is a state-administered program. See below for further information on Medicaid. Both Medicare and Medicaid are complicated and confusing programs, with health literacy issues in enrollment, making choices, patient rights, and terminology (Hudman, 2003; Scala, 2002).

Because CMS runs the Medicare program, it is directly responsible for communication with people covered under Medicare about health insurance coverage, their rights and protections in Medicare, and their health plan options. Communication about the Medicaid program is a function of each state, and CMS works with the states to ensure that people in Medicaid receive the information they need (see below for further information on Medicaid). In both cases, CMS works to ensure that these communications are accurate, reliable, relevant, understandable, and, to the extent possible, culturally appropriate. One way it does so is through the provision of agency-wide communication guidelines and training materials such as "Writing and Designing Print Materials for Beneficiaries: A Guide for State Medicaid Agencies." CMS also uses consumer research and training, consultation with literacy experts, and communication guidelines to develop materials for consumers that are intended to be easy to navigate and understand through format, design, and wording modifications. Consumer research and testing includes target audience members with lower education levels, from a variety of ethnic, racial, income, and health experience backgrounds.

The Food and Drug Administration   The FDA regulates and provides information about drugs, biological products, medical and radiological devices, the food supply, and cosmetics. Three general areas of FDA activity related to health literacy are advertising, outreach, and labeling.

•   **Advertising.** Advertising for prescription drugs is regulated by the Code of Federal Regulations (21 CFR 202) and is enforced by the FDA. Criteria indicate that both print and broadcast advertisements must not be misleading, must provide balanced information about risks and benefits, must state the major risks, and, for print advertisements, must contain a brief summary statement of effectiveness. Broadcast advertisements also are required to include "adequate provision" for methods to obtain more detailed information, such as through a print ad, a toll-free telephone number, or by asking a health-care provider.

•   **Outreach.** Outreach to consumers and patients is a central activity for the FDA. The FDA develops public service campaigns and announcements, maintains web information for consumers, and carries out educational programs on specific topics. Challenges to successful consumer outreach at the FDA include: getting information to a wide variety of consumers with different needs, abilities, and desires; encouraging consumers to use the information; simplifying information without losing meaning or becoming too lengthy; and ensuring balance between risks and benefits (Lechter, 2002).

•   **Labeling.** The FDA approves and has legal jurisdiction over the content of labels for prescription and over-the-counter medications as well as biologics and medical devices. Aspects of medication labeling overseen by the FDA include medication guides, patient package inserts, and the standardized over-the-counter Drug Facts format. The FDA also performs research on label comprehension and the actual use of labels by consumers, monitors the prescription information provided to consumers by the private sector, carries out consumer outreach, and monitors prescription drug advertising.

An FDA regulation requires that over-the-counter medication labels be written: ". . . in such terms as to render them likely to be read and understood by the ordinary individual, including individuals of low comprehension, under customary conditions of purchase and use."[17] The sponsor or

---

[17]21 CFR 330.10(a)(4)(v).

manufacturer of a medication is responsible for producing labels that comply with this requirement, and may conduct label comprehension studies that require the participants to apply the label information in hypothetical situations. The FDA reviews the results of these studies in order to strengthen the label, and to determine whether the medication can safely and effectively be used without professional guidance. Participants in the studies include individuals with "low comprehension" as required by the regulation mentioned above. Low comprehension is typically defined as having an eighth-grade reading level or below, and the Rapid Estimate of Adult Literacy in Medicine (REALM) is frequently used to make this determination.

The Centers for Disease Control and Prevention   As the lead public health agency of the United States, the CDC has a central role in successfully communicating information on health and illness to all members of the public. The CDC identifies "Providing credible information to enhance health decisions" (CDC, 2003) as one of the central goals of its mission. Related to health literacy, the CDC's focus has encompassed efforts around plain language including training, testing and pre-testing materials, surveys, and the provision of health information to TV shows, networks, writers, and producers. The CDC has addressed issues of culture in several of its programs. For example, the National Institute for Occupational Safety and Health added a Spanish-language section to its web site in 2001, and the National Immunization Program developed educational material for American Indians and Native Alaskans in 2003. Currently, CDC is redesigning its web site based on a CDC web evaluation completed in 2002. The evaluation showed that consumers looking for basic health information regarding disease and disease prevention are the largest segment of visitors to the CDC web site.

The National Institutes of Health   The National Institutes of Health (NIH) play the crucial role of determining federal funding for health literacy research, and thus in large part set the research agenda on the topic in the United States. Figure 6-3 shows NIH funding of health literacy over the past 6 years.[18] These data were derived from a search of the NIH CRISP database from 1993 to 2002 using the following operands: "health literacy," "health and literacy," "health and readability," and "literacy and readability." The grants retrieved were examined for relevance to the field

---

[18]The committee thanks Patrick Weld and K. Visnawath, Ph.D., of the National Cancer Institute for their contributions to this section of the report. Mr. Weld and Dr. Viswanath performed this search and analysis of the CRISP database. An expanded description of the methods of their work can be found in Appendix A.

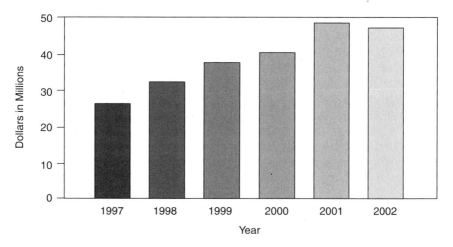

FIGURE 6-3 National Institutes of Health grant funding over the 1997–2002 period.

of health literacy. A total of 906 grants for a 10-year period were identified, but 229 of the grants from 1993–1996 contain missing financial data. The figure shows the funding totals from the 565 grants that remained after eliminating grants that were not funded, and grants for which data were missing.

"Low-literacy" components were included in studies in cancer, childhood development and reading, arthritis, asthma, diabetes, HIV, mental health, Alzheimer's, health disparities, and studies in Spanish-speaking populations. In addition, "low literacy" was included in seven Requests for Applications since 2000, in studies such as Environmental Justice (sponsored by the National Institute of Environmental Health Sciences), Adult and Family Literacy (sponsored by the National Institute of Child Health and Human Development), Native American Research Centers for Health, oral health disparities, diet and physical activity assessment, and cancer communications.

Although the increase in funding over the past decade clearly represents a positive trend, the amount funded by NIH for programs and projects that examine health literacy is a small segment of the NIH budget. This amount, which is equivalent to $20 to $50 million per year, has consistently been less than half of 1 percent of the annual grant funding by NIH.

The Health Resources and Services Administration   The Health Resources and Services Administration (HRSA) of HHS provides both service and educational programs intended to improve access to health care, the quality of health care, and health outcomes. HRSA's programs serve millions of diverse people from multiple racial and ethnic groups with differing educational levels who are frequently of low-income socioeconomic status. Educational programs provide training in interpretation, cultural competence, and communication for health-care providers, while HRSA's service programs provide funding and direction for health-care delivery sites across the nation. Health-care delivery sites focused on various populations and types of care are administered by the various bureaus of HRSA, including the HIV/AIDS Bureau, the Bureau of Primary Health Care, and the Maternal and Child Health Bureau. The service programs utilize community health workers (also known as promotoras, outreach workers, or lay health workers) who are lay members of the community and work in association with the local health-care system, providing health education, interpreting health information, and assisting in obtaining access to services.

Agency for Healthcare Research and Quality The AHRQ is the part of HHS that sponsors, carries out, and disseminates research on health-care quality, medical errors and patient safety, health-care cost, and health disparities. AHRQ recently sponsored an evidence-based review of health literacy research to answer the following questions:

- What is the relationship between literacy and health outcomes, use of health services, and resources?
- What is the relationship between health literacy and racial disparities in health and health care?
- What are effective interventions to reduce the impact of health literacy?
- What are effective literacy-related interventions for reducing racial disparities in health and health care?

Although the results of this project were not available at the time of publication of this report, AHRQ worked with the IOM to provide preliminary information that was valuable in informing the work of the Committee.

The Department of Veterans Affairs The Department of Veterans Affairs (VA) is responsible for providing federal benefits, including health care, to the nation's veterans and their dependents. The VA's National Center for Health Promotion and Disease Prevention (NCP) uses patient education and health promotion techniques in order to increase quality of life and reduce health-care costs. The VA patient population is a vast heterogeneous group—6 million "enrolled" veterans, and over 25 million "eligible" vets.

They span all races, numerous cultures, all levels of education, all socioeconomic strata, and both genders, with approximately 85 percent males. The VA patient population also shows a wide age range of 18 years and up, with two basic spikes—20- to 30-year-old veterans with short military stints, and those over 50 years, representing retired military. The heterogeneity of the population points to the need for awareness of differences in attitudes, perceptions, and level of technological adeptness. Disabilities in the veteran population (including blindness, deafness, and mental disorders) also present barriers to access and communication. The NCP uses various techniques to ensure that educational and health promotional materials respond to all of these issues and needs.

Roles of State Governments

State governments have also identified health literacy as a critical issue. In 2002, the Council of State Governments undertook a national research project with the goals of (1) gathering data from the latest findings on health literacy, (2) determining what states are doing to make it easier for someone with low health literacy to navigate the health-care system, and (3) preparing a report providing information and tools necessary for state leaders to determine what appropriate action they might take. They sent a National Survey on Health Literacy Initiatives to state governor's offices, departments of heath, Medicaid and State Children's Health Insurance Program offices, departments of education, and offices of heath literacy. This resulted in a 2002 publication, *The State Officials Guide to Health Literacy* (Matthews and Sewell, 2002).

The most important finding from this survey is that health literacy is an emerging issue that few states have addressed specifically and directly. They report that while no state is addressing health literacy in a comprehensive, multifaceted manner, individual agencies in a handful of states—including Georgia, Illinois, Massachusetts, and Virginia—have established programs, hired staff, or created task forces to respond to low health literacy and its effects on health-care delivery. A number of states are involved in activities that make it easier for someone with low health literacy to navigate public assistance programs—such as simplifying enrollment materials and procedures—or to increase health literacy by setting health education standards in both K-12 and adult literacy classes. Examples of some of these efforts are discussed further below in the section on approaches to health literacy.

As discussed briefly above, Medicaid, the health-care assistance program for low-income individuals and families, is a state-run program. Each state sets its own guidelines for eligibility and services for Medicaid, under the general guidance of CMS. As reviewed in Chapter 3, individuals with lower income or resources are more likely than those with higher incomes or resources to have limited literacy skills. Those enrolled in Medicaid, therefore, may be more likely to encounter barriers to care related to health literacy. Box 6-2 discusses the differences across states in dealing with health literacy and related issues in contracts with managed care providers of health care to those enrolled in Medicaid.

Roles of Regulatory Agencies

There are two main private organizations in the United States for accreditation and review of health-care facilities and providers: the Joint Commission on Accreditation of Healthcare Organizations (JCAHO) and the National Committee for Quality Assurance (NCQA).

Joint Commission on Accreditation of Healthcare Organizations   The private, nonprofit JCAHO is the oldest and largest health accreditation organization in the United States, providing accreditation to over 17,000 organizations including hospitals, health-care networks, home care agencies, and nursing homes. Its mission is "to continuously improve the safety and quality of care provided to the public through the provision of health care accreditation and related services that support improvement in health care organizations" (JCAHO, 2003). JCAHO approaches health literacy through its standards on patients' rights and on patient and family education and responsibilities. These standards include assessing patient and family involvement in care and care decisions, the informed consent process, and hospital patient education tailored to patients' assessed needs, abilities, learning preferences, and readiness to learn. Compliance with these standards is assessed through document review, staff interviews, and review of patient complaints. However, it is not clear how effective these standards are in improving organizational performance regarding health literacy issues, and significant changes in this process are planned for 2004.

National Committee for Quality Assurance   NCQA is a private, not-for-profit organization dedicated to improving health-care quality, best known for its work in assessing and reporting on the quality of the nation's managed care plans through their accreditation and performance programs. NCQA identifies health literacy as a critical step in ensuring patient participation in their health care. Testimony to the Committee from NCQA indicates that thus far it has been unable to create a valid and reliable measure that is feasible to apply at either the health plan or provider level. Such a measure is critical in trying to hold health-care providers and insurers accountable for both initial health literacy and improvement in health literacy (personal communication, L. Gregory Pawlson, M.D., M.P.H., NCQA, June 13, 2003). Regardless, there are a few provisions related to

BOX 6-2
State Medicaid Managed Care Contracts

Information from the Center for Health Services Research and Policy's database on Medicaid managed care contracts (Rosenbaum et al., 2001) indicates that guidelines and requirements for Medicaid managed care providers vary across the states. Language in medicaid managed care contracts, valid as of 2001, shows that although a number of states' contracts do address some literacy- and language-related issues, there are no specific requirements related to health literacy in any state, and many states do not address these issues at all or do so inconsistently.

Among the 42 states with risk contracts that are captured in the Medicaid Managed Care database, 33 states and the District of Columbia included in their Medicaid managed care contracts some type of requirement pertaining to the provision of easily understood information. There is a great deal of variability across the states in how this is defined, and the method of determining if the requirement is being met. Notably, in most states, the requirement refers to the understanding of written material only. An exception is California, which requires that both verbal and written information be provided in a manner that can be easily understood.

In some cases, the Medicaid managed care contract includes general language about patient comprehension such as the statement in the Massachusetts Medicaid Contract that requires that "written information...[be provided]...in a format and manner that is easily readable, comprehensible to its intended audience..." (Rosenbaum et al., 2001). Frequently, states indicate that written information must be readable at a specific reading grade level (see Chapter 2 for a discussion of reading grade levels). The reading grade level indicated varies significantly across states, ranging from as high as grade 8 in Montana and North Dakota, to grade 4 in a number of states, to a less-specific "suitable reading comprehension level" in Maryland. Still other states require that "plain language" be used. Overall, a sixth-

health literacy issues that are currently part of the NCQA standards for managed care organizations, such as:

- Quality Improvement Standard 4, which determines whether the organization assesses the cultural, ethnic, racial, and linguistic needs of its members and adjusts the availability of practitioners within its network, if necessary.
- Patient Rights and Responsibilities 4, which assesses whether the organization provides translation services within its member services telephone function based on the linguistic needs of its members.

In addition, there is an indirect assessment of clinical function in the Consumer Assessment of Health Plan Survey. This survey includes a query grade reading level is the most frequently cited requirement among the states that mention a reading level.

A related issue is that some of the information provided to patients must be provided "as written" in federal law, and Medicaid managed contracts may specifically exclude such language from requirements to be easily understood. For example, in Texas, patient information about advance directives is excluded from its general readability requirement since certain language is required by federal law.

Methods to determine readability level or whether information is easily understood also vary across states. Some states name specific programs, indices, or tests that must be used to determine reading grade level; these include methods such as the Fry Readability Index, Flesch Scale Analysis, or the McLaughlin Simplified Measure of Gobbledygook Index. Other states' contracts simply state the desired reading grade level. Some states require that the managed care organization itself determine if its patient information meets the requirements, while in other states this task is reserved for the state or its designee.

Clearly, much of this language such as that referring to the intended audience implies that attention should be given to individuals who do not speak English or who speak English as a second language, but less frequently is this explicitly stated. A few states do, however, require that information be provided in the other languages when the minority-language group makes up greater than 10 percent of the population. However, contracts more frequently include provisions for translation services and cultural competence. The Medicaid managed care contracts of 12 states do not include a requirement for services to be provided to persons whose primary language is not English. Although 25 states include a requirement that Medicaid managed care providers must insure cultural competence, only 10 of these states explicitly define what is meant by cultural competence.

NOTE: The information presented in this section was obtained from Rosenbaum et al. (2001).

which asks whether the member looked for any information about how a health plan works in written materials or on the Internet, and asks how much of a problem, if any, it was to find or understand this information.

OPPORTUNITIES IN HEALTH SYSTEMS

The understanding that no one size fits all is fundamental to the understanding of health literacy. There is not a simple solution to a complex problem. Determinants and approaches for health literacy are complex, dynamic, and require unique know-how, strategic thinking, and understanding of the audience. While we have stressed the importance of contributions of three contexts (the educational system, culture and society, and the health system) for improving health literacy, in Finding 2-1 we highlight that the health-care system "carries significant opportunity and responsibility to improve health literacy." This section explores options for how the health-care system can approach this responsibility to limit the negative impact that limited health literacy has on health care and health outcomes.

The strategies discussed in this section are based on current knowledge of interventions for limited literate individuals in health-care settings and on the small but growing evidence about how health literacy might be affected by various interventions. There are a few examples of interventions specifically designed to incorporate health literacy into health systems, and some information is available from the literature regarding interventions in other related fields such as health communication and health education. However, scientific investigation of interventions to minimize the impact of limited health literacy and promote the development of health literacy skills in the context of the health-care system is in its infancy. Conclusions about the success of health literacy programs based on these areas should be made cautiously. Research to evaluate the efficacy of these interventions is needed, and the committee's discussions represent the present consensus of experts in the field.

Overview of Current Efforts

There are limited systematic approaches to health literacy and some of the organizations addressing health literacy are not based in academic institutions. It is important to be aware of approaches not yet evaluated or published in the peer-reviewed literature. Therefore, the committee commissioned an overview of approaches to health literacy currently being used in the United States that have not appeared in the peer-reviewed literature.[19]

The commissioned authors conducted a survey of organizations that "could make a difference" with health literacy. The types of organizations were identified first, and then the individuals most likely to be aware of health literacy issues and activities in that organization were contacted. The survey was a 5-minute, 15-question, web-based survey based on a previous survey to assess health literacy activities at the state level (Matthews and Sewell, 2002).

Information collected included: whether health literacy is considered in program development and service activities; the degree to which organiza-

---

[19]The committee thanks Terry Davis, Ph.D.; Julie Gazmararian, M.P.H., Ph.D.; and Estela Marin, M.A., for their contributions to this section of the report. Drs. Davis and Gazmararian and Ms. Marin designed, carried out, and analyzed the survey. An expanded description of the methods of their work can be found in Appendix A.

tions follow health literacy principles in their programs; target audience(s) for activities; whether organizations pilot test materials for comprehension or cultural competence; evaluation of materials; which activities people associate with health literacy and lessons learned. Of the 101 individuals e-mailed, completed surveys were received from 95 individuals from a variety of government agencies, public and private interest groups, as well as related business groups.

Eighty-one percent of respondents indicated that they consider health literacy in their program development and service activities. Almost all of the respondents associated health literacy with "comprehension" (94 percent) or "clear language" (92 percent). The majority associated health literacy with "cultural competence" (80 percent), "no jargon" (72 percent), or "readability testing" (71 percent) and "self-management" (67 percent). In addition to the pre-coded categories, respondents had the opportunity to provide other areas they associated health literacy with. A few other topics identified included issues of autonomy, empowerment, decision-making; patient safety and error reduction; numeracy and computation; provider responsibility for patient understanding; and quality of care. Table 6-2

TABLE 6-2 Frequency of Doing Health Literacy-Related Activities

	Regularly	Sometimes	Do not do	Don't know	No response
Simplify language and check readability	77%	18%	2%	0	3%
Reformat materials to make them more user-friendly	74%	19%	3%	0	4%
Confirm patient/client understanding	50%	25%	17%	3%	5%
Train agency, staff, or health-care providers about health literacy	46%	32%	14%	2%	6%
Use audiovisual aids	44%	36%	14%	1%	5%
Provide materials in multiple languages	43%	30%	18%	3%	6%
Use pictographs, cartoons, etc. to instruct and inform	39%	40%	19%	0	3%
Test for reading levels in clients	25%	20 (21%)	42 (44%)	5%	4%
Use interactive computer or kiosk	16%	25 (26%)	45 (47%)	7%	3%

NOTE: Respondents could select more than one activity.

summarizes the type of health literacy activities that respondents reported they or their organization were involved in. Almost 95 percent of respondents indicated that they simplified language and checked readability, and 93 percent indicated that they reformatted materials to make them more user-friendly either regularly or sometimes. Minority (e.g., Hispanic, African American, etc.) and low-income populations were the primary target group for these health literacy activities.

It is important to view the information gained from this survey with caution. The survey was sent to a limited number of organizations and individuals. The respondents are not generally representative of their respective organizations. Some of the nonrespondents may have wished to avoid confusion between personal opinion and institutional goals and policy, avoiding the possibility that their response would be interpreted as an institutional statement of policy rather than a personal view.

Approaches to Health Literacy in the Health System

Given the newness of the field, it is not surprising that little empirical work exists at this time. Much more needs to be done to provide solid guidance to all stakeholders for the most effective interventions in a variety of settings. However, as the survey above indicates, many different approaches that show promise are currently being tried; such innovations need to be encouraged and evaluated. In this section, we review different categories of approaches, look at some of the studies that have evaluated such approaches, consider what is already known about that approach from other fields, and showcase a number of promising efforts that are examples of the kind of work being done in this field.

For heuristic purposes, we have structured the following discussion around six categories of interventions under which most efforts appear to fall. These categories are as follows:

- Provision of Simplified/More Attractive Written Materials
- Technology-Based Communication Techniques
- Personal Communication and Education
- Combined Approaches
- Tailored Approaches
- Partnerships

In addition, it is important to note that training of educators and providers is one of the most important areas of current activity in the health literacy field. Because training cuts across nearly all of the intervention categories above, we have chosen not to break it out as a separate area, but will mention particularly notable efforts in this area where appropriate.

Table 6-3 summarizes results from a sample of studies that have examined interventions taking place in, or sponsored by, health-care organizations. They are organized into the categories listed above, although we acknowledge that there is necessarily some overlap among categories with some types of interventions. These studies were gleaned from a review of the database on health literacy performed by Michael Pignone and colleagues as a commissioned project for AHRQ,[20] as well as from recently published abstracts and testimony. This selection of studies was chosen to represent an array of various types of interventions in different populations and is not intended to be comprehensive. Studies included here did not have to measure the literacy level of participants. Overall, the studies displayed in Table 6-3 reflect the early state of the field. Pignone and colleagues evaluated the strength of the available evidence for health literacy interventions as part of the above-mentioned project for AHRQ (Pignone, 2003). The four criteria used to determine reliability were (1) the study was randomized, (2) the study design minimized confounding, (3) literacy was measured, and (4) the result of the intervention was reported by literacy level.

Five of the studies in Table 6-3 have been identified by Pignone (2003) as the most methodologically reliable of those that have been published (Davis et al., 1998b; Meade et al., 1994; Michielutte et al., 1992; Murphy et al., 2000; Wydra, 2001). Wydra and colleagues (2001) found that their interactive videodisc intervention increased reported self-care ability among cancer patients, but that the literacy level of the patients had no effect on this increase. Meade and colleagues (1994) examined the effectiveness of conveying information about colon cancer via videotape versus a printed booklet. Compared to controls, participants receiving any information demonstrated increased knowledge, but the difference between the two modes of communication was not significant. Davis and colleagues (1998b) found that those with the lowest literacy levels, after receiving a simplified and more appealing brochure, did not show a similar increase in comprehension similar to those with higher literacy skills. In contrast, Michielutte and colleagues (1992) also provided two different brochures—one with text and one illustrated—and found that even while two brochures had no influence on comprehension in the total research sample, those in the lowest literacy levels showed increased comprehension with the illustrated format. It is possible that a larger sample would show a different effect.

---

[20]The committee would like to thank AHRQ for its assistance with this segment of the report.

TABLE 6-3   Samples of Published Studies of Interventions in
Health-Care Settings

Citation	Setting	Study Design	Population
Provision of Simplified/More Attractive Written Materials			
Davis et al., 1998c	Private and university oncology clinics, and a low-income housing complex	Nonrandomized trial	n = 183 53 patients with cancer or another medical condition and 130 apparently healthy participants
Davis et al., 1998b	Three pediatric care facilities in Louisiana	Randomized controlled trial	n = 610 Parents bringing children to pediatric care facility
Eaton and Holloway, 1980	Outpatient clinic at Veterans Administration hospital in Minneapolis, MN	Randomized controlled trial	n = 108 Outpatients who could read English, see normal size type, and were not receiving warfarin therapy
Hussey, 1994	Geriatric outpatient clinic in a county hospital in the southwestern U.S.	Controlled trial (nonrandomized)	n = 80 Patients of clinic 65 years or older with at least one chronic health problem, and either of low socioeconomic status or indigent

Intervention	Outcome
Simplified informed consent form versus standard form. 69 participants given Standard Southwestern Oncology Group (SWOG) consent form (16th grade level) and 114 participants given simplified form (7th grade level) developed for study.	Participants preferred simplified form over the SWOG form, and 97% thought the simplified form was easier to read than the SWOG form ($p < 0.0001$). However, there was no significant difference in degree of understanding of the two forms.
Polio vaccine information brochures: 304 parents received simplified LSU version, 306 received CDC version	Overall, readers of LSU brochure showed significantly higher comprehension (65% vs. 60%, $p < 0.01$); however, comprehension for most items did not achieve clinical significance and parents in the two lowest reading levels did not demonstrate increased comprehension with the LSU brochure. LSU brochure was preferred over CDC version.
Patient drug information guide about warfarin written at either 5th- or 10th-grade reading levels.	Comprehension was greater for 5th-grade-level information compared to 10th-grade-level information ($p < 0.001$), and for patients with a higher reading ability compared to those with a lower reading ability ($p < 0.001$). Reading ability explained 24% of variance and grade level of materials explained 8% of variance. Participants' perception of level of difficulty, understandability, and clarity of the material was more favorable for the group receiving the 5th-grade material as compared with those receiving the 10th-grade material.
Color-coded method to increase medication compliance. Group 1 received verbal teaching about medications only; Group 2 received verbal teaching and color-coded medication schedule.	Significant increase in knowledge in both Groups 1 and 2 ($p < 0.001$), with no difference between the groups in knowledge increase. Significant increase in compliance in both Groups 1 and 2 ($p = 0.007$), with a greater increase in compliance for Group 2 (color-coded schedule) among those with low compliance scores at baseline.

Continued

TABLE 6-3 Continued

Citation	Setting	Study Design	Population
Jacobson et al., 1999	Ambulatory clinic at Grady Memorial Hospital, Atlanta, GA	Randomized controlled trial	n = 433 Primary care patients that had not previously been vaccinated, and had one of the following: diabetes, heart failure, other chronic illness, 65 years or older
Michielutte et al., 1992	A private family practice and three public health clinics —OB/GYN, family planning, and sexually transmitted diseases	Randomized trial	n = 217 Women age 18 or older Women who reported no ability to read or who reported "serious illness" were excluded
Powell et al., 2000	Pediatric clinic at Northwestern University Medical Center, Chicago, IL	Prospective cohort	n = 66 families Parents of children 6 years or younger who obtained primary care from the clinic

Technology-Based Communication Techniques

Kim et al., 2001	Urology clinics in two VA hospitals in Chicago	Uncontrolled trial	n = 30 100% male
Meade et al., 1994	Cancer clinic	Randomized trial	n = 1100

Intervention	Outcome
Low-literacy (below 5th-grade) handout to increase patient–physician dialogue about pneumococcal vaccination and increases rates of immunization. Intervention group received handout encouraging patients to "ask your doctor about the pneumonia shot" and control group received a low-literacy handout about nutrition.	Intervention group significantly more likely than control group (p < 0.001 for all variables) to discuss vaccine with clinician, to receive vaccine, to show brochure to clinician, and for the clinician to recommend vaccine. When adjusted for race, sex, age, education, health status, insurance status, clinician training, and vaccine indication, intervention group significantly more likely than control group (p < 0.001 for all variables) to discuss vaccine with clinician and to receive vaccine.
Cervical cancer information brochures: 112 women received illustrated brochure, 105 received nonillustrated version.	No difference overall in comprehension with the two brochures. When results were analyzed by reading level, the illustrated brochure was better comprehended by lower literacy patients.
Injury prevention information provided by pictorial anticipatory guidance (PAG) sheet requiring limited reading skills or TIPP (The Injury Prevention Program).	No significant differences in caretaker recall of injury prevention information assessed by telephone 2–4 weeks later.
Evaluate the knowledge, satisfaction level, and treatment preferences of men newly diagnosed with prostate cancer after intervention of CD-ROM about prostate cancer.	Satisfaction with information and likelihood of following treatment preference not significantly different by literacy or educational background.
Colon cancer information presented in printed and videotaped formats. Subjects received either a booklet, viewed a videotape, or received no intervention.	Participants receiving any intervention showed increased knowledge compared with controls (booklet = 23% and videotape = 26%, no intervention = 3%).

Continued

TABLE 6-3 Continued

Citation	Setting	Study Design	Population
Murphy et al., 2000	Sleep clinic at Louisiana State University Health Sciences Center	Controlled trial (nonrandomized)	n = 192 (20 of which were caregivers) Patients at sleep clinic 18 years or older If younger than 18, caregiver participated
Pepe and Chodzko-Zajko, 1997	Urban health department in the Midwest	Uncontrolled trial	n = 20 Low-income, inner-city adults aged 60–80
Wydra, 2001	Four comprehensive cancer centers	Randomized trial	86 intervention patients, 88 controls Patients over age 18 who were receiving outpatient cancer treatment Those with less than 5th-grade reading level or brain or visual dysfunction were excluded

Personal Communication and Education

Mulrow et al., 1987	Diabetes clinic in London	Randomized trial	n = 120 Patients with diabetes who were overweight and not taking insulin Patients with a history of diabetic ketoacidosis, diabetes onset prior to age 29, or over the age of 70 where excluded.
Paasche-Orlow, 2003	Two urban medical centers	Uncontrolled	n = 80 Adults hospitalized for asthma exacerbation

Intervention	Outcome
Information about sleep apnea from an instructional videotape or a simple brochure.	Short-term knowledge about sleep apnea was less accurate for those with reading levels less than 8th grade than for those with reading levels at or above 9th grade. Video intervention significantly improved only two areas of knowledge for readers below grade 8 ($p < 0.05$).
Cholesterol information videotape shown on follow-up visit.	Increase in cholesterol knowledge score from baseline (62%) to two-week follow-up after videotape (77%). 6 week follow-up scores at 72%. Change in time in cholesterol knowledge was not significantly different between reading groups.
Interactive videodisc program designed to improve self-care with respect to fatigue symptoms for patients with cancer.	Intervention patients reported greater self-care ability after the intervention ($p < 0.0001$). Literacy level did not affect the amount of self-care ability gained ($p = 0.31$).
Education program for patients with non-insulin-dependent diabetes to improve and sustain glucose and weight control. Subjects were assigned to (1) monthly group sessions with videotapes for diabetic persons with low literacy skills; (2) monthly group sessions without videotapes; or (3) no monthly sessions after first introductory section like Group 2.	No statistically significant differences in change in HbA1C levels within or between groups at either 7 or 11 months. Differences in weight change were significant ($p < 0.05$) at 7 months but no change at 11 months. No significant change in knowledge score with intervention.
One-on-one oral and written intervention at discharge covering medication schedule and metered dose inhaler technique	After instruction, about 1 in 3 high-risk adults required additional instruction about medication regimen. Higher acute care utilization, not low health literacy, predicted the need for additional instruction.

Continued

TABLE 6-3 Continued

Citation	Setting	Study Design	Population
Rothman et al., 2003	University-based general internal medicine practice	Randomized trial	n = 206 Patients with diabetes and poor glucose control
Schillinger et al., 2003b	Two primary care clinics in San Francisco	Uncontrolled trial	n = 74 Patients with type 2– diabetes mellitus
Combined Approaches			
Davis et al., 1998a	Public hospital in Shreveport, LA	Randomized controlled trial	n = 445 Women 40 years old or over, attending ambulatory or eye clinic, and no mammogram in the past year
Tailored Approaches			
Hayes, 1998	Emergency departments, Midwestern rural area	Randomized trial	n = 60 Elderly emergency room patients

Intervention	Outcome
Comprehensive disease management intervention.	Literacy levels predicted improvement in glucose control among a control group with usual care, but not among the intervention group in the disease management program.
A measure of the extent to which physicians assess patient recall and comprehension in a public hospital setting.	Higher health literacy and physician application of interactive communication strategy were associated with good glycemic control (p < 0.01).
3 different interventions to increase mammography usage. Group 1: personal recommendation from one of the investigators. Group 2: recommendation and easy-to-read National Cancer Institute brochure. Group 3: recommendation, brochure, and 12-minute interactive educational and motivational program, including video based on focus groups from the target population.	At 6 months after intervention, Group 3 showed significant increase (p = 0.05) in mammography utilization as compared to Groups 1 or 2. This increase was no longer significant at 2 years. In a multivariate analysis with age, race, literacy and mammography knowledge at baseline, the only significant predictor of mammography use at 6 months was the Group 3 intervention.
Comparison of the level of reading knowledge from either preprinted discharge instructions (control) or individualized computer generated discharge instructions (intervention). Contacted by telephone for follow-up interview.	Intervention group did better on Knowledge of Medication Subtest (p = 0.05).

Provision of Simplified/More Attractive Written Materials

Most of the approaches to improving health literacy that the committee has encountered involve producing patient information materials that are written with simplified language, have improved format (for example, more white space and friendlier layout), or use pictograms or other graphic devices (see information from survey above). It should be recognized that although creating patient information at readability levels that match patient and family reading levels may achieve limited positive patient outcomes, it may not achieve improved comprehension in all situations. For example, while simplification of informed consent information resulted in less intimidation (Davis et al., 1998c) and lower consent anxiety and higher satisfaction (Coyne et al., 2003), it did not improve patient comprehension. An example of an effort in this category is a project of the Geriatrics Section at the University of California–San Francisco that is seeking to increase the accessibility of advance directives to individuals with limited literacy skills. An advance directive form has been developed that incorporates culturally appropriate text-enhancing graphics appropriate for individuals with limited literacy skills. The form, available in both Spanish and English, not only describes what an advance directive is, but also walks patients through the process of filling out the form. It is written at a fifth-grade reading level and is currently being pilot tested and compared to other standard advance directive forms.

Graphics and other visual devices (also referred to as pictograms) are often used to replace or supplement text in health information communications. Pharmacies or patient educators may use pictograms as part of patient education handouts, or as stickers to be placed on prescription medication packaging. These types of uses are not considered part of the official packaging, and thus are not regulated by the FDA. Concerns have been expressed that some of the pictograms currently in use do not accurately convey the intended information (Rother et al., 2002). They may be open to interpretation, and interpretation may vary by an individual's background and experiences. Pictograms are thought to be particularly beneficial for communicating information to consumers who speak English as a second language and to those with lower reading ability levels (USP, 2003). However, research suggests that individuals with limited health literacy may have particular difficulties correctly interpreting pictograms (Price et al., 2003). A research projected funded by Pfizer, Inc. entitled "Pictograms: A Tool for Enhancing Health Care Outcomes Among Underserved Patients in Primary Care?" is currently examining whether pictograms affixed to medication bottles enhance long-term recall of medication knowledge in patients identified as having difficulty with their medications; however, no data are as yet available from this 200-patient study. The nonprofit organization

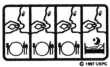

Take 4 times a day, with meals and at bedtime.   This medicine may make you drowsy.

Take by mouth.   Store in refrigerator.

FIGURE 6-4   Examples of pictograms for patient education.
SOURCE: United States Pharmacopeial Convention, Inc. Reprinted with permission. Copyright © 2004 United States Pharmacopeial Convention, Inc. All rights reserved.

U.S. Pharmacopeial Convention, Inc. (USP) maintains a free library of 81 pictograms that may be downloaded from the Internet. Figure 6-4 shows several examples of pictograms from the USP pictogram library.

Guidelines, templates, and tools are available that inform investigators and clinicians about ways to rewrite consent documents and other communications so that they are easier to understand. For example, Philipson and others (1999) evaluated a writing improvement intervention program implemented at Hartford Hospital to help the research writer produce more comprehensible informed consent documents and determined that the program increased the percentages of consent documents that were readable and at the target reading grade level. The National Cancer Institute (1998) has prepared a set of templates and recommendations for the development of easy-to-understand informed consent documents for cancer clinical trials that are available online and were distributed to IRBs, hospitals, cancer centers, patient groups, and researchers. These templates are currently in use among cooperative cancer clinical trial groups across the United States. While such guidelines and tools are helpful aids, solutions must also support changes in policies at the institutional and national level and become part of ongoing federal regulatory and monitoring activities of local compliance and IRBs. Box 6-3 displays two versions of an informed consent document: the original and simplified versions.

Technology-Based Communication Techniques

A number of the interventions displayed in Table 6-3 tested the effectiveness of technology-based communication techniques such as videos,

BOX 6-3
Example of a Consent Form for Participation in
Smoking Cessation Study

Original Consent Document

Women are being invited to participate in a research investigation to determine the efficacy of two methods of assisting pregnant women in their smoking cessation attempts. A comparison of the effectiveness of educational media in combination with a counseling method on smoking habits is being examined. It cannot be guaranteed that women may personally benefit from this investigation, but in some instances, the knowledge gained might be beneficial to others. It is important to recognize that participation in this study is entirely voluntary. Individuals may withdraw from the study at any time without penalty or loss of benefits to which they are otherwise entitled. Such withdrawal will not compromise any individual's ability to receive medical care at this institution.

Revised Simplified Consent Document

Introduction

You are being asked to take part in a study that looks at ways to help pregnant women stop smoking. We want to know if booklets can help you to stop smoking. We also want to find out how nurses can help you to stop smoking. We cannot be sure that this study will help you, but it may help others. Taking part in this study is up to you. You can stop taking part in it at any time. It will not get in the way of your care at this clinic.

SOURCE: Doak et al. (1996). Reprinted with permission of the Oncology Nursing Society.

CD-ROMs, and interactive multimedia programs. Findings from these studies are equivocal. Some show positive outcomes such as increased knowledge or self-care ability, while others show no effect. Two of these studies found no interaction between the technology-based intervention and the literacy level of the individuals in the studies (Kim et al., 2001; Wydra, 2001). Simply transforming text versions of disease-specific education to more visually oriented media (for example, CD-ROM), while associated with improvements in satisfaction, does not appear to increase knowledge among patients with limited health literacy (Kim et al., 2001).

Although there is not yet clear evidence about the effectiveness of these types of technology-based communication techniques for improving health literacy or mitigating the effects of limited health literacy, such techniques are supported by research in the fields of commercial and social marketing, health education, and health communication. *Speaking of Health* (IOM, 2002c) provides an overview of this evidence base. In addition, evaluation of interventions to improve the informed consent process provide support for technology-based communication techniques such as computerized decision aids (Rostom et al., 2002), videotape plus physician communication (Agre et al., 1997), telephone-based nursing interventions (Aaronson et al., 1996), and audiovisual documentation of oral consent (video + audiotape + photography) (Benitez et al., 2002).

The Foundation for Informed Medical Decision Making has produced education videos intended to aid in patient decision-making as part of shared decision-making programs in clinics, managed care organizations, and other settings (Kasper et al., 1992). Based on studies indicating which patient preferences are most likely to affect treatment choices, these products incorporate testimonials about patient experiences and describe the consequences of different choices. A systematic review of this approach indicated that such decision aids improve knowledge, reduce decisional conflict, and stimulate patients to be more active in decision-making without increasing anxiety, while having variable effects on decisions and outcomes of decisions (O'Connor et al., 1999). Because health literacy is important to the shared decision-making process, this type of approach is important to consider but, unfortunately, has not yet been evaluated with patients with limited health literacy or limited literacy.

One widely used type of technology-based communication technique is telephone-delivered interventions (TDIs) in which health-related counseling and reminders are delivered using the telephone. *Speaking of Health* (IOM, 2002c) reports that the efficacy of such interventions is strongly supported by the evidence base but that they are underused by diverse populations. TDIs can vary by the type of service provider, the extent to which the call is scripted and varies based on characteristics and responses of the individual, and the extent to which subsequent calls take into account information

BOX 6-4
Examples of Ongoing Approaches Using Technology-Based Communication Techniques

- The Florida/Caribbean AIDS Education and Training Center, funded by HRSA, is developing a CD-ROM and web site that can be accessed at a computer in the provider's office to present patient information to women who are neither literate nor fluent in English. The draft format includes pictures with simultaneous narration in Creole or Spanish, and includes presentations for each commonly used antiretroviral medication that demonstrate how to take the medications as well as how to administer them to a child.
- The HRSA HIV/AIDS Bureau provides technical assistance and funding to the Northwest AIDS Education & Training Center's Minority AIDS Initiative called Building Effective AIDS Response. This program developed a video centered on increasing health literacy about HIV-infection in Native American communities in Washington, Oregon, Idaho, and Montana, and addressing the fear and shame barriers to accessing health care.
- The *Improving Diabetes Efforts across Language and Literacy* project, developed at San Francisco General Hospital, intends to implement and evaluate disease management programs tailored to the language and literacy levels of patients with diabetes. The project will test the feasibility and acceptability of health communication interventions in a public delivery system and compare the effects of technologically oriented vs. interpersonally oriented chronic disease support. Diabetes patients will be randomized to receive (1) weekly phone calls via an automated telephone diabetes management system that was developed with the assistance of patients with limited literacy, (2) monthly group medical visits, or (3) usual care.
- CDC's Health Communication Division has a cooperative agreement with the University of Southern California's Norman Lear Center to provide information to TV shows, networks, writers, and producers. The Center develops tip sheets on priority topics for CDC, arranges biannual briefings for the Hollywood Writer's Guild, and responds to requests from Hollywood producers for accurate and timely information. Television programming can provide accurate, timely information about disease, injury, and disability in their storylines for millions of people in a format available and understood by everybody.

from other encounters with the individual (IOM, 2002c). In addition, TDIs can be initiated by the individual through calls to helplines or services, or by the health system, through outbound calls (IOM, 2002c). The effect of these variable characteristics is yet to be evaluated among individuals with low literacy and low health literacy.

Testimony to the committee has revealed a wide array of activities in the category of technology-based communication techniques that are currently being used. Some of these are summarized in Box 6-4.

Personal Communication and Education

Approaches in the category of personal communication and education include efforts such as classes or health education sessions for patients or other individuals, communication techniques used by health-care providers, and patient navigator programs. Although a review of the field of health education programs is beyond the scope of this report, several studies in Table 6-3 evaluated the effectiveness of education programs or one-on-one communication for individuals with low literacy skills. The study by Paasche-Orlow and colleagues (2003) found that among a groups of adults hospitalized for asthma exacerbation, all of the patients benefited from the one-on-one instruction regarding medications and inhaler technique, and that low health literacy as determined by the Short Test of Functional Health Literacy in Adults (S-TOFHLA) was not related to the need for additional instruction before understanding was achieved (see Table 6-3). In contrast, a study of patients with diabetes by Rothman and colleagues (2003) found that among the control group receiving no intervention, those with higher health literacy as measured by the REALM were more likely to achieve glucose control after 6 months than patients with low literacy, and among the intervention group, there was no difference in glucose control improvement between those with higher and lower health literacy (see Table 6-3). These findings suggest that the intervention was successful at mitigating the adverse effects of limited health literacy. The evaluation by Schillinger and others (2003b) of physician's use of an interactive communication strategy in which the physician assessed patient recall and comprehension is another promising approach for individuals with limited health literacy. They found that the use of this strategy was associated with better glycemic control, although higher health literacy as measured by the S-TOFHLA was also associated with good glycemic control.

Programs using community health workers and patient navigators use one-on-one interaction to assist patients in navigating the health-care system. Such programs show promise for helping to mitigate the effects of limited health literacy since health system navigation has been noted as a particular problem for individuals with limited health literacy. Community health workers are known by various names (including lay health workers, outreach workers, and *promotoras*) and are lay members of the community who work in association with the local health-care system to provide health education, interpret health information, and assist in obtaining access to services. HRSA's Bureau of Primary Health Care plays a large role in training and providing support to community health workers in a number of settings, including farm worker *promotoras* at its Migrant Health Centers.

Patient navigator programs are often run by hospitals or other health-care systems, and many historically have been designed for patients with cancer. One of the first patient navigator programs was initiated by Harold P. Freeman in 1990 at what was then Harlem Hospital Center in New York City. The impetus for the program came from findings by the American Cancer Society that poor people face specific barriers when attempting to seek diagnosis and treatment of cancer and that these barriers result in failure to seek care, or diagnosis at a later—and less treatable—stage of disease. This program seeks to alleviate financial barriers, communication and information barriers, medical system barriers (such as missed appointments and lost results), and fear and emotional barriers by providing a navigator to patients with suspicious results from initial screening tests. The navigator acts as the patient's advocate in the interval between the screening and further diagnosis or treatment, assisting with such practical issues as paperwork for financial support, childcare, or transportation problems. The navigator also may translate medical jargon into understandable language, provide education about the disease and its treatment, assist the patient in communicating with and asking questions of his or her doctor, and be available to listen to fears and concerns (Health Care Association of New York, 2002). Follow-up from the first two years of the program showed that 87.5 percent of patients with navigators completed recommended breast biopsies, while the rate in patients without a navigator was 56.6 percent. Patients with navigators also completed the biopsy in significantly less time than those without navigators (Freeman et al., 1995). The Patient Navigator Program continues at the newly established Ralph Lauren Center for Cancer Care and Prevention in Harlem, and similar programs have since been established in other settings such as Solano County, California, where a Patient Navigator Program was founded in 1999 by the Solano Coalition for Better Health–Community Cancer Task Force (CancerActionNOW.org, 2003) and at the Washington Cancer Institute in Washington, DC.

Combined Approaches

Some approaches to health literacy have incorporated a number of the different types of approaches discussed above into one intervention. A study by Davis and colleagues (1998a) at a public hospital in Louisiana (shown in Table 6-3 above) sought to increase mammography usage in women attending ambulatory and eye clinics. One of the interventions provided a personal recommendation from one of the investigators, an easy-to-read brochure, and a 12-minute education program using a video based on focus groups. Results of this randomized controlled trial showed that this combined approach intervention was the only significant predictor of increased mammography usage at 6 months after controlling for literacy, age, race, and baseline knowledge; patients who received only a recommendation or only a brochure did not show increased mammography usage. Similarly, some promising interventions that have sought to improve understanding for informed consent involve the combined use of simplified written and verbal presentation to help patients better understand and concentrate on the information (Chan et al., 2002; Langdon et al., 2002; Muss et al., 1979; Sorrell, 1991; Tindall et al., 1994; Young et al., 1990). Research about the effectiveness of combining tailored print communications with TDIs remains equivocal, with some studies supporting increased effectiveness while others showed no effect. This research is reviewed in *Speaking of Health* (IOM, 2002c). Molina Healthcare, a managed care organization that focuses on low-income and Medicaid populations, conducted an evaluation of a low-literacy program of this combined type. Families with a child younger than six years of age were randomly assigned to either the control group (n = 13,737 and 5,614 at 2 years) or an intervention group (n = 28,366 and 12,079 at 2 years) that received a self-help book in the mail, plus follow-up reminders. The self-help book was appropriate for low-literacy populations and was intended to supplement information provided by advice nurses that are available by phone to all plan members. Results after two years showed decreases among the intervention group in parents taking their child to the emergency department for fever, rash, and diarrhea/vomiting and increases in parental self-efficacy for the same symptoms. The intervention group also demonstrated a decrease in calls to the advice nurse, and were more likely to still be members of the plan after two years than those in the control group (Ryan, 2003).

Box 6-5 describes a promising combined approach to health literacy that uses written materials, patient educators, provider communication techniques, and follow-up telephone calls.

Tailored Materials

As Chapter 4 emphasizes, culture gives significance to health information and messages and thus approaches to health literacy should consider the background and experiences of people. Patient viewpoints can provide important insights about what, how, when, where, and in what manner information can best be presented. Research on the informed consent process that has looked at the experience from the perspective of the patient has found that this can aid in untangling the complex dynamics associated with the process (Albrecht et al., 2003; Cox, 2002; Ruckdeschel et al., 1996). As Ratzan (2001) points out, the challenge in designing effective and understandable health communications is to determine the optimal context, channels, and content which reflect the realities of people's everyday lives, situations, and communication practices. In this way, messages are

BOX 6-5
Chronic Disease Management Program

Researchers and practitioners at the University of North Carolina have developed several chronic disease management programs that are designed to identify and overcome literacy-related barriers to care. The programs, which include interventions for diabetes, heart failure, chronic pain, and anticoagulation, are led by mid-level providers, mainly clinical pharmacist practitioners, who use evidence-based algorithms, a computerized patient registry, and literacy-independent teaching techniques to facilitate effective self-care and assure receipt of effective services and medications. The teaching techniques are used by clinical pharmacists and trained health educators in a one-on-one interaction with the patient during clinic visits, and feature:

- A teach-back method in which the patient teaches the content back to the educator
- Practical skills rather than complex physiology
- Written educational materials designed for low-literacy users that the educator reviews with the patient
- Follow-up telephone calls and quick visits by the educator when the patient returns to the clinic that serve to reinforce the education
- A collaborative learning environment based on sensitivity to the role of literacy in communication with patients

In each area, the program organizers have systematically measured literacy as well as relevant health outcomes. For diabetes and anticoagulation, completed studies have found that these programs can mitigate the adverse effects of low literacy. Studies in heart failure and chronic pain are ongoing. Their success in improving outcomes has led to stable funding for these programs from the hospital's quality improvement department.

grounded within the sociopolitical and environmental structures of the community and can better reflect the everyday lives of people. Furthermore, health information that is developed from an interdisciplinary approach is more likely to be effective, adopted, and successfully diffused within individual communities (Allen, 2001; Manderson, 1999; Watters, 2003). Project Toolbox is one example of an approach that used the viewpoints and experiences of the intended population to design the program; it is described in Box 6-6.

Similarly, characteristics of the individual patient or the target population can be used to tailor existing materials to fit specific situations. This is frequently done using computer-based algorithms that take various patient characteristics into account. These characteristics might include language, age, gender, ethnicity, reading ability, health literacy level, and the specific

---

BOX 6-6
Description of Project Toolbox

Project Toolbox, funded by the State of Florida in 1999, represented a communication initiative of the H. Lee Moffitt Cancer Center & Research Institute. This project aimed to develop culturally, linguistically, and literacy relevant educational tools for community health-care providers and lay health educators for reaching medically underserved African-American and Hispanic migrant and seasonal farm workers with breast, cervical, and prostate cancer early detection and screening information. Four English and Spanish language toolboxes were created using social marketing and community-participatory research processes (Meade et al., 2002; Meade et al., 2003). Each toolbox contained a videotape, flipchart, educational brochures, and facilitator guide. Materials were written at a grade 3–4 reading level. Concepts were communicated using visuals, testimonials, and pictures that fit the everyday realities of the intended audiences.

---

questions, needs, and goals of the patient at that time. Research on tailored print communications has typically shown that they can improve health outcomes (for review, see Revere and Dunbar, 2001) but research also suggests that they are less effective at influencing individuals who are not thinking about making a behavior change (IOM, 2002c). Hayes (1998) found that patients who received easily readable tailored discharge instructions subsequently performed better on a test of medication knowledge than patients given the standard preprinted instructions (see Table 6-3). Some current approaches that have come to the attention of the committee also use this strategy. For example, the Veterans Administration designed and distributes a "Flu Toolkit" that can be tailored to the educational and cultural needs of specific locales. Another example is currently being investigated by researchers at the University of California–San Francisco. They have developed a simple new communication tool that allows clinicians to print for their patients an individualized, visual medicine schedule (VMS). The VMS is a computer-generated, single page of paper that contains the names and digital images of the prescribed doses of medication, with symbols signifying the daily dosing schedule. The VMS displays the doses on a weekly calendar to accommodate participants with medication doses that differ from day to day. It can be updated and printed by the provider using a color printer and can include instructions in Spanish and Chinese in addition to English.

However, such approaches may not meet the needs of those with limited health literacy. Investigators from the Department of Obstetrics and Gynecology at the University of California–San Francisco have developed and evaluated a computerized, prenatal-testing, decision-assisting tool ("PT

Tool"), which is designed to inform pregnant women (and their partners) about prenatal testing options, and to assist them in making informed choices regarding prenatal testing for chromosomal disorders. The PT Tool provides background information about chromosomal abnormalities and other birth defects, highlighting the personal nature of prenatal testing decisions and the important role of individual preferences and values. The information is tailored for the individual patient, providing individualized risk estimates and allowing women to assess their own preferences and select testing options and strategies about which they would like more information. In a recently completed randomized controlled trial, it was found that women who viewed PT Tool had significantly greater knowledge, more satisfaction, and less decisional conflict than women who viewed a computerized version of the educational pamphlets distributed to pregnant women by the State of California. Furthermore, women viewing PT Tool differed in their testing inclination toward and utilization of prenatal testing. That these effects were particularly strong in college-educated women, raises questions about whether the tool would be effective for individuals with limited health literacy. The investigators are now developing a new, lower-literacy version of PT Tool that will be more engaging and accessible through the use of narrated animations and visual displays.

Partnerships

The increasing complexity of health systems—including new definitions of health, evolution of new media and the discovery of innovative biologic and genomic interventions, as well as the needs of diverse audiences—demands broad, interdisciplinary, multisectoral approaches. An IOM report, *Bridging Disciplines in the Brain: Behavioral and Clinical Sciences*, observes that "Solutions to existing and future health problems will likely require drawing on a variety of disciplines and approaches in which interdisciplinary efforts characterize not only the cutting edge of research but also the utilization of knowledge" (IOM, 2000a: 1).

To advance health literacy, it will be necessary to develop coordinated activities with local programs and institutions that improve quality and access to services, strengthen systems, and formulate effective policies. This includes fostering broad, interdisciplinary approaches to health literacy and supporting the design and management processes necessary to make them successful. Additionally, this requires involvement beyond the traditional health-care system with universities, training institutions, private- and public-sector media, and governmental social service departments.

A number of promising approaches brought to the committee's attention have featured interdisciplinary partnerships. Among the longest running and most well-known of these is the National Literacy and Health Program in Canada which currently involves a partnership among 27 national organizations in Canada and is coordinated by the Canadian Public Health Association. In existence for more than a decade, its objectives are to (1) raise awareness among health professionals about the links between literacy and health; (2) build commitment among participating national health associations to promote literacy and health; and (3) establish links between national health associations and the federal government, literacy organizations, and provincial health associations in order to coordinate action on literacy and health. The program has undertaken a number of major projects such as producing a multimedia training resource for health professionals, providing a literacy and health curriculum for youth, and producing guidelines for prescription medication manufacturers. Although the National Literacy and Health Program has not as yet been evaluated formally (such an evaluation is currently under way), it appears to have had a major impact on both the health professional and literacy community in Canada.

In the United States, federal-level collaborative efforts have revolved around *Healthy People 2010* (HHS, 2000). *Healthy People 2010*, as previously discussed, includes an objective on health literacy which is "to improve the health literacy of persons with marginal or inadequate literacy skills." The Office of the Secretary, ODPHP is the lead agency for this objective, and has been working to identify and coordinate health literacy activities across HHS, to convene HHS agencies to work collaboratively on health literacy, and to identify external partners. In 2000, ODPHP established a partnership with the National Center for Education Statistics, U.S. Department of Education, to develop health literacy measures that are included in the 2003 National Assessment of Adult Literacy. This assessment will provide the first national measures of health literacy. ODPHP has also collaborated with outside organizations on health literacy including the AMA and the Academy of General Dentistry.

Some state- and local-level partnerships also currently exist. For example, the Santa Clara (California) Medical Center, Santa Clara County Library, and Plane Tree Health Library have partnered since 2001 to operate a center for health literacy on the Medical Center campus. The community learning center provides information on a variety of medical topics and conditions in English, Spanish, and Vietnamese in a variety of formats (print, audio, and video) with a focus on easy-to-read materials. The Medical Center provides space readily accessible to patients, the Plane Tree Library provides supervision and expertise in resource development, and the Santa Clara Library recruits adult literacy students to visit the Center and provide literacy support to patrons referred by health-care providers. Since May 2001, more than 2,000 clients have been served.

Summary of Approaches

It can be seen that, as in the survey, most of the examples and studies cited above fall into the category of "simplifying materials," which includes issues of multiple languages and translation, and can be used for enhanced provider–patient communication as well as in other settings. Several of them include the dimension of testing materials with the intended users for understanding and subsequently making appropriate modifications, which the committee has noted is very important. Some work is now in progress to develop nonprint approaches, such as visual aids, computer instruction, and entertainment programs. Many of the federal and some state efforts are in the training area, most notably many of the programs in the multiple bureaus of the HRSA. The emerging partnerships in both the public and private sectors will be critical if sustained and systematic progress is to be made.

When respondents to the survey discussed above were asked an open-ended question about lessons learned from their health literacy activities, three fairly consistent themes about lessons learned emerged:

1. Organizational support and policies are lacking
2. Quality standards are needed
3. A variety of health literacy modalities are needed to be effective

Some comments from survey responders that correspond to each of these themes appear in Box 6-7 to illustrate current sentiment in the field.

This glimpse of ongoing activities from the literature, from the survey, and from testimony and Committee knowledge indicates that concerned organizations and individuals have recognized the complexity of the health literacy problem and have begun to simplify and pilot test materials, and to acknowledge the need to test a wide variety of health literacy approaches. This is a substantial improvement from the 1980s and early 1990s. However, it also highlights the lack of national- and organizational-level policy. Health literacy activities seemed to be based on the interest and determination of a few people within organizations who frequently are not policy makers. Increased awareness and activities related to health literacy appear to spread anecdotally rather than as a result of policy. This type of approach to the problem of limited health literacy is not sufficient to ensure continued interest and improvement in health literacy interventions. The next decade must see a significant increase in the number of programs and approaches that are developed and evaluated, as well as more systematic approaches and partnerships within and across both the public and private sectors.

BOX 6-7
Comments from Respondents to Survey

1. Organizational support and policies are lacking; health-literacy approaches are typically led by a few individuals within organizations.
   - "The most pressing thing in the field right now is that many individuals are trying to make health literacy an issue in their organizations but they lack organizational/management support."
   - "Too many roadblocks exist; policy shifts are needed locally and nationally."
   - "Executive leadership/attention is needed."
   - "Visible department level support is needed for health literacy."
   - "We WANT to serve the American public well . . . but there are certainly a lot of extra bureaucratic hurdles that make this a lot harder than it should be."
   - "As long as consumer communication is marginalized within organizations (an afterthought to the main agenda) health literacy will be ignored."
   - "Healthcare organizations will not invest in health-literacy interventions until someone shows them the business case for doing so."
   - "Having a pharmaceutical company (Pfizer) take ownership is not sufficient and privatized the agenda."
2. Quality standards are needed.
   - "There need to be quality standards for training in this field."
   - "Health literacy needs to be part of staff orientation—at all levels."
   - "Quality standards for designing materials and learning approaches need to be established."
   - "Quality standards are needed to provide the support necessary to make a difference in health-literacy initiatives."
   - "Most health professionals don't know about the issues of health literacy and plain language and can't define either term."
   - "We find that staff develop material that tells too much 'why' when patients need the 'what'."
3. A variety of health-literacy modalities are needed to be effective.
   - "In order to be effective, health messages need to audience-specific and use various modalities."
   - "Developing materials for consumers is a science. Unfortunately, there is not one solution that fits everyone."
   - "Information is only useful if it is appropriate for the intended audience."
   - "Sending a message is not enough, you need to be sure that your message has been conveyed properly."
   - "To be effective health communication needs to involve the intended audience in the development of information/education products."
   - "Language and cultural competence and varied strategies and methods appropriate to the identified audience are key to creating useful materials."

Finding 6-1 Demands for reading, writing, and numeracy skills are intensified because of health-care systems' complexities, advancements in scientific discoveries, and new technologies. These demands exceed the health-literacy skills of most adults in the United States.

Finding 6-2 Health literacy is fundamental to quality care, and relates to three of the six aims of quality improvement described in the IOM *Crossing the Quality Chasm* report: safety, patient-centered care, and equitable treatment. Self-management and health literacy have been identified by IOM as cross-cutting priorities for health-care quality and disease prevention.

Finding 6-3 The readability levels of informed consent documents (for research and clinical practice) exceed the documented average reading levels of the majority of adults in the United States. This has important ethical and legal implications that have not been fully explored.

Recommendation 6-1 Health-care systems, including private systems, Medicare, Medicaid, the Department of Defense, and the Veterans Administration should develop and support demonstration programs to establish the most effective approaches to reducing the negative effects of limited health literacy. To accomplish this, these organizations should:
  • Engage consumers in the development of health communications and infuse insights gained from them into health messages.
  • Explore creative approaches to communicate health information using printed and electronic materials and media in appropriate and clear language. Messages must be appropriately translated and interpreted for diverse audiences.
  • Establish methods for creating health information content in appropriate and clear language using relevant translations of health information.
  • Include cultural and linguistic competency as an essential measure of quality of care.

Recommendation 6-2 HHS should fund research to define the needed health-literacy tasks and skills for each of the priority areas for improvement in health-care quality. Funding priorities should include participatory research that engages the intended populations.

Recommendation 6-3 Health literacy assessment should be a part of health-care information systems and quality data collection. Public and private accreditation bodies, including Medicare, NCQA, and JCAHO, should clearly incorporate health literacy into their accreditation standards.

Recommendation 6-4 HHS should take the lead in developing uniform standards for addressing health literacy in research, service, and training applications. This includes addressing the appropriateness of research design and methods and the match among the readability of instruments, the literacy level, and the cultural and linguistic needs of study participants. In order to achieve meaningful research outcomes in all fields:

- Investigators should involve patients (or subjects) in the research process to ensure that methods and instrumentation are valid and reliable and in a language easily understood.
- NIH should collaborate with appropriate federal agencies and institutional review boards to formulate the policies and criteria to ensure that appropriate consideration of literacy is an integral part of the approval of research involving human subjects.
- NIH should take literacy levels into account when considering informed consent issues in human subjects research. IRBs should meet existing standards related to the readability of informed consent documents.

REFERENCES

Aaronson NK, Visser-Pol E, Leenhouts GH, Muller MJ, van der Schot AC, van Dam FS, Keus RB, Koning CC, ten Bokkel Huinink WW, van Dongen JA, Dubbelman R. 1996. Telephone-based nursing intervention improves the effectiveness of the informed consent process in cancer clinical trials. *Journal of Clinical Oncology.* 14(3): 984–996.

Agre P, McKee K, Gargon N, Kurtz RC. 1997. Patient satisfaction with an informed consent process. *Cancer Practice.* 5(3): 162–167.

Albrecht TL, Ruckdeschel JC, Riddle DL, Blanchard CG, Penner LA, Coovert MD, Quinn G. 2003. Communication and consumer decision making about cancer clinical trials. *Patient Education and Counseling.* 50(1): 39–42.

Allen CE. 2001. 2000 presidential address: Eliminating health disparities. *American Journal of Public Health.* 91(7): 1142–1143.

Appelbaum PS. 1997. Rethinking the conduct of psychiatric research. *Archives of General Psychiatry.* 54(2): 117–120.

Baker LM, Wilson FL. 1996. Consumer health materials recommended for public libraries: Too tough to read? *Public Libraries.* 35: 124–130.

Baker DW, Parker RM, Williams MV, Pitkin K, Parikh NS, Coates W, Imara M. 1996. The health care experience of patients with low literacy. *Archives of Family Medicine.* 5(6): 329–334.

Benitez O, Devaux D, Dausset J. 2002. Audiovisual documentation of oral consent: A new method of informed consent for illiterate populations. *Lancet.* 359(9315): 1406–1407.

Bennett CL, Ferreira MR, Davis TC, Kaplan J, Weinberger M, Kuzel T, Seday MA, Sartor O. 1998. Relation between literacy, race, and stage of presentation among low-income patients with prostate cancer. *Journal of Clinical Oncology.* 16(9): 3101–3104.

Benson JG, Forman WB. 2002. Comprehension of written health care information in an affluent geriatric retirement community: Use of the test of functional health literacy. *Gerontology.* 48(2): 93–97.

Berland GK, Elliott MN, Morales LS, Algazy JI, Kravitz RL, Broder MS, Kanouse DE, Munoz JA, Puyol JA, Lara M, Watkins KE, Yang H, McGlynn EA. 2001. Health information on the Internet: Accessibility, quality, and readability in English and Spanish. *Journal of the American Medical Association.* 285(20): 2612–2621.

Bertakis KD. 1977. The communication of information from physician to patient: A method for increasing patient retention and satisfaction. *Journal of Family Practice.* 5(2): 217–222.

Bodenheimer T. 1999. Disease management—Promises and pitfalls. *New England Journal of Medicine.* 340(15): 1202–1205.

Bray JK, Yentis SM. 2002. Attitudes of patients and anaesthetists to informed consent for specialist airway techniques. *Anaesthesia.* 57(10): 1012–1015.

CancerActionNOW.org. 2003. *CancerActionNOW.org: Compassionate Use for Cancer Patients.* [Online]. Available: http://canceractionnow.org/ [accessed: September, 2003].

CDC (Centers for Disease Control and Prevention). 2003. *About CDC.* [Online]. Available: http://www.cdc.gov/aboutcdc.htm [accessed: October, 2003].

Chan Y, Irish JC, Wood SJ, Rotstein LE, Brown DH, Gullane PJ, Lockwood GA. 2002. Patient education and informed consent in head and neck surgery. *Archives of Otolaryngology–Head and Neck Surgery.* 128(11): 1269–1274.

Cole SA, Bird J. 2000. *The Medical Interview: The Three-Function Approach.* 2nd edition. St Louis: Mosby.

Cooper LA, Roter DL. 2003. Patient-provider communication: The effect of race and ethnicity on process and outcomes in health care. In: *Unequal Treatment: Confronting Racial and Ethnic Disparities in Health Care.* Smedley BD, Stith AY, Nelson AR, Editors. Washington, DC: The National Academies Press. Pp. 336–354.

Cox K. 2002. Informed consent and decision-making: Patients' experiences of the process of recruitment to phases I and II anti-cancer drug trials. *Patient Education and Counseling.* 46(1): 31–38.

Coyne CA, Xu R, Raich P, Plomer K, Dignan M, Wenzel LB, Fairclough D, Habermann T, Schnell L, Quella S, Cella D, Eastern Cooperative Oncology Group. 2003. Randomized, controlled trial of an easy-to-read informed consent statement for clinical trial participation: A study of the Eastern Cooperative Oncology Group. *Journal of Clinical Oncology.* 21(5): 836–842.

Crane JA. 1997. Patient comprehension of doctor-patient communication on discharge from the emergency department. *Journal of Emergency Medicine.* 15(1): 1–7.

Criscione LG, Sugarman J, Sanders L, Pisetsky DS, St Clair EW. 2003. Informed consent in a clinical trial of a novel treatment for rheumatoid arthritis. *Arthritis and Rheumatism.* 49(3): 361–367.

Davis TC, Mayeaux EJ, Fredrickson D, Bocchini JA Jr, Jackson RH, Murphy PW. 1994. Reading ability of parents compared with reading level of pediatric patient education materials. *Pediatrics.* 93(3): 460–468.

Davis TC, Bocchini JA Jr, Fredrickson D, Arnold C, Mayeaux EJ, Murphy PW, Jackson RH, Hanna N, Paterson M. 1996. Parent comprehension of polio vaccine information pamphlets. *Pediatrics.* 97(6 Pt 1): 804–810.

Davis TC, Fredrickson DD, Arnold C, Murphy PW, Herbst M, Bocchini JA. 1998a. A polio immunization pamphlet with increased appeal and simplified language does not improve comprehension to an acceptable level. *Patient Education and Counseling.* 33(1): 25–37.

Davis TC, Holcombe RF, Berkel HJ, Pramanik S, Divers SG. 1998b. Informed consent for clinical trials: A comparative study of standard versus simplified forms. *Journal of the National Cancer Institute.* 90(9): 668–674.

Davis TC, Berkel HJ, Arnold CL, Nandy I, Jackson RH, Murphy PW. 1998c. Intervention to increase mammography utilization in a public hospital. *Journal of General Internal Medicine.* 13(4): 230–233.

Doak LG, Doak CC, Meade CD. 1996. Strategies to improve cancer education materials. *Oncology Nursing Forum.* 23(8): 1305–1312.

Eaton ML, Holloway RL. 1980. Patient comprehension of written drug information. *American Journal of Hospital Pharmacy.* 37(2): 240–243.

Edlin M. 2002. Consumer-Directed Health Care—The goals: More choice, more control. *Healthplan Magazine.* 43(2): 12–17.

Elswick, J (BenefitNews.com). 2003. *Consumer-Driven Health on a Roll.* [Online]. Available: http://www.benefitnews.com/detail.cfm?id=4734&terms=|elswick| [accessed: August, 2003].

FACCT (Foundation for Accountability). 2002. *Who's in the Drivers Seat? Increasing Consumer Involvement in Health Care.* [Online]. Available: http://www.facct.org/facct/doc libFiles/documentFile_528.pdf [accessed: August, 2003].

Federman AD, Cook EF, Phillips RS, Puopolo AL, Haas JS, Brennan TA, Burstin HR. 2001. Intention to discontinue care among primary care patients: Influence of physician behavior and process of care. *Journal of General Internal Medicine.* 16(10): 668–674.

Fiscella K, Franks P, Gold MR, Clancy CM. 2000. Inequality in quality: Addressing socioeconomic, racial, and ethnic disparities in health care. *Journal of the American Medical Association.* 283(19): 2579–2584.

Flores G, Laws MB, Mayo SJ, Zuckerman B, Abreu M, Medina L, Hardt EJ. 2003. Errors in medical interpretation and their potential clinical consequences in pediatric encounters. *Pediatrics.* 111(1): 6–14.

Freda MC, DeVore N, Valentine-Adams N, Bombard A, Merkatz IR. 1998. Informed consent for maternal serum alpha-fetoprotein screening in an inner city population: How informed is it? *Journal of Obstetric, Gynecologic, and Neonatal Nursing.* 27(1): 99–106.

Freeman HP, Muth BJ, Kerner JF. 1995. Expanding access to cancer screening and clinical follow-up among the medically underserved. *Cancer Practice.* 3(1): 19–30.

Gaba AG, Grossman SA. 2003. Braine Readability of informed consent forms at Johns Hopkins Hospital clinical oncology research protocols (1991–1999). *Proceedings of the American Society for Clinical Oncology.* 22: 524.

Gardner AW, Jones JW. 2002. An audit of the current consent practices of consultant orthodontists in the UK. *Journal of Orthodontics.* 29(4): 330–334.

Gerteis M, Edgman-Levitan S, Walker JD, Stoke DM, Cleary PD, Delbanco TL. 1993. What patients really want. *Health Management Quarterly.* 15(3): 2–6.

Goldstein AO, Frasier P, Curtis P, Reid A, Kreher NE. 1996. Consent form readability in university-sponsored research. *Journal of Family Practice.* 42(6): 606–611.

Good BJ, Good MJD. 1981. The meaning of symptoms: A cultural hermeneutic model for clinical practice. In: *The Relevance of Social Science for Medicine.* Eisenberg L, Kleinman A, Editors. Dordecht, Holland: Reidel. Pp. 165–196.

Graber MA, Roller CM, Kaeble B. 1999. Readability levels of patient education material on the World Wide Web. *The Journal of Family Practice.* 48(1): 58–61.

Gribble JN. 1999. Informed consent documents for BRCA1 and BRCA2 screening: How large is the readability gap? *Patient Education and Counseling.* 38(3): 175–183.

Grossman SA, Piantadosi S, Covahey C. 1994. Are informed consent forms that describe clinical oncology research protocols readable by most patients and their families? *Journal of Clinical Oncology.* 12(10): 2211–2215.

Grundner TM. 1980. On the readability of surgical consent forms. *New England Journal of Medicine.* 302(16): 900–902.

Hammerschmidt DE, Keane MA. 1992. Institutional Review Board (IRB) review lacks impact on the readability of consent forms for research. *The American Journal of the Medical Sciences.* 304(6): 348–351.

Hayes KS. 1998. Randomized trial of geragogy-based medication instruction in the emergency department. *Nursing Research.* 47(4): 211–218.

Health Care Association of New York. 2002. *HANYS Breast Cancer Demonstration Project.* [Online]. Available: www.hanys.org/quality_index/Breast_Cancer_Project/pnresourcekit. htm [accessed: September, 2003].

Heffler S, Smith S, Won G, Clemens MK, Keehan S, Zezza M. 2002. Health spending projections for 2001–2011: The latest outlook. Faster health spending growth and a slowing economy drive the health spending projection for 2001 up sharply. *Health Affairs.* 21(2): 207–218.

Hewlett S. 1996. Consent to clinical research—Adequately voluntary or substantially influenced? *Journal of Medical Ethics.* 22(4): 232–237.

HHS (U.S. Department of Health and Human Services). 2000. *Healthy People 2010: Understanding and Improving Health.* Washington, DC: U.S. Department of Health and Human Services. [Online]. Available: http://www.health.gov/healthypeople [accessed: January 15, 2003].

Hochhauser M. 1997. Can your HMO's documents pass the readability test? *Managed Care.* 6(9): 60A, 60G–60H.

Hopper KD, TenHave TR, Hartzel J. 1995. Informed consent forms for clinical and research imaging procedures: How much do patients understand? *American Journal of Roentgenology.* 164(2): 493–496.

Hopper KD, TenHave TR, Tully DA, Hall TE. 1998. The readability of currently used surgical/procedure consent forms in the United States. *Surgery.* 123(5): 496–503.

Horng S, Emanuel EJ, Wilfond B, Rackoff J, Martz K, Grady C. 2002. Descriptions of benefits and risks in consent forms for phase 1 oncology trials. *New England Journal of Medicine.* 347(26): 2134–2140.

Hudman J. 2003. *Understanding the Medicaid and Low-Income Populations: Implications for Health Literacy.* Presentation given at a workshop of the Institute of Medicine Committee on Health Literacy. April 30, 2003, Washington, DC.

Hussey LC. 1994. Minimizing effects of low literacy on medication knowledge and compliance among the elderly. *Clinical Nursing Research.* 3(2): 132–145.

IOM (Institute of Medicine). 1999. *The Unequal Burden of Cancer: An Assessment of NIH Research and Programs for Ethnic Minorities and the Medically Underserved.* Haynes MA, Smedley BD, Editors. Washington, DC: National Academy Press.

IOM. 2000a. *Bridging Disciplines in the Brain, Behavioral, and Clinical Sciences.* Pellmar TC, Eisenberg L, Editors. Washington, DC: National Academy Press.

IOM. 2000b. *To Err Is Human: Building a Safer Health System.* Washington, DC: National Academy Press.

IOM. 2001. *Crossing the Quality Chasm: A New Health System for the 21st Century.* Washington, DC: National Academy Press.

IOM. 2002a. *Care Without Coverage: Too Little, Too Late.* Washington, DC: National Academy Press.

IOM. 2002b. *Health Insurance Is a Family Matter.* Washington, DC: The National Academies Press.

IOM. 2002c. *Speaking of Health: Assessing Health Communication Strategies for Diverse Populations.* Washington, DC: The National Academies Press.

IOM. 2003a. *Unequal Treatment: Confronting Racial and Ethnic Disparities in Health Care.* Smedley BD, Stith AY, Nelson AR, Editors. Washington, DC: The National Academies Press.

IOM. 2003b. *Priority Areas for National Action: Transforming Healthcare Quality.* Adams K, Corrigan JM, Editors. Washington, DC: The National Academies Press.

Jacobson TA, Thomas DM, Morton FJ, Offutt G, Shevlin J, Ray S. 1999. Use of a low-literacy patient education tool to enhance pneumococcal vaccination rates: A randomized controlled trial. *Journal of the American Medical Association.* 282(7): 646–650.

JCAHO (Joint Commission on Accreditation of Healthcare Organizations). 2003. *Facts about the Joint Commission on Accreditation of Healthcare Organizations.* [Online]. Available: http://www.jcaho.org/about+us/index.htm [accessed: October, 2003].

Jubelirer SJ. 1991. Level of reading difficulty in educational pamphlets and informed consent documents for cancer patients. *The West Virginia Medical Journal*. 87(12): 554–557.

Kaiser Commission on Medicaid and the Uninsured. 2003a. *Access to Care for the Uninsured: An Update*. Pub. No. 4142. Washington, DC: The Henry J. Kaiser Family Foundation.

Kaiser Commission on Medicaid and the Uninsured. 2003b. *The Uninsured: A Primer. Key Facts about Americans Without Health Insurance*. Washington, DC: The Henry J. Kaiser Family Foundation.

Kalichman SC, Rompa D. 2000. Functional health literacy is associated with health status and health-related knowledge in people living with HIV-AIDS. *Journal of Acquired Immune Deficiency Syndromes and Human Retrovirology*. 25(4): 337–344.

Kalichman SCP, Ramachandran BB, Catz SP. 1999. Adherence to combination antiretroviral therapies in HIV patients of low health literacy. *Journal of General Internal Medicine*. 14(5): 267–273.

Kasper JF, Mulley AG Jr, Wennberg JE. 1992. Developing shared decision-making programs to improve the quality of health care. *Quality Review Bulletin*. 18(6): 183–190.

Kaufer DS, Steinberg ER, Toney SD. 1983. Revising medical consent forms: An empirical model and test. *Law, Medicine, and Health Care*. 11(4): 155–162.

Kerka S. 2000. *Health and Adult Literacy*. Practice Application Brief No. 7. Columbus, OH: ERIC Clearinghouse on Adult, Career, and Vocational Education.

Kim SP, Knight SJ, Tomori C, Colella KM, Schoor RA, Shih L, Kuzel TM, Nadler RB, Bennett CL. 2001. Health literacy and shared decision making for prostate cancer patients with low socioeconomic status. *Cancer Investigation*. 19(7): 684–691.

King J. 2001. Consent: The patients' view—A summary of findings from a study of patients' perceptions of their consent to dental care. *British Dental Journal*. 191(1): 36–40.

Kleinman A. 1980. *Patients and Healers in the Context of Culture: An Exploration of the Borderland Between Anthropology, Medicine, and Psychiatry*. Berkeley, CA: University of California Press.

Langdon IJ, Hardin R, Learmonth ID. 2002. Informed consent for total hip arthroplasty: Does a written information sheet improve recall by patients? *Annals of the Royal College of Surgeons of England*. 84(6): 404–408.

Lawson SL, Adamson HM. 1995. Informed consent readability: Subject understanding of 15 common consent form phrases. *IRB; A Review of Human Subjects Research*. 17(5–6): 16–19.

Lechter K. 2002. *Patient Information Activities at the FDA*. Presentation given at a workshop of the Institute of Medicine Committee on Health Literacy. December 10, 2002, Washington, DC.

Levit K, Smith C, Cowan C, Lazenby H, Martin A. 2002. Inflation spurs health spending in 2000. *Health Affairs*. 21(1): 172–181.

Levit K, Smith C, Cowan C, Lazenby H, Sensenig A, Catlin A. 2003. Trends in U.S. health care spending, 2001. *Health Affairs*. 22(1): 154–64.

Linzer M, Konrad TR, Douglas J, McMurray JE, Pathman DE, Williams ES, Schwartz MD, Gerrity M, Scheckler W, Bigby JA, Rhodes E. 2000. Managed care, time pressure, and physician job satisfaction: Results from the physician worklife study. *Journal of General Internal Medicine*. 15(7): 441–450.

Lorig KR, Sobel DS, Stewart AL, Brown BW Jr, Bandura A, Ritter P, Gonzalez VM, Laurent DD, Holman HR. 1999. Evidence suggesting that a chronic disease self-management program can improve health status while reducing hospitalization: A randomized trial. *Medical Care*. 37(1): 5–14.

LoVerde ME, Prochazka AV, Byyny RL. 1989. Research consent forms: Continued unreadability and increasing length. *Journal of General Internal Medicine*. 4(5): 410–412.

MacKinnon JR. 1984. Health professionals' patterns of communication: Cross-purpose or problem-solving? *Journal of Allied Health.* 13(1): 3–12.

Mader TJ, Playe SJ. 1997. Emergency medicine research consent form readability assessment. *Annals of Emergency Medicine.* 29(4): 534–539.

Manderson L. 1999. New perspectives in anthropology and cancer control, disease and palliative care. *Anthropology and Medicine.* 6(3): 317–322.

Martin A, Whittle L, Levit K, Won G, Hinman L. 2002. Health care spending during 1991–1998: A fifty-state review. *Health Affairs.* 21(4): 112–126.

Mathew J, McGrath J. 2002. Readability of consent forms in schizophrenia research. *Australian and New Zealand Journal of Psychiatry.* 36(4): 564–565.

Matthews TL, Sewell JC. 2002. *State Official's Guide to Health Literacy.* Lexington, KY: The Council of State Governments.

McCulloch DK, Price MJD, Hindmarsh M, Wagner EH. 2000. Improvement in diabetes care using an integrated population-based approach in a primary care setting. *Disease Management.* 3(2): 75–82.

McManus PL, Wheatley KE. 2003. Consent and complications: Risk disclosure varies widely between individual surgeons. *Annals of the Royal College of Surgeons of England.* 85(2): 79–82.

Meade CD, Byrd JC. 1989. Patient literacy and the readability of smoking education literature. *American Journal of Public Health.* 79(2): 204–206.

Meade CD, Howser DM. 1992. Consent forms: How to determine and improve their readability. *Oncology Nursing Forum.* 19(10): 1523–1528.

Meade CD, Byrd JC, Lee M. 1989. Improving patient comprehension of literature on smoking. *American Journal of Public Health.* 79(10): 1411–1412.

Meade CD, McKinney WP, Barnas GP. 1994. Educating patients with limited literacy skills: The effectiveness of printed and videotaped materials about colon cancer. *American Journal of Public Health.* 84(1): 119–121.

Meade CD, Calvo A, Cuthbertson D. 2002. Impact of culturally, linguistically and literacy relevant cancer information among Hispanic migrant and seasonal farmworkers. *Journal of Cancer Education.* 17: 50–54.

Meade CD, Calvo A, Rivera M, Baer R. 2003. Focus groups in the design of prostate cancer screening information for Hispanic farmworker and African American men. *Oncology Nursing Forum.* 30(6): 967–975.

Meeuwesen L, Bensing J, van den Brink-Muinen A. 2002. Communicating fatigue in general practice and the role of gender. *Patient Education and Counseling.* 48(3): 233–242.

Michielutte R, Bahnson J, Dignan MB, Schroeder EM. 1992. The use of illustrations and narrative text style to improve readability of a health education brochure. *Journal of Cancer Education.* 7(3): 251–260.

Molina C, Zambrana RE, Aguirre-Molina M. 1994. The influence of culture, class, and environment on health care. In: *Latino Health in the U.S.: A Growing Challenge.* Molina C, Aguirre-Molina M, Editors. Washington, DC: American Public Health Association. Pp. 23–43.

Morales LS, Weidmer BO, Hays RD. 2001. Readability of CAHPS® 2.0 Child and Adult Core Surveys. In: *Seventh Conference on Health Survey Research Methods.* Lynamon ML, Kulka RA, Editors. Pub. No. (PHS) 01-1013. Hyattsville, MD: Department of Health and Human Services.

Mulrow C, Bailey S, Sonksen PH, Slavin B. 1987. Evaluation of an Audiovisual Diabetes Education Program: Negative results of a randomized trial of patients with non-insulin-dependent diabetes mellitus. *Journal of General Internal Medicine.* 2(4): 215–219.

Murphy PW, Chesson AL, Walker L, Arnold CL, Chesson LM. 2000. Comparing the effectiveness of video and written material for improving knowledge among sleep disorders clinic patients with limited literacy skills. *Southern Medical Journal.* 93(3): 297–304.

Muss HB, White DR, Michielutte R, Richards F 2nd, Cooper MR, Williams S, Stuart JJ, Spurr CL. 1979. Written informed consent in patients with breast cancer. *Cancer.* 43(4): 1549–1556.

NCI (National Cancer Institute). 1998. *Simplification of Informed Consent Documents.* U.S. Department of Health and Human Services. [Online]. Available: http://www.cancer.gov/clinicaltrials/understanding/simplification-of-informed-consent-docs/ [accessed: September 30, 2003].

Norris SL, Nichols PJ, Caspersen CJ, Glasgow RE, Engelgau MM, Jack L, Isham G, Snyder SR, Carande-Kulis VG, Garfield S, Briss P, McCulloch D. 2002a. The effectiveness of disease and case management for people with diabetes. A systematic review. *American Journal of Preventive Medicine.* 22(4 Supplement): 15–38.

Norris SL, Nichols PJ, Caspersen CJ, Glasgow RE, Engelgau MM, Jack L, Snyder SR, Carande-Kulis VG, Isham G, Garfield S, Briss P, McCulloch D. 2002b. Increasing diabetes self-management education in community settings. A systematic review. *American Journal of Preventive Medicine.* 22(4 Supplement): 39–66.

NRC (National Research Council). 2003. *Safety Is Seguridad: A Workshop Summary.* Washington, DC: The National Academies Press.

O'Connor AM, Rostom A, Fiset V, Tetroe J, Entwistle V, Llewellyn-Thomas H, Holmes-Rovner M, Barry M, Jones J. 1999. Decision aids for patients facing health treatment or screening decisions: Systematic review. *British Medical Journal.* 319(7212): 731–734.

Ogloff JR, Otto RK. 1991. Are research participants truly informed? Readability of informed consent forms used in research. *Ethics and Behavior.* 1(4): 239–252.

Ordovas BJP, Lopez BE, Urbieta SE, Torregrossa S.R., Jimenez TNV. 1999. An analysis of patient information sheets for obtaining informed consent in clinical trials. *Medicina Clinica.* 112(3): 90–94.

Osborne H, Hochhauser M. 1999. Readability and comprehension of the introduction to the Massachusetts Health Care Proxy. *Hospital Topics.* 77(4): 4–6.

Osuna E, Perez-Carceles MD, Perez-Moreno JA, Luna A. 1998. Informed consent. Evaluation of the information provided to patients before anaesthesia and surgery. *Medicine and Law.* 17(4): 511–518.

Osuna E, Lorenzo MD, Perez-Carceles MD, Luna A. 2001. Informed consent: Evaluation of the information provided to elderly patients. *Medicine and Law.* 20(3): 379–384.

Paasche-Orlow M. 2003. Education of patients with asthma and low literacy. Abstract. *Journal of General Internal Medicine.* 18(Supplement 1).

Paasche-Orlow MK, Taylor HA, Brancati FL. 2003. Readability standards for informed-consent forms as compared with actual readability. *New England Journal of Medicine.* 348(8): 721–726.

Pepe MV, Chodzko-Zajko WJ. 1997. Impact of older adults' reading ability on the comprehension and recall of cholesterol information. *Journal of Health Education.* 28(1): 21–27.

Philipson SJ, Doyle MA, Gabram SG, Nightingale C, Philipson EH. 1995. Informed consent for research: A study to evaluate readability and processability to effect change. *Journal of Investigative Medicine.* 43(5): 459–467.

Philipson SJ, Doyle MA, Nightingale C, Bow L, Mather J, Philipson EH. 1999. Effectiveness of a writing improvement intervention program on the readability of the research informed consent document. *Journal of Investigative Medicine.* 47(9): 468–476.

Piette JD. 1999. Satisfaction with care among patients with diabetes in two public health care systems. *Medical Care.* 37(6): 538–546.

Piette JD. 2000. Interactive voice response systems in the diagnosis and management of chronic disease. *The American Journal of Managed Care.* 6(7): 817–827.

Pignone M. 2003. *Literacy and Health: Findings from the Systematic Review for AHRQ. Presentation at the Pfizer Health Literacy Initiative 6th National Conference. Key Advances in Health Literacy: Models for Action.* September 18–19, 2003, Washington, DC.

Pope JE, Tingey DP, Arnold JM, Hong P, Ouimet JM, Krizova A. 2003. Are subjects satisfied with the informed consent process? A survey of research participants. [Comment]. *Journal of Rheumatology.* 30(4): 815–824.

Powell EC, Tanz RR, Uyeda A, Gaffney MB, Sheehan KM. 2000. Injury prevention education using pictorial information. *Pediatrics.* 105(1): e16.

Price S, Raynor DK, Knapp P. 2003. *Developing Effective Medicine Pictograms for the UK. Abstract. Presentation at the Health Services Research and Pharmacy Practice Conference, Belfast.* [Online]. Available: http://hsrpp.org.uk/abstracts/2003_41.shtml [accessed: December 15, 2003].

Raich PC, Plomer KD, Coyne CA. 2001. Literacy, comprehension, and informed consent in clinical research. *Cancer Investigation.* 19(4): 437–445.

Ratzan SC. 2001. Health literacy: Communication for the public good. *Health Promotion International.* 16(2): 207–214.

Reicken HW, Ravich R. 1982. Informed consent to biomedical research in Veterans Administration Hospitals. *Journal of the American Medical Association.* 248: 344–348.

Reid JC, Klachko DM, Kardash CAM, Robinson RD, Scholes R, Howard D. 1995. Why people don't learn from diabetes literature: Influence of text and reader characteristics. *Patient Education and Counseling.* 25(1): 31–38.

Revere D, Dunbar PJ. 2001. Review of computer-generated outpatient health behavior interventions: Clinical encounters "in Absentia." *Journal of the American Medical Informatics Association.* 8: 62–79.

Rivera R, Reed JS, Menius D. 1992. Evaluating the readability of informed consent forms used in contraceptive clinical trials. *International Journal of Gynecology and Obstetrics.* 38(3): 227–230.

Root J, Stableford S. 1999. Easy to read consumer communication: A missing link in medicaid managed care. *Journal of Health Politics, Policy and Law.* 24(1): 1–26.

Rosenbaum S, Sonosky CA, Shaw K, Zakheim MH. 2001. *Negotiating the New Health System: A Nationwide Study of Medicaid Managed Care Contracts.* Shin P, Repasch L, Managing Editors. Center for Health Services Research and Policy, George Washington University.

Ross R. 1996. *Returning to the Teachings: Exploring Aboriginal Justice.* Toronto: Penguin Books.

Rost K, Roter D. 1987. Predictors of recall of medication regimens and recommendations for lifestyle change in elderly patients. *Gerontologist.* 27(4): 510–515.

Rostom A, O'Connor A, Tugwell P, Wells G. 2002. A randomized trial of a computerized versus an audio-booklet decision aid for women considering post-menopausal hormone replacement therapy. *Patient Education and Counseling.* 46(1): 67–74.

Roter DL. 2000. The outpatient medical encounter and elderly patients. *Clinics in Geriatric Medicine.* 16(1): 95–107.

Roter DL, Hall JA. 1992. *Doctors Talking with Patients/Patients Talking with Doctors: Improving Communication in Medical Visits.* Westport, CT: Auburn House.

Roter DL, Stewart M, Putnam SM, Lipkin M Jr, Stiles W, Inui TS. 1997. Communication patterns of primary care physicians. *Journal of the American Medical Association.* 277(4): 350–356.

Roter DL, Stashefsky-Margalit R, Rudd R. 2001. Current perspectives on patient education in the US. *Patient Education and Counseling.* 44(1): 79–86.

Rother HA, London L, Maruping M, Miller S. 2002. *Hazard Communication for Pesticide Safety in Developing Countries: When is the Message Adequate?* Bethesda, MD: Society for Occupational and Environmental Health Conference: Pesticide Exposure and Health.

Rothman RL, Pignone M, Malone R, Bryant B, DeWalt DA, Crigler B. 2003. A longitudinal analysis of the relationship between literacy and metabolic control in patients with diabetes. Abstract. *Journal of General Internal Medicine.* 18(Supplement 1).

Ruckdeschel JC, Albrecht TL, Blanchard C, Hemmick RM. 1996. Communication, accrual to clinical trials, and the physician-patient relationship: implications for training programs. *Journal of Cancer Education.* 11(2): 73–79.

Rudd RE. 2003. Objective 11-2: Improvement of Health Literacy. In: *Communicating Health: Priorities and Strategies for Progress.* Washington, DC: Office of Disease Prevention and Health Promotion, U.S. Department of Health and Human Services.

Rudd RE, DeJong W. 2000. *In Plain Language: The Need for Effective Communication in Medicine and Public Health* [Video]. Cambridge, MA: Harvard University.

Rudd RE, Colton T, Schacht R. 2000. *An Overview of Medical and Public Health Literature Addressing Literacy Issues: An Annotated Bibliography. Report #14.* Cambridge, MA: National Center for the Study of Adult Learning and Literacy

Ryan M. 2003. *Demand Management. Presentation for Molina Healthcare.*

Scala M. 2002. *Linking Health Literacy and Medicare Education.* Presentation given at a workshop of the Institute of Medicine Committee on Health Literacy. December 10, 2002, Washington, DC.

Scandlen, G. (Galen Institute). 2003. *Consumer Driven Health Care: New Tools for a New Paradigm.* [Online]. Available: http://www.galen.org/news/New_Tools.pdf [accessed: August, 2003].

Schillinger D, Grumbach K, Piette J, Wang F, Osmond D, Daher C, Palacios J, Sullivan GaD, Bindman AB. 2002. Association of health literacy with diabetes outcomes. *Journal of the American Medical Association.* 288(4): 475–482.

Schillinger D, Machtinger E, Win K, Wang F, Chan L-L, Rodriguez ME. 2003a. Are pictures worth a thousand words? Communication regarding medications in a public hospital anticoagulation clinic. Abstract. *Journal of General Internal Medicine.* 18(Supplement 1): 187.

Schillinger D, Piette J, Grumbach K, Wang F, Wilson C, Daher C, Leong-Grotz K, Castro C, Bindman AB. 2003b. Closing the loop: Physician communication with diabetic patients who have low health literacy. *Archives of Internal Medicine.* 163(1): 83–90.

Schillinger D, Bindman A, Stewart A, Wang F, Piette J. 2004. Functional health literacy and the quality of physician-patient communication among diabetes patients. *Patient Education and Counseling.* 52(3): 315–323.

Schopp A, Valimaki M, Leino-Kilpi H, Dassen T, Gasull M, Lemonidou C, Scott PA, Arndt M, Kaljonen A. 2003. Perceptions of informed consent in the care of elderly people in five European countries. *Nursing Ethics: An International Journal for Health Care Professionals.* 10(1): 48–57.

Scott TL, Gazmararian JA, Williams MV, Baker DW. 2002. Health literacy and preventive health care use among Medicare enrollees in a managed care organization. *Medical Care.* 40(5): 395–404.

Scrimshaw SC, Hurtado E. 1987. *Rapid Assessment Procedures for Nutrition and Primary Health Care: Anthropological Approaches to Improving Program Effectiveness.* Los Angeles, CA: University of California at Los Angeles, Latin American Center.

Shook EV. 1985. *Ho'oponopono: Contemporary Uses of a Hawaiian Problem-solving Process.* Honolulu, HI: East-West Center, University of Hawaii Press.

Shortell SM, Kaluzny AD, Editors. 2000. *Health Care Management: Organization, Design, and Behavior.* 4th edition. Albany, NY: Delmar Publishers.

Smith H, Gooding S, Brown R, Frew A. 1998. Evaluation of readability and accuracy of information leaflets in general practice for patients with asthma. *British Medical Journal*. 317(7153): 264–265.

Sorrell JM. 1991. Effects of writing/speaking on comprehension of information for informed consent. *Western Journal of Nursing Research*. 13(1): 110–122.

Street RL Jr. 1991. Information-giving in medical consultations: The influence of patients' communicative styles and personal characteristics. *Social Science and Medicine*. 32(5): 541–548.

Sugarman J, McCrory DC, Hubal RC. 1998. Getting meaningful informed consent from older adults: A structured literature review of empirical research. *Journal of the American Geriatrics Society*. 46(4): 517–524.

Sugarman J, Kurtzberg J, Box TL, Horner RD. 2002. Optimization of informed consent for umbilical cord blood banking. *American Journal of Obstetrics and Gynecology*. 187(6): 1642–1646.

Tait AR, Voepel-Lewis T, Malviya S. 2003. Do they understand? (Part II): Assent of children participating in clinical anesthesia and surgery research. *Anesthesiology*. 98(3): 609–614.

Tarnowski KJ, Allen DM, Mayhall C, Kelly PA. 1990. Readability of pediatric biomedical research informed consent forms. *Pediatrics*. 85(1): 58–62.

Tindall B, Forde S, Ross MW, Goldstein D, Barker S, Cooper DA. 1994. Effects of two formats of informed consent on knowledge amongst persons with advanced HIV disease in a clinical trial of didanosine. *Patient Education and Counseling*. 24(3): 261–266.

Triantafyllou K, Stanciu C, Kruse A, Malfertheiner P, Axon A, Ladas SD, European Society of Gastrointestinal Endoscopy. 2002. Informed consent for gastrointestinal endoscopy: A 2002 ESGE survey. *Digestive Diseases*. 20(3–4): 280–3.

USP. 2003. *Drug Information: USP Pictograms*. [Online]. Available: http://www.usp.org/drugInformation/pictograms/. [accessed: June, 2003].

Vinicor F, Burton B, Foster B, Eastman R. 2000. Healthy people 2010: Diabetes. *Diabetes Care*. 23(6): 853–855.

Vohra HA, Ledsham J, Vohra H, Patel RL. 2003. Issues concerning consent in patients undergoing cardiac surgery—The need for patient-directed improvements: A UK perspective. *Cardiovascular Surgery*. 11(1): 64–69.

Von Korff M, Gruman J, Schaefer J, Curry SJ, Wagner EH. 1997. Collaborative management of chronic illness. *Annals of Internal Medicine*. 127(12): 1097–1102.

Wagner EH. 1995. Population-based management of diabetes care. *Patient Education and Counseling*. 26(1–3): 225–230.

Wagner EH, Glasgow RE, Davis C, Bonomi AE, Provost L, McCulloch D, Carver P, Sixta C. 2001. Quality improvement in chronic illness care: A collaborative approach. *The Joint Commission Journal on Quality Improvement*. 27(2): 63–80.

Wallerstein N. 1992. Health and safety education for workers with low-literacy or limited-English skills. *American Journal of Industrial Medicine*. 22(5): 751–65.

Warde C. 2001. Time is of the essence. *Journal of General Internal Medicine*. 16(10): 712–713.

Watters EK. 2003. Literacy for health: An interdisciplinary model. *Journal of Transcultural Nursing*. 14(1): 48–54.

Williams BF, French JK, White HD, HERO-2 consent substudy investigators. 2003. Informed consent during the clinical emergency of acute myocardial infarction (HERO-2 consent substudy): A prospective observational study. *Lancet*. 361(9361): 918–922.

Williams MV, Parker RM, Baker DW, Parikh NS, Pitkin K, Coates WC, Nurss JR. 1995. Inadequate functional health literacy among patients at two public hospitals. *Journal of the American Medical Association*. 274(21): 1677–1682.

Williams MV, Baker DW, Honig EG, Lee TM, Nowlan A. 1998a. Inadequate literacy is a barrier to asthma knowledge and self-care. *Chest*. 114(4): 1008–1015.

Williams MV, Baker DW, Parker RM, Nurss JR. 1998b. Relationship of functional health literacy to patients' knowledge of their chronic disease. A study of patients with hypertension and diabetes. *Archives of Internal Medicine*. 158(2): 166–172.

Wydra EW. 2001. The effectiveness of a self-care management interactive multimedia module. *Oncology Nursing Forum*. 28(9): 1399–1407.

Young DR, Hooker DT, Freeberg FE. 1990. Informed consent documents: increasing comprehension by reducing reading level. *IRB: A Review of Human Subjects Research*. 12(3): 1–5.

7

A Vision for a
Health-Literate America

> My best advice to others with poor reading skills is to not presume but to ask questions. Poor readers need to take responsibility also. We need to learn how to ask questions better. I would recommend more training for us. Remember, we [adult learners] want to be part of the solution.
>
> My best advice to health providers is to think of us as partners. Treat us like partners. Tell us that you need our help too. You might think about setting up training sessions to help staff know how to ask questions that get the best answers. Make sure compassion is part of the training and include us in the training. We can teach along with you. When talking with us, use pictures (those drawn by you are just as good as the fancy ones—even stick figures). Use plain language not medicalese.
>
> Personal story graciously provided by Toni Cordell, Adult Learner and Literacy Advocate, as told to C.D. Meade, September 2003.

The evidence and judgment presented in this report indicate how important improving heath literacy is to improving the health of individuals and populations. This is why the Institute of Medicine identified improving health literacy as one of two cross-cutting issues needing attention in its recent Priority Areas for National Action in Quality Improvement (IOM, 2003), and why the Surgeon General recently stated that "health literacy can save lives, save money, and improve the health and well-being of millions of Americans . . . health literacy is the currency of success for everything I am doing as Surgeon General" (Carmona, 2003).

As the report also indicates, much more needs to be known about the causal pathways between education and health and the more specific role of literacy, as well as the discrete contribution of health literacy. As a result, we will then be in a position to understand which interventions and approaches are the most appropriate and effective. This Committee believes that a health-literate America is an achievable goal. We envisage a society in which people have the skills that they need to obtain, interpret, and use health information effectively, and within which a wide variety of health systems and institutions take responsibility for providing clear communication and adequate support to facilitate health-promoting actions. Specifically, we believe a health-literate America would be a society in which:

- everyone has the opportunity to improve their health literacy.
- everyone has the opportunity to use reliable, understandable information that could make a difference in their overall well-being, including everyday behaviors such as how they eat, whether they exercise, and whether they get checkups.
- health and science content would be basic parts of K-12 curricula,
- people are able to accurately assess the credibility of health information presented by health advocate, commercial, and new media sources.
- there is monitoring and accountability for health literacy policies and practices.
- public health alerts, vital to the health of the nation, are presented in everyday terms so that people can take needed action.
- the cultural contexts of diverse peoples, including those from various cultural groups and non-English-speaking peoples, are integrated into all health information.
- health practitioners communicate clearly during all interactions with their patients, using everyday vocabulary.
- there is ample time for discussions between patients and health-care providers.
- patients feel free and comfortable to ask questions as part of the healing relationship.
- rights and responsibilities in relation to health and health care are presented or written in clear, everyday terms so that people can take needed action.
- informed consent documents used in health care are developed so that all people can give or withhold consent based on information they need and understand.

While achieving this vision is a profound challenge, we believe that significant progress can and must be made over the coming years so that the potential of optimal health can benefit all individuals and populations in our society.

REFERENCES

Carmona RH. 2003. *Health Literacy in America: The Role of Health Care Professionals. Prepared Remarks given at the American Medical Association House of Delegates Meeting.* Saturday, June 14, 2003. [Online]. Available: http://www.surgeongeneral.gov/news/speeches/ama061403.htm [accessed: August 2003].

IOM (Institute of Medicine). 2003. *Priority Areas for National Action: Transforming Healthcare Quality.* Adams K, Corrigan JM, Editors. Washington, DC: The National Academies Press.

A

Data Sources and Methods

In order to respond to the study charge, several steps were undertaken to define the scope of the problem of limited health literacy, identify obstacles to creating a health-literate public, assess the approaches that have been attempted, and identify goals for health literacy efforts. Sources of data and information included the expertise of the committee members, literature reviews and Internet searches of principal concepts, informal interviews, commissioned works, hosting of several public workshops, and other invited presentations.

STUDY COMMITTEE

An 11-member study committee was convened to assess available data and respond to the study charge. The committee included members with expertise in public health, primary medical care, health communication, sociology, anthropology, adult literacy education, and K-12 education. The committee convened for six 2-day meetings on October 21–22, 2002; December 10–11, 2002; February 13–14, 2003; April 29–30, 2003; June 16–17, 2003; and September 11–12, 2003. Biographies of individual committee members appear in Appendix D.

LITERATURE REVIEW

The committee conducted extensive literature reviews and Internet searches regarding health literacy and related topics. The literature reviewed in this report represents diverse fields and academic disciplines. In particular, Institute of Medicine (IOM) staff used in-house databases, including Academic Premier Search, Medline, ERIC,[1] PsychInfo, Sociological Abstracts, and CINAHL[2] to identify relevant peer-reviewed literature. Keyword searches include the following: "health literacy," "literacy and health," and "reading and health." Additional studies for consideration were identified through testimony to the committee by experts in the field.

PUBLIC WORKSHOPS

The study committee hosted three 1-day public workshops in order to obtain input from various stakeholders, consumers, and researchers. These workshops were held in conjunction with three of the six committee meetings mentioned above.

The first public workshop of the committee was held on December 10–11, 2002 in Washington, DC. This workshop focused on health literacy-related activities in federal government agencies, academia, and other relevant organizations. Michael Pignone, M.D., M.P.H., Assistant Professor of Medicine at the University of North Carolina, Chapel Hill, School of Medicine, presented information about an ongoing research project sponsored by the Agency for Health Care Research and Quality intended to review the evidence base of health literacy research. Arlene S. Bierman, M.D., M.S., from the Center of Outcomes and Effectiveness Research, Agency for Healthcare Research and Quality, spoke about health disparities and health literacy. Lawrence J. Fine, M.D., Dr. P.H., of the Office of Behavioral and Social Science Research at the National Institutes of Health, discussed how health literacy relates to other areas in health such as health disparities, behavioral change, and socioeconomic determinants of health such as education. Cynthia Baur, Ph.D., of the U.S. Department of Health and Human Services, spoke about federal involvement in health literacy efforts and how to leverage existing work that is relevant to the field. Anthony Tirone, J.D., from the Joint Commission on Accreditation of Healthcare Organizations (JCAHO), discussed some of the work of JCAHO that has implications for how health systems respond to health literacy. Marisa Scala, M.G.S., from the Center for Medicare Education of the American Association of Homes and Services for the Aging, talked about the specific needs of the Medicare population as they relate to health literacy. Karen Lechter, J.D., Ph.D., from the Center for Drug Evaluation and Research of the U.S. Food and Drug Administration (FDA) provided an

---

[1]Educational Resources Information Center.
[2]Cumulative Index to Nursing and Allied Health Literature.

overview of the activities of the FDA and their relevance to health literacy. Lauren Schwartz, M.P.H., from the New York City Poison Control Center shared background about and lessons from a program educating adult learners about medications. Linda Morse, R.N., M.A., from the New Jersey Office of Academic and Professional Standards discussed current activity in the educational sector to improve health literacy, including efforts specific to New Jersey, such as the New Jersey Core Curriculum Content Standards for Comprehensive Health and Physical Education, which are currently being implemented. Judy A. Shea, Ph.D., from the University of Pennsylvania School of Medicine, shared findings about a recent research project looking at the interplay between health literacy and patient satisfaction with different modes of health-related communication. Finally, Tina Tucker, M.A., M.Ed., RTC, from the National Program in Literacy, American Foundation for the Blind, discussed the health needs and desires of individuals who are visually impaired and low literate. The agenda for this workshop is shown in Box A-1.

The third meeting of the committee was held on February 13–14, 2003, at the Arnold and Mabel Beckman Center of the National Academies in Irvine, California, and a public workshop was held in conjunction with this meeting. On the afternoon of February 13, the committee heard from representatives of consumer and advocacy groups, as well as several experts in the areas of literacy, communication, and chronic diseases. Dean Schillinger, M.D., from the University of California–San Francisco spoke about the relationships between care for patients with chronic diseases, health literacy, and quality of care, with a specific emphasis on the role of patient–physician communication in determining quality of care. Tetine Sentell, M.A., of the University of California–Berkeley presented new analyses of data from the National Adult Literary Survey. Susan M. Shinagawa, from the Asian and Pacific Islander National Cancer Survivors Network, and Heng L. Foong, of the Pacific Asian Language Services for Health, highlighted the most critical health literacy issues facing Asian Americans and Pacific Islanders today, with an emphasis on issues of health and doctor-patient communication in populations with limited English that represent native speakers of diverse languages. Rita Hargrave, M.D., of the University of California–Davis and Veterans Medical Center of Northern California, discussed mental health care, ethnicity, and health literacy, and the influence of physician and patient communication styles and preferences. Alvin Billie, of the Family Learning Center and the Gathering Place in New Mexico, discussed the unique health literacy issues facing Native Americans, and addressed the effect of large cultural differences on doctor-patient communication, as well as approaches to the problems created by these cultural differences. Francis Prado and Francisco Para, from Latino Health Access based in Santa Ana, California, described health literacy

BOX A-1
First Workshop Hosted by the Committee on Health Literacy

Date: December 10–11, 2003
Location: Keck Center of the National Academies
             500 5th Street, NW
             Washington, D.C.

December 10, 2003

1:00 p.m.   **Report from the AHRQ Evidence-Based Practice Center Report**
             on Health Literacy
             Michael Pignone, M.D., M.P.H.
             Assistant Professor of Medicine, University of North Carolina at
             Chapel Hill School of Medicine

1:20 p.m.   **Health Literacy and Health Disparities: Assessing Health**
             Outcomes and Quality of Care
             Arlene S. Bierman, M.D., M.S.
             Senior Research Physician, Center of Outcomes and Effectiveness
             Research, Agency for Healthcare Research and Quality

1:50 p.m.   **Education Pathways to Health: Health Literacy**
             Lawrence J. Fine, M.D., Dr.Ph., Medical Advisor
             Office of Behavioral and Social Science Research, National
             Institutes of Health

2: 00 p.m.   **The Federal Sector and Health Literacy**
             Cynthia Baur, Ph.D.
             Health Communication and e-Health Advisor, U.S. Department of
             Health and Human Services

2:30 p.m.   **Activities of the Joint Commission to Improve Health Literacy**
             Anthony Tirone, J.D.
             Director of Federal Relations, Joint Commission on Accreditation of
             Healthcare Organizations

3:00 p.m.   **Break**

challenges in Latin American populations based on their experiences as community health workers, emphasizing how the different experiences of patients and doctors affect the meaning in their communication, resulting in less effective health care. The agenda for this meeting is presented in Box A-2.

At the fourth meeting of the committee, a public workshop was held with representatives of health-care system organizations and consumer groups, as well as experts on the research base on health literacy and on the legal issues surrounding health literacy. This workshop took place on April

3:15 p.m.   **Linking Health Literacy and Medicare Education**
            Marisa Scala, M.G.S.
            Executive Director, Center for Medicare Education, American
            Association of Homes and Services for the Aging

3:45 p.m.   **Patient Information Activities at the FDA**
            Karen Lechter, J.D., Ph.D.
            Social Science Analyst, Center for Drug Evaluation and Research,
            U.S. Food and Drug Administration

4:15 p.m.   **General Discussion and Public Comment**

5:00 p.m.   **Adjourn**

December 11, 2003

8:30 a.m.   **Health Education Literacy Program: A Medicine Safety Program
            for Adult Learners**
            Lauren Schwartz, M.P.H.
            Community Health Educator, New York City Poison Control Center

9:15 a.m.   **Improving Health Literacy: An Educational Response to a
            Public Health Problem**
            Linda Morse
            Director, New Jersey Office of Academic and Professional Standards

10:00 a.m. **Development of Patient Satisfaction Survey Materials for
            Low-Literacy Consumers**
            Judy A. Shea
            University of Pennsylvania School of Medicine

10:45 a.m. **Health Management Solutions for Adults Who Are Visually
            Impaired and Have Low Literacy Skills**
            Tina Tucker
            American Foundation for the Blind

11:30 a.m. **Discussion**

12:30 a.m. **Adjourn**

29, 2003, at the Keck Center of the National Academies in Washington, DC. Michael Pignone, Ph.D., of the University of North Carolina at Chapel Hill presented updated information about an ongoing study on the health literacy research database sponsored by the Agency for Healthcare Research and Quality. Julie Hudman, Ph.D., from the Kaiser Commission on Medicaid and the Uninsured of the Henry J. Kaiser Family Foundation spoke about the health literacy issues confronting Medicaid and low-income individuals. Joanne Schwartzberg, M.D., of the American Medical Association (AMA), discussed the ongoing efforts of the AMA to educate

---

BOX A-2
Second Workshop Hosted by the
Committee on Health Literacy

Date: February 13, 2003
Location: Arnold and Mabel Beckman Center of the National Academies,
            Irvine, CA

3:00 p.m.   **Literacy and Chronic Disease Care: New Research Insights and**
            Reflections on Quality Standards
            Dean Schillinger, M.D.
            Associate Professor of Medicine, University of California–San
                Francisco, San Francisco General Hospital Medical Center

3:45 p.m.   **Relationships Between Literacy, Race, Age, Education, and**
            Health in a National Sample: An Extension of NALS Analyses
            Tetine Sentell, M.A.
            Ph.D. Candidate, University of California, Berkeley

4:00 p.m.   **Health Literacy Concerns for Asian Americans & Pacific**
            Islanders: Challenges and Opportunities
            Susan M. Shinagawa
            Patient Advocate and Founder, Asian and Pacific Islander National
                Cancer Survivors Network

            Heng L. Foong
            Patient Advocate and Program Director, Pacific Asian Language
                Services for Health

4:15 p.m.   **The Interplay of Ethnicity and Health Literacy in Mental Health-**
            care
            Rita Hargrave, M.D.
            Assistant Professor of Psychiatry, Department of Psychiatry,
                University of California, Davis, Veterans Medical Center of
                Northern California System of Clinics

4:30 p.m.   **Health and Literacy—A Native American Point of View**
            Alvin Billie
            Program Manager, The Gathering Place, Thoreau, NM

4:45 p.m.   **Health Care Barriers in the Latino Community of Orange County**
            Francis Prado, Francisco Para
            Health Educators and Promotoras, Latino Health Access

5:00 p.m.   **Discussion**

5:30 p.m.   **Adjourn**

---

health professionals about health literacy. Frank M. McClellan, J.D., a professor at the Temple University James E. Beasley School of Law, provided background on the legal precedents and legal and ethical implications of health literacy and informed consent. Joyce Dubow, M.U.P., of

AARP, spoke about health literacy issues related to Medicare beneficiaries. L. Natalie Carroll, M.D., of the National Medical Association, presented information on African Americans and health literacy, and described the positions and efforts of the National Medical Association in the area. Finally, Eduardo Crespi, R.N., from Centro Latino de Salud in Missouri, discussed health literacy needs of the Latin American population served by Centro Latino, and described some of the programs available to address those needs. The agenda for this workshop is presented in Box A-3.

BOX A-3
Third Workshop Hosted by the Committee on Health Literacy

Date: April 29, 2003
Location: Keck Center of the National Academies, Washington, DC

2:00 p.m. **Understanding the Medicaid and Low-Income Population: Implications for Health Literacy**
Julie Hudman, Ph.D.
Associate Director, Kaiser Commission on Medicaid and the Uninsured, Henry J. Kaiser Family Foundation

2:30 p.m. **Low Health Literacy: Increasing Physician Awareness of an Emerging Issue**
Joanne Schwartzberg, M.D.
Director of Aging and Community Health, American Medical Association

3:00 p.m. **Legal Implications of Health Literacy**
Frank M. McClellan, J.D.
I. Herman Stern Professor of Law, Temple University James E. Beasley School of Law

3:30 p.m. **Break**

3:45 p.m. **Health Literacy Among Medicare Beneficiaries**
Joyce Dubow, M.U.P.
Senior Policy Advisor, Public Policy Institute, AARP

4:15 p.m. **African Americans and Health Literacy**
L. Natalie Carroll, M.D.
President, National Medical Association

4:45 p.m. **Health Literacy and the Midwestern Latino Community**
Eduardo Crespi, R.N.
Executive Director, Centro Latino de Salud, Columbia, MO

5:15 p.m. **Discussion**

5:45 p.m. **Adjourn**

COMMISSIONED PAPERS AND BACKGROUND INFORMATION

The committee commissioned several papers and research projects in order to fill gaps in the available evidence base. Three of the papers can be found in Appendix B, and input from other consultants has been integrated into the report. The committee commissioned work from Terry Davis of Louisiana State University, Julie Gazmararian of Emory University, David H. Howard of Emory University, Frank McClellan of Temple University School of Law, Dean Schillinger of University of California–San Francisco, and Barry D. Weiss of the University of Arizona College of Medicine. Davis and Gazmararian collaborated to examine some promising approaches to health literacy; background and methodology of their work is discussed further below. Howard was commissioned to look at the economic implications of limited health literacy in a Medicare population. His paper is included in Appendix B, and provides important information for the discussion in Chapter 3 concerning the associations of limited health literacy. McClellan spoke to the committee and provided information about legal issues that are important to consider with health literacy. This information provides the basis for the section on health law that appears in Chapter 6. Schillinger examined chronic disease care for patients with limited health literacy from a health systems perspective. His work on informed consent is cited in Chapter 6, and can be found in Appendix B. Weiss provided a piece considering the different stakeholders in the health literacy discussion; this work can also be found in Appendix B.

This section presents the methodology used for two of the research activities commissioned by the committee from outside consultants that are not separately presented in a paper: (1) a review of approaches to health literacy not found in the published literature, and (2) a compilation of the federal funding for health literacy projects over the past 10 years.

Approaches to Improving Health Literacy: Lessons from the Field

The committee commissioned a project from Terry Davis, M.D., Louisiana State University Health Sciences Center, and Julie Gazmararian, Ph.D., Emory University, to look at approaches to improving health literacy that are currently being used and may not be reflected in the peer-reviewed literature. Findings from this project are discussed in Chapter 6. Drs. Davis and Gazmararian, and IOM staff, identified key individuals or organizations that should be contacted to inquire about health literacy activities in which they were involved. The selection process was not intended to result in a complete survey of approaches to health literacy, but rather to identify a sample of key organizations that could make a difference in the field of health literacy. The types of organizations that were targeted included federal and state government agencies, pharmaceutical companies, national organizations, foundations, and local service providers. IOM staff identified a contact person to respond from each organization. Individuals identified for possible participation in the survey were those who were aware of health literacy. We also decided to elicit information on health literacy activities from the National Institute for Literacy (NIFL)-health listserv (see www.nifl.gov for more information).

Terry Davis and Julie Gazmararian developed a 5-minute, 15-question, web-based survey to send to selected individuals. This instrument was developed on the basis of a previous survey by the Council of State Governments to assess health literacy activities at the state level (Matthews and Sewell, 2002). Information collected included: whether health literacy is considered in program development and service activities; the degree to which organizations follow health literacy principles in their programs; target audience(s) for activities; whether organizations pilot test materials for comprehension or cultural competence; evaluation of materials; which activities people associate with health literacy and lessons learned.

The Internet service www.zoomerang.com was used to create the web-based survey because it provides low-cost, web-based survey implementation tools. IOM staff sent an e-mail message with a web link to the original list of 101 individuals identified, and to the NIFL-health listserv, which has 568 members. The survey was open for 10 days. No follow-up reminders were sent to the designated individuals or the listserv.

Figure A-1 outlines the response to the survey. Of the 101 individuals e-mailed, 7 e-mails were undeliverable, leaving 94 individuals directly contacted. Including respondents from the listserv, we received completed surveys from 95 individuals; 33 of these were from the initial list of individuals, and 62 were from the listserv.

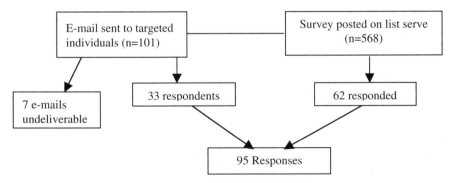

FIGURE A-1   Response to web-based survey.

Respondents came from state and federal government agencies, associations, foundations, health-care organizations, institutes of higher education, community/advocacy groups, adult education programs, and literacy businesses (see Table A-1).

TABLE A-1   Summary of Respondents and Nonrespondents to Survey

E-mailed Survey Respondents	NIFL Listserv Respondents
Asian American Network for Cancer Awareness, Research and Training	American Institutes for Research
American Academy of Family Physicians Foundation	American Society on Aging
	Ball Memorial Family Practice Residency
American Academy of Neurology	Blue Cross Blue Shield of Michigan
American Medical Association	Bronson Healthcare Group
Agency for Toxic Substances and Disease Registry (CDC)	Brown University, Center for Environmental Studies
California HealthCare Foundation	Butler University–College of Pharmacy
California Literacy, Inc.	Cambridge Health Alliance
Center for Medicare Education	Centers for Disease Control and Prevention
Centers for Disease Control and Prevention	Center for Health Care Strategies
Centro Latino de Salud	CHOICE Regional Health Network
Food and Drug Administration	Clear Language Group
Martinez VA Outpatient Clinic	Dartmouth-Hitchcock Medical Center
Mettger Communications	Eastern Massachusetts Literacy Council
National Cancer Institute	EasyRead Copywriting
National Program Office, Hablamos Juntos	Emory University School of Medicine/ Grady Hospital
National Cancer Institute's Cancer Information Service of New York	En Memphis, Hablamos Juntos
National Institute on Deafness and Other Communication Disorders (NIH)	Environmental Toxicology Program, Maine Bureau of Health
New York City Poison Control Center	Family Health Research
Pfizer, Inc.	Georgia Department of Technical & Adult Education
The Gathering Place	Hablamos Juntos
U.S. Department of Health and Human Services	Harris School of Nursing, Texas Christian University
U.S. Food and Drug Administration, Los Angeles District	Health Literacy Center, University of New England
University of North Texas Health Science Center	Health Literacy Consulting
University of Virginia School of Medicine	Home Health VNA
	Health Resources and Services Administration
	Inova Health System
	Kootenai Medical Center Medical Library
	Literacy Assistance Center
	Literacy Volunteers of Santa Fe

TABLE A-1 Continued

E-mailed Survey Respondents	NIFL Listserv Respondents
	Massachusetts Department of Public Health
	Mayfield Adult Basic and Literacy Education
	Molina Healthcare, Inc.
	National Alliance for the Mentally Ill (NAMI)
	National Institutes of Health
	National Marrow Donor Program
	National Cancer Institute—Office of Education and Special Initiatives
	Neighborhood Health Plan of Rhode Island
	National Institute of Neurological Disorders and Stroke (NIH)
	New York City Department of Health and Mental Hygiene
	Parma Adult Basic and Literacy Education
	Queens Library
	Rancho Los Amigos National Rehabilitation Center
	Saint Eugene Medical Center
	Santa Clara Valley Medical Center
	Section of Patient Education Mayo Clinic Rochester
	Southwest Washington Medical Center
	St. Joseph Regional Health Center
	Temple University Health System
	The Catholic University of America School of Nursing
	The Ohio State University
	The Robert Wood Johnson Foundation
	University of Texas
	University of North Carolina School of Medicine
	University of Pennsylvania
	University of South Carolina School of Medicine
	University of Tennessee Extension Service
	University of Texas Health Science Center
	Virginia Adult Learning Resource Center
	Vision Literacy
	Wayne State University

NOTE: The same organization can be found in different categories because separate individuals may or may not have completed the survey.

Federal Funding for Health Literacy over a 10-Year Period

Patrick Weld, M.S.W., M.P.A., L.G.S.W., of the National Cancer Institute (NCI), with the assistance of K. Vish Visnawath, Ph.D., also of NCI, provided the committee with a table of federal funding of health literacy-related projects over the past 10 years. The data were derived from a search of the NIH CRISP database; searches for each fiscal year from 1993 to 2002 used the following operands: "health literacy," "health and literacy," "health and readability," and "literacy and readability." The grants retrieved were examined for relevance to the field of health literacy, and financial information was obtained.

Results were then downloaded into Portfolio Management Application software developed by Department of Cancer Control and Population Science of the National Institutes of Health for identification and deletion of duplicate grants, and linkage to financial data. A total of 906 grants for the 10-year period were identified. Because of a technology change in 1995–1996, 229 of the grants could not be linked to financial data. Thus, the early years of the search results (1993–1996) contain missing financial data. While Drs. Weld and Viswanath were able to identify all of the missing grants, further work to access the financial data for those grants was not successful.

The information for the remaining 667 grants available was downloaded into an Excel spreadsheet for further manipulation. The awarded grants were identified, and unawarded grants were excluded, bringing the final count of grants to 565. This information has been compiled into yearly federal grant funding (new and continuing grants) over a 10-year period, and is presented in Chapter 6.

REFERENCE

Matthews TL, Sewell JC. 2002. *State Official's Guide to Health Literacy*. Lexington, KY: The Council of State Governments.

B

Commissioned Papers

CONTENTS

255

The Relationship Between
Health Literacy and Medical Costs

David H. Howard, Ph.D.

INTRODUCTION

Past research has shown that individuals with low levels of health literacy are more likely to be hospitalized and have worse disease outcomes (Baker et al., 1998, 2002; Schillinger et al., 2002). The major obstacle to extending these results by examining the relationship between health literacy and spending is the lack of data containing measures of both. Some insight about the impact of health literacy on costs can be gleaned from studies that examine the impact of years of schooling on medical costs, but health literacy is a fundamentally different concept from educational attainment (Davis et al., 1994; Stedman and Kaestle, 1991). At least one study has examined the association between general literacy and costs (Weiss et al., 1994). It found no relationship, though the sample size was small (N = 402) and not representative of the overall U.S. population (over half the study subjects qualified for Medicaid because of disability). Furthermore, inpatient and outpatient costs were not analyzed separately and the analysis did not control for confounding patient characteristics. Another paper by the same author (Weiss) shows large differences in costs by grade reading level in a Medicaid population (Weiss, 1999), but descriptions of the methods and data are not available. This study examines the relationship between health literacy and costs using a unique dataset combining cost information from an administrative claims file and a health literacy measure from a beneficiary survey. Multivariate techniques are used to adjust for underlying differences in respondents' characteristics.

Data Description

Health literacy data were collected as part of a survey of persons enrolling in a Prudential Medicare health maintenance organization between December of 1996 and August of 1997 in one of four locations: Cleveland, Ohio; Houston, Texas; South Florida (including Fort Lauderdale, Miami, and nearby areas); and Tampa, Florida. New Prudential Medicare members were contacted three months after enrollment, and those meeting the eligibility criterion were asked to complete an in-person survey. In order to be included in the study, members had to be comfortable speaking either English or Spanish, living in the community, and possess adequate visual and cognitive function. The survey included the Short Test of Functional

Health Literacy in Adults (S-TOFHLA) (Parker et al., 1995), a series of questions designed to measure health literacy. A detailed description of the survey and data has been published elsewhere (Gazmararian et al., 1999).

Prudential administrative claims databases were used to compute annual health expenditures from the date of enrollment for all eligible enrollees by site of service (inpatient, outpatient, emergency room, and pharmacy). The claims database includes costs for all medical services used by enrollees associated with insurance reimbursement. The cost for each service is the sum of Prudential's reimbursement and the beneficiary's out-of-pocket payment.

Table B-1 presents evidence on how closely the study sample represents the U.S. population of health-care consumers. The first column of the table presents summary statistics for the 3,260 responders, the second for the 3,245 nonresponders, and the third for participants of comparable age in the household component of the 1997 Medical Expenditure Panel Survey (MEPS) (for a description see Cohen et al., 1996–1997). Differences between samples were assessed using one-way analysis of variance (ANOVA) tests by group for three-sample comparisons of continuous variables and chi-squared tests for two-sample comparisons of binary variables. ANOVA tests for differences in the cost variables were performed on the natural

TABLE B-1 Representativeness of the Study Sample

| | Prudential | | | |
	Responders	Nonresponders	MEPS 97	P-value
Inpatient costs	$5,321	$4,512	$2,276	<0.01
Outpatient costs	$1,837	$1,547	$1,203	<0.01
ER costs	$131	$115	$124	<0.01
Pharmacy costs	$677	$655	$743	<0.01
Age	72.8±6.4	73.3±6.8	74.6±6.8	<0.01
Schooling				
12 years	34%	no data	31%	0.03
>12 years	31%	no data	28%	0.03
Need help				
with ADLs	5%	no data	9%	<0.01
Need help with				
IADLs	31%	no data	16%	<0.01
N	3,260	3,245	3,833	

NOTE: Age row reports mean ± standard deviation.

logarithm of costs to make the variable conform to the normality assumption underlying the F-test.

Compared to nonresponders and the MEPS sample, responders incurred higher inpatient, outpatient, emergency room, and pharmacy expenditures. There were also small differences in average age (0.5 years) and the proportion with more than 12 years of schooling. Compared to MEPS respondents, Prudential respondents were less likely to need assistance with at least one activity of daily living but more likely to need assistance with at least one instrumental activity of daily living. Differences in survey administration may account for some of these inconsistencies (Wiener et al., 1990).

Spending differences between the Prudential population and the MEPS sample, which is nationally representative, may reflect the fact that study participants reside primarily in large urban areas, where reimbursement rates tend to be higher. South Florida, one of the locales from which respondents were drawn, is known to have the highest level of per beneficiary Medicare spending in the country (Center for Evaluative Clinical Sciences, 1998). The study population may also differ in health status. While Medicare managed care plans tend to enroll a healthier mix of beneficiaries compared to the traditional Medicare program (Hellinger and Wong, 2000), managed care plans that offer generous prescription drug coverage or require little in the way of cost-sharing may attract beneficiaries with chronic conditions. A final explanation for the cost differences is that MEPS fails to capture a large portion of spending for Medicare beneficiaries due to restrictive sampling criteria (Selden et al., 2001).

Raw S-TOFLHA score were converted to a discreet categorical variable for purposes of analysis (Baker et al., 1999). Persons scoring 67 and above on the S-TOFHLA were classified as having "adequate" health literacy and those scoring 66 or below were classified as having "inadequate" health literacy. Previous studies have distinguished between a "marginal" health literacy group, with scores between 56 and 66, and an "inadequate" group, with scores 55 or below (Baker et al., 2000). This study combined data from the marginal and inadequate groups to increase statistical power, as no significant cost differences were found between these two groups in preliminary analyses.

Table B-2 displays detailed summary statistics by health literacy level for the responders. Differences between groups were assessed using chi-squared tests for binary variables and t-tests for continuous variables. Persons with inadequate health literacy had lower incomes and fewer years of schooling. More Caucasian subjects had adequate than inadequate health literacy, while more African Americans and Spanish-speaking Hispanics had inadequate health literacy. Physical and mental quality-of-life, as mea-

TABLE B-2 Characteristics of the Study Sample

	Literacy		
	Adequate	Inadequate	P-value
Age	71.6±5.6	75.1±6.9	<0.01
Female	58%	57%	n.s.
Race			
White	84%	61%	<0.01
Black	7%	22%	<0.01
Hispanic, English speaking	2%	2%	n.s.
Hispanic, Spanish speaking	7%	14%	<0.01
Other	1%	1%	n.s.
Income			
No response	14%	20%	<0.01
<$10K	12%	29%	<0.0
$10K–$25K	50%	42%	<0.01
>$25K	24%	9%	<0.01
Schooling			
<8 years	7%	36%	<0.01
9–11 years	15%	25%	<0.01
12 years	38%	25%	<0.01
>12 years	40%	14%	<0.01
Smoking			
Never	38%	55%	<0.01
Former	49%	43%	<0.01
Current	13%	12%	n.s.
Drinking			
None	59%	72%	<0.01
Light to Moderate	37%	26%	<0.01
Heavy	4%	2%	<0.01
Physical health SF-12 score	46.4±10.7	42.6±11.8	<0.01
Mental health SF-12 score	55.6±8.0	53.1±10.4	<0.01
Chronic conditions			
High blood pressure	45%	50%	0.01
Arthritis	50%	58%	<0.01
Depression	6%	5%	n.s.
N	2,094	1,166	

NOTE: Age and SF-12 score rows report mean ± standard deviation; n.s. = not significant.

sured by SF-12 scores (Ware et al., 1996) and chronic condition indicators, were higher in those with inadequate health literacy, indicating worse health status overall. Somewhat surprisingly, persons with inadequate health literacy are less likely to smoke or have smoked previously and less likely to consume alcohol.

Statistical Analysis

Costs by site of service were compared between the adequate and inadequate health literacy groups using a two-part regression model of medical spending. The two-part model is the standard statistical framework in empirical health economics for measuring the impact an individual characteristic on medical costs (Diehr et al., 1999). It is designed to account for the unique distribution of medical spending found in most samples; a sizeable minority of individuals do not use medical care, many use small amounts, and a few individuals incur substantial medical bills that account for a large percentage of aggregate spending. Because of the highly skewed distribution and presence of a large number of "0" values, standard statistical methods that assume the dependent variable is normally distributed yield inaccurate predictions of costs (Duan et al., 1983). The two-part model attempts to more accurately mimic the empirical distribution of medical spending by splitting the distribution into two parts and allowing the impact of independent variables, such as health literacy, on the probability of using medical care to be independent of their impact on the costs of medical care for those who use it.

The first stage of the model measures the probability of using medical care as a function of individual characteristics. Typically, logistic or probit regression is used, where the dependent variable equals one if costs are strictly positive and zero otherwise. Probit (or probability unit) regression was used in this case. Health literacy was included as an independent variable, along with controls for age, sex, race, income, schooling, smoking, and alcohol consumption. The second stage of the model estimates the relationship between independent variables and costs among those who use medical care. Parameters are estimated via least squares regression, where the dependent variable is the logarithm of costs and the independent variables are the same as in the first stage but the sample includes only individuals who received care (i.e., those with strictly positive values for the relevant cost category).

Coefficient estimates for the two-part model are difficult to interpret in isolation, since the dependent variable of the second stage is in log, rather than constant, dollars, and it is customary to state results in terms of predicted spending levels. These are constructed by computing predicted probabilities from the first stage and then multiplying these predicted probabilities by the exponentiated second-stage predicted values and a "smearing factor" (Duan, 1983), which is needed to transform logged dollars back to constant dollars, and averaging the predicted spending levels over the entire sample. Transforming log to constant dollars via this method may produce misleading results if the variance of spending in the upper part of the distribution differs from the variance in the lower part (Manning, 1998).

To address this issue, costs were also analyzed using the modified two-part model proposed by Mullahy (1998). In this model, the first stage is the same as in the standard two-part model, but the second stage is a nonlinear equation where cost equals the exponentiated sum of dependent variables and coefficients. This modified two-part model produced estimates within 5 percent of the predicted values from the standard two-part model. Therefore, only the results from the standard two-part model are presented below.

Two values are used to summarize the effect of a binary independent variable on spending. The first is the average predicted spending level with the variable indicating inadequate health literacy set equal to zero for every respondent; the second is the average predicted spending level with the health literacy variable set equal to one. Computed predicted values in this manner nets out the impact of observable individual characteristics, such as age, on spending.

Confidence intervals for predicted values were computed via simulation; the first- and second-stage coefficients were drawn from their respective multivariate normal distributions and predicted values were computed following the steps outlined above. Repeating this routine 1,000 times produced distributions of predicted values, and the lower and upper bounds of the confidence intervals were set equal to the 2.5th percentiles and the 97.5th percentiles of the distributions, respectively.

Two models were estimated. The first (or basic) model includes controls for sex, age, income, schooling, smoking, and alcohol consumption. The second includes additional controls for physical and mental status (from the SF-12) and chronic conditions (high blood pressure, arthritis, and depression). This model does not include the 66 observations for which no physical or mental health SF-12 scores were reported, for a sample of 3,192 observations (= 3,260 − 66).

Results

Results from the two-part model are displayed in Table B-3. Inpatient costs are the largest component of total medical spending. Predicted inpatient spending for persons with inadequate health literacy is $993 higher than that of persons with adequate health literacy (difference in raw means: $1,859). Controlling for health status, predicted inpatient spending for persons with inadequate health literacy is about $450 higher than that of persons with adequate health literacy. The confidence intervals for inpatient spending from the basic model overlap slightly, while the confidence intervals for inpatient spending from the model that includes controls for health status display a greater degree of overlap. Examining separately the results from each stage of the two-part model helps illuminate the reasons

TABLE B-3   Predicted Health-Care Spending

Cost Category	Health Literacy		Difference
	Adequate	Inadequate	
Basic Model			
Inpatient	$5,093 [$4,593 – $5,656]	$6,086 [$5,424 – $6,806]	$993
Outpatient	$1,910 [$1,816 – $2,017]	$1,795 [$1,681 – $1,914]	($115)
Emergency room	$110 [$97 – $124]	$174 [$154 – $196]	$64
Pharmacy	$700 [664 – $739]	$686 [$629 – $741]	($14)
Model with Controls for Health Status			
Inpatient	$5,352 [$4,832 – $5,945]	$5,794 [$5,042 – $6,573]	$442
Outpatient	$1,989 [$1,881 – $2,118]	$1,709 [$1,589 – $1,854]	($280)
Emergency room	$115 [$102 – $130]	$166 [$144 – $193]	$51
Pharmacy	$778 [$729 – $832]	$695 [$633 – $765]	($83)

NOTE: 95% confidence intervals are in brackets. Difference column displays the mean cost in the Inadequate column subtracted from the mean cost in the Adequate column. Negative values are in parentheses.

for spending differences. According to the first part of the two-part model for inpatient spending (results not shown; complete regression results are available from the author upon request), persons with inadequate health literacy are more likely to use inpatient services (p < 0.05), but, among those who used inpatient care, spending did not differ by health literacy status.

In contrast to the results for inpatient spending, the predicted outpatient spending level from the basic model for persons with adequate health literacy is higher than the predicted value for persons with inadequate health literacy. Predicted spending on emergency room care is lower for persons with adequate health literacy, while the predicted values for pharmacy spending from the basic model are comparable.

These results are shown in terms of total spending by the study sample in Table B-4. The first column shows predicted total spending under the assumption that the proportion of individuals with adequate health literacy is 64 percent, the actual proportion in the study sample. The second column shows predicted total spending under the assumption that the proportion of individuals with adequate health literacy is 100 percent, representing the maximum attainable level of health literacy in the population.

TABLE B-4   In-Sample Prediction of Health Literacy and Total Costs

	Percent with Adequate Literacy		
	64% (actual)	100%	Difference
Inpatient	17,877,000	$16,616,000	$1,261,000
Outpatient	6,079,400	$6,227,300	($147,900)
Emergency room	438,480	$359,910	$78,570
Pharmacy	$2,263,400	$2,277,700	($14,300)

NOTE: Difference column displays the mean cost in the inadequate column subtracted from the mean cost in the adequate column. Negative values are in parentheses.

Discussion

When assessing the causality of the results presented in Tables B-3 and B-4, it is important know whether health literacy, like ethnicity, is a constant, fixed characteristic of individuals or, like income, is associated with changes in health. Health literacy declines sharply with age in the study cohort (Baker et al., 2000), suggesting the latter. If so, then the relationship between health and health literacy is bidirectional; health literacy affects health and vice versa. To take an extreme example, an individual who experiences a severe stroke may lose the ability to read. It would be incorrect in such a case to attribute the costs associated with post-stroke care to illiteracy, since the stroke caused illiteracy and not the other way around. Controlling for health status, as is done in the extended model, removes the effect of health on health literacy but also removes the effect of health literacy on disease incidence, leading to estimates of the impact of health literacy on spending that are systematically lower than the true effect. Declines in health literacy by age are unrelated to the onset of chronic conditions (Baker et al., 2000), suggesting that the bias due to reverse causality is not large. Nevertheless, future studies could address this issue by taking two or more measurements of health literacy from the same respondent at different points in time.

Another caveat to this study is that though the analysis included fairly extensive controls for individual characteristics, including income, education, smoking, and alcohol consumption, there still may be unobserved individual characteristics correlated with both health literacy and spending that confound the results. For example, if individuals with low health literacy are also distrustful of the medical care system and are reluctant to seek medical attention, then the results will understate the impact of health literacy on costs.

Some insight on the validity of these results may be gained by examining differences in spending by site of service. Studies have shown that patients with low levels of health literacy receive fewer preventive services (Lindau et al., 2002; Scott et al., 2002), frequently fail to follow medication instructions (Andrus and Roth, 2002), and have worse health outcomes (Schillinger et al., 2002). The results of this study are consistent with these findings; individuals with inadequate health literacy make greater use of services designed to treat complications and advanced cases of disease, as indicated by higher spending for inpatient and emergency room care. Simultaneously, they use fewer services designed to manage disease, as evidenced by lower spending for outpatient care.

In conclusion, these results lend support to the hypothesis that individuals with low levels of health literacy incur higher medical costs, but, because of the limitations discussed above, no definitive conclusions can be drawn from the analysis. Results were sensitive to the inclusion of controls for health status, and the confidence intervals around predicted inpatient spending from the basic model overlapped by a small amount. Although it is impossible to prove causality, future studies should take advantage of statistical methods, such as propensity score estimators (Coyte et al., 2000; Rubin, 1997), designed to estimate treatment effects efficiently and the diagnostic information contained on claims to determine if expenditures are higher for persons with the conditions thought to be most responsive to patient knowledge. Data with repeated measurements of health literacy over time would also be helpful, especially for assessing the responsiveness of health literacy to health. For the time being, researchers should be cautious in terms of justifying interventions to improve health literacy based on potential cost savings.

REFERENCES

Andrus MR, Roth MT. 2002. Health literacy: A review. *Pharmacotherapy.* 22(3): 282–302.

Baker DW, Parker RM, Williams MV, Clark WS. 1998. Health literacy and the risk of hospital admission. *Journal of General Internal Medicine.* 13(12): 791–798.

Baker DW, Williams MV, Parker RM, Gazmararian JA, Nurss J. 1999. Development of a brief test to measure functional health literacy. *Patient Education and Counseling.* 38: 33–42.

Baker DW, Gazmararian JA, Sudano J, Patterson M. 2000. The association between age and health literacy among elderly persons. *Journals of Gerontology Series B—Psychological Sciences & Social Sciences.* 55B(6): S368–S374.

Baker DW, Gazmararian JA, Williams MV, Scott T, Parker RM, Green D, Ren J, Peel J. 2002. Functional health literacy and the risk of hospital admission among Medicare managed care enrollees. *American Journal of Public Health.* 92(8): 1278–1283.

Center for Evaluative Clinical Sciences. 1998. *The Dartmouth Atlas of Health Care.* Chicago, IL: American Hospital Publishing.

Cohen JW, Monheit AC, Beauregard KM, Cohen SB, Lefkowitz DC, Potter DE, Sommers JP, Taylor AK, Arnett RH 3rd. 1996–1997. The Medical Expenditure Panel Survey: A national health information resource. *Inquiry*. 33(4): 373–389.

Coyte PC, Young W, Croxford R. 2000. Costs and outcomes associated with alternative discharge strategies following joint replacement surgery: Analysis of an observational study using a propensity score. *Journal of Health Economics*. 19(6): 907–929.

Davis TC, Mayeaux EJ, Fredrickson D, Bocchini JA Jr, Jackson RH, Murphy PW. 1994. Reading ability of parents compared with reading level of pediatric patient education materials. *Pediatrics*. 93(3): 460–468.

Diehr P, Yanez D, Ash A, Hornbrook M, Lin DY. 1999. Methods for analyzing health care utilization and costs. *Annual Review of Public Health*. 20: 125–144.

Duan N. 1983. Smearing estimate: A nonparametric retransformation method. *Journal of the American Statistical Association*. 78: 605–610.

Duan N, Manning WG Jr, Morris CN, Newhouse JP. 1983. A comparison of alternative models for the demand for medical care. *Journal of Business and Economic Statistics*. 1: 115–126.

Gazmararian JA, Baker DW, Williams MV, Parker RM, Scott TL, Green DC, Fehrenbach SN, Ren J, Koplan JP. 1999. Health literacy among Medicare enrollees in a managed care organization. *Journal of the American Medical Association*. 281(6): 545–551.

Hellinger FJ, Wong HS. 2000. Selection bias in HMOs: A review of the evidence. *Medical Care Research and Review*. 57(4): 405–439.

Lindau ST, Tomori C, Lyons T, Langseth L, Bennett CL, Garcia P. 2002. The association of health literacy with cervical cancer prevention knowledge and health behaviors in a multiethnic cohort of women. *American Journal of Obstetrics & Gynecology*. 186(5): 938–943.

Manning WG. 1998. Much ado about two: Reconsidering retransformation and the two-part model in health economics. *Journal of Health Economics*. 48: 375–391.

Mullahy J. 1998. Much ado about two: Reconsidering retransformation and the two-part model in health econometrics. *Journal of Health Economics*. 17(3): 247–281.

Parker RM, Baker DW, Williams MV, Nurss JR. 1995. The Test of Functional Health Literacy in Adults: A new instrument for measuring patients' literacy skills. *Journal of General Internal Medicine*. 10(10): 537–541.

Rubin DB. 1997. Estimating causal effects from large data sets using propensity scores. *Annals of Internal Medicine*. 127(8 Pt 2): 757–763.

Schillinger D, Grumbach K, Piette J, Wang F, Osmond D, Daher C, Palacios J, Sullivan GAD, Bindman AB. 2002. Association of health literacy with diabetes outcomes. *Journal of the American Medical Association*. 288(4): 475–482.

Scott TL, Gazmararian JA, Williams MV, Baker DW. 2002. Health literacy and preventive health care use among Medicare enrollees in a managed care organization. *Medical Care*. 40(5): 395–404.

Selden TM, Levit KR, Cohen JW, Zuvekas SH, Moeller JF, McKusick D, Arnett RH 3rd. 2001. Reconciling medical expenditure estimates from the MEPS and the NHA, 1996. *Health Care Financing Review*. 23(1): 161–178.

Stedman L, Kaestle C. 1991. *Literacy and Reading Performance in the United States from 1880 to Present*. New Haven, CT: Yale University Press. Pp. 75–128.

Ware J Jr, Kosinski M, Keller SD. 1996. A 12-Item Short-Form Health Survey: Construction of scales and preliminary tests of reliability and validity. *Medical Care*. 34(3): 220–233.

Weiss BD. 1999. How common is low literacy? In: *20 Common Problems in Primary Care*. Weiss BD, Editor. New York: McGraw-Hill. Pp. 468–481.

Weiss BD, Blanchard JS, McGee DL, Hart G, Warren B, Burgoon M, Smith KJ. 1994. Illiteracy among Medicaid recipients and its relationship to health care costs. *Journal of Health Care for the Poor & Underserved.* 5(2): 99–111.

Wiener JM, Hanley RJ, Clark R, Van Nostrand JF. 1990. Measuring the activities of daily living: Comparisons across national surveys. *Journal of Gerontology.* 45(6): S229–S237.

Improving Chronic Disease Care for Populations with Limited Health Literacy

Dean Schillinger, M.D.

The problem with communication is the assumption that it has occurred.

—*George Bernard Shaw*

Introduction

Chronic disease management is one of the major challenges facing health-care systems and patients in industrialized nations. Nearly three-quarters of all health-care resources are devoted to the treatment of chronic diseases, and nearly one-half of the U.S. population has one or more chronic condition (Institute for Health and Aging, 1996). The collaboration between the system of care, providers, patients, and the community to provide the best health outcomes adds a layer of complexity to the delivery of health care to individuals with chronic disease. Effective disease management is based on systematic, interactive communication between patients and the providers and health system with whom they interact (Norris et al., 2002a, b; Von Korff et al., 1997), all occurring in the context of a community whose resources meet patients' needs (Wagner, 1995).

This paper uses the definition of disease management provided by the Task Force on Community Preventive Services, a nonfederal Task Force convened in 1996 by the Department of Health and Human Services (HHS) to provide leadership in the evaluation of community, population, and health-care system strategies to address a variety of public health and health promotion topics, and appointed by the Director of the Centers for Disease Control and Prevention (Norris et al., 2002a, b). Disease management is an organized, proactive, multicomponent approach to health-care delivery that involves all members of a population with a specific disease, is focused on the spectrum of the disease and its complications (including the prevention of co-morbid conditions), and is integrated across the relevant aspects of the delivery system.

The last few decades have seen tremendous advances in the care of chronic conditions, including an array of new therapeutic options, risk-factor modification for secondary prevention of co-morbid conditions, the availability of home monitoring tools, and the growth of disease manage-

The research reported herein was supported, in part, through grants from the National Center for Research Resources (K-23 RR16539), the Soros Open Society Institute, and The Commonwealth Fund.

ment programs (Bodenheimer, 1999; Diabetes Control and Complications Trial Research Group, 1993, 1996; McCulloch et al., 2000; United Kingdom Prospective Diabetes Study Group, 1998). Despite these advances, health quality and clinical outcomes of patients with chronic diseases vary across sociodemographic lines (American Diabetes Association, 1998; CDC, 2000; Fiscella et al., 2000; Piette, 1999; Vinicor et al., 2000). Much of the burden of chronic disease falls on the elderly and those of low socioeconomic status, populations that have also been shown to have disproportionately high rates of health literacy problems (Gazmararian et al., 1999a; Williams et al., 1995b). It is increasingly apparent that the health-care system has not evolved to serve those with limited health literacy. The prevalence of limited health literacy, compounded by a health-care system in which scientific advances and market forces place greater technical and self-management demands on patients and their families, may help to create unequal outcomes despite what some consider equal access (IOM, 2001, 2003).

There currently is a lack of precision and uniformity regarding the meaning of the term "health literacy" (American Medical Association, 1999; Davis et al., 1991; HHS, 2000; Nutbeam, 2000) and little consensus as to the extent to which literacy equates with health literacy (see Chapter 2 in this report). There is general agreement, however, that (1) literacy and numeracy skills are deeply embedded in the construct of health literacy and (2) the problems associated with having limited health literacy are most intense for those individuals with limited literacy skills. The ensuing discussion in this chapter is based on these two assumptions.

The purpose of this article is to (1) briefly review the elements of the most well-accepted model to restructure chronic disease care delivery, the Chronic Care Model of Wagner and others (1995), (2) describe the ways in which limited health literacy may lead to worse chronic disease outcomes, (3) use the Chronic Care Model to consider opportunities to reduce health literacy-related disparities, and (4) reflect on strategies to develop quality-of-care indicators to promote improvement in chronic disease care for patients with limited health literacy.

The Chronic Care Model

Health-care delivery is poorly organized to meet the needs of patients with chronic diseases. Rushed practitioners find it difficult to follow established practice guidelines, limited coordination hampers multidisciplinary care, inadequate training leaves many patients ill-equipped to manage their illnesses, and lack of active follow-up leads to preventable deterioration in function. Some managed care organizations and integrated delivery systems have attempted to correct deficiencies in management of chronic diseases.

To guide the reorganization of chronic disease care, Dr. Ed Wagner and others developed the Chronic Care Model (see Figure B-1), which summarizes the basic elements for improving care in health systems at multiple levels (Wagner, 1998, 2003). These include the health system, health-care delivery system design, decision support, clinical information systems, the community, and self-management support. For example, a *community* that has the infrastructure and resources to facilitate patients' self-care activities (transportation to appointments, safe recreational spaces for exercise, adequate produce for healthy food choices, opportunities for educational or communal engagement); a health system that trains patients to be active participants through *self-management* educational activities (such as group medical visits or other organized, skill-building activities); a clinic that restructures its *care delivery* through multidisciplinary teams, planned visits, or home visits; or a practice that uses *disease registries* to track patients' progress, stratify intensity of care, promote outreach, and maintain continuity—all would represent efforts consistent with the Chronic Care Model. Focusing on these components could foster interactions between patients

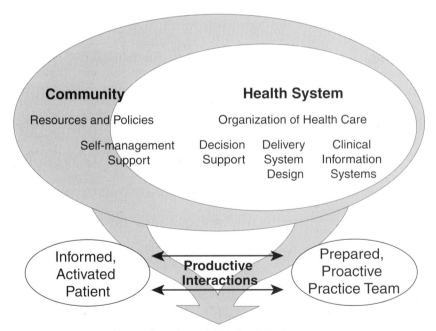

FIGURE B-1 Model for improvement of chronic illness care.
SOURCE: Wagner (1998). Reprinted with permission of the American College of Physicians.

who take an active part in their care and providers who are backed up by resources and expertise. The Chronic Care Model integrates the published evidence in chronic disease management, including the importance of executive leadership and incentives to promote quality, systems to track and monitor patients' progress and support timely provider decision-making (Piette, 2000), patient self-management training (Lorig et al., 1999; Von Korff et al., 1997), and community-oriented care. Patients and providers prepared in these ways are likely more able to engage in productive interactions that promote system efficiency and patient well-being (Norris et al., 2002a).

A growing body of research demonstrates that self-management practices and clinical outcomes in chronic disease care vary by patients' level of health literacy (Kalichman and Rompa, 2000; Schillinger et al., 2002; Williams et al., 1998b). The Chronic Care Model and similar comprehensive, population-based disease management approaches may offer insights into the ways in which limited health literacy affects chronic disease care and identify potential points of intervention. Preliminary evidence from a small randomized trial suggests that disease management strategies can reduce health literacy-related disparities in diabetes care (Rothman et al., 2003) and that tailoring communication to those with limited health literacy might affect outcomes in chronic anticoagulation and diabetes care (Schillinger et al., 2002, 2003b). However, we were unable to locate published results of any comprehensive disease management systems specifically designed to improve chronic disease care for individuals with limited health literacy. Developing such a system would likely benefit not only those with limited health literacy, but all chronic disease patients, as many of the barriers faced by those with limited health literacy are also experienced, albeit it a somewhat lesser extent, by those with adequate health literacy.

How Limited Health Literacy Affects Chronic Disease Outcomes

Limited health literacy has been shown to be associated with worse health status (Weiss et al., 1992), higher utilization of services (Baker et al., 1997, 1998) and worse clinical outcomes (Kalichman and Rompa, 2000; Schillinger et al., 2002). Whether limited health literacy is a marker for other determinants of health, such as socioeconomic status, or is in the causal pathway to poor health is currently a matter of some debate. For chronic disease care, which relies on self-management, self-advocacy, ongoing monitoring, and interactive communication, it is reasonable to hypothesize that health literacy may be one determinant of health outcomes.

Limited health literacy may affect many aspects of chronic disease care. It may influence the interaction between provider and patient, impact the ability of the health system to communicate successfully with the patient, and affect the availability of community resources for chronic disease patients and their families (Figure B-2). By reviewing this framework, we can begin to generate a set of priorities for targeted study and intervention that reflects a blending of what we have learned from the Chronic Care Model and what is known about empowering low-literacy adults from the field of adult education (Roter et al., 1998, 2001).

Office-Based Clinician–Patient Communication

Much of chronic disease care takes place in the context of a medical office visit. Communication about chronic diseases during outpatient visits may be hampered by several factors. These include the relative infrequency and brevity of visits, language barriers and limited literacy, differences between providers' and patients' agendas and communication styles, lack

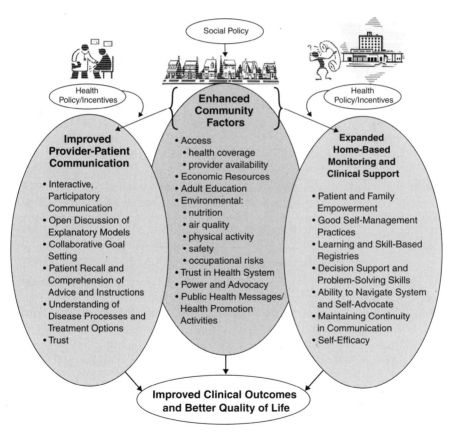

FIGURE B-2 Improving chronic disease care: a framework based on health literacy and related research.

of trust between the patient and provider, overriding or competing clinical problems, lack of timeliness of the visit in relation to disease-specific problems, and the complexity and variability of patients' reporting of symptoms and progress of their disease.

Patients with chronic diseases and limited health literacy have been shown to have less knowledge of their condition and of its management (Williams et al., 1998a, b) often despite having received standard self-management education. Patients with limited health literacy have greater difficulties accurately reporting their medication regimens and describing the reasons for which their medications were prescribed (Schillinger et al., 2003b; Williams et al., 1995a; Win and Schillinger, 2003) and more frequently have explanatory models that may interfere with adherence (Kalichman et al., 1999). While patients with limited health literacy clearly have problems with literacy and numeracy skills in the health-care setting, patients also experience difficulties with oral communication. A recent study among patients with diabetes demonstrated that those patients with limited health literacy (as measured by the Short Test of Functional Health Literacy in Adults [S-TOFHLA] [Nurss et al., 1995]) appear to have particular problems with both the decision-making and the explanatory, technical components of dialogue (Schillinger et al., 2004). Patients with limited health literacy may also be less likely to challenge, ask questions of the provider (Baker et al., 1996; Street, 1991), or disclose poor understanding (Baker et al., 1996), and may cope by being passive or appearing uninterested (Cooper and Roter, 2003; Roter, 2000; Roter and Hall, 1992; Roter et al., 1997). Clinicians tend to underestimate the information needs of patients (Cegala, 1997) and underuse interactive teaching strategies that may be especially useful for patients with limited health literacy (Schillinger et al., 2003b). Clinicians' frequent use of jargon in clinical encounters may be particularly problematic for patients with limited health literacy. This jargon can range from technical jargon (words that have meaning only in the clinical context, e.g., "*glucometer*"), quantitative jargon (words for which clinical judgment is required to accurately interpret, e.g., "*excessive wheezing*"), to lay jargon (words for which two meanings exist, one with clinical meaning and the other with lay meaning, e.g., "your weight is *stable*"). Clinicians are often unaware of the mismatch between their process of giving information and patients' process of recalling, understanding, and acting on the information (Davis et al., 2002b; Doak et al., 1998; Williams et al., 2002).

Home-Based Monitoring and Clinical Support

Chronic care involves an ongoing process of patient assessments, adjustments to treatment plans, and reassessments to measure change in patient health status. Without timely and reliable information about patients' health status, symptoms, and self-care, the necessary health education, treatments, or behavioral adjustments may come late or not at all. This can compromise patients' health and increase the likelihood of poor outcomes.

To best manage chronic disease, patients must remember any self-care instructions they have received from their provider, be able to correctly interpret symptoms or results of self-monitoring, and appropriately solve problems regarding adjustments to the treatment regimen, as well as when and how to contact the provider should the need arise. A number of studies demonstrate that patients remember and understand as little as half of what they are told by their physicians (Bertakis, 1977; Cole and Bird, 2000; Crane, 1997; Rost and Roter, 1987; Roter, 2000) and the more information provided, the less the patient is able to recall (Chow, 2003). Patients with limited health literacy are likely to understand and remember at even lower rates (Schillinger et al., 2004). In addition, they may be less equipped to overcome gaps when they are at home due to knowledge deficits (Williams et al., 1998a, b) and difficulties reading or interpreting instructions (Crane, 1997; Williams et al., 1998b). Cross-sectional studies involving patients with diabetes suggest that traditional self-management education may not eliminate health literacy-related disparities in chronic disease outcomes (Schillinger et al., 2002; Williams et al., 1998b).

Only a minority of clinical practices provide any form of care management that involves outreach and support in the patient's home (Casalino et al., 2003). In addition, home-based disease-specific education, monitoring, and clinical support increasingly rely on patients and providers interacting via web-based or "e-health" interfaces (Robert Wood Johnson Foundation and the National Cancer Institute, 2002). While these interfaces have been suggested as a potential method of increasing interaction between patients and providers (Robert Wood Johnson Foundation and the National Cancer Institute, 2002), they may present overwhelming barriers to patients with limited health literacy. Individuals with limited health literacy may have trouble accessing the web (Fox and Fallows, 2003), difficulties reading from web sites (Berland et al., 2001), and problems with navigation once they get online (Robert Wood Johnson Foundation, 2002; Zarcadoolas et al., 2002). Accreditation of health-related web sites (such as the Health on the Net Foundation Code of Conduct) does little to improve readability of diabetes web sites (Kusec et al., 2003).

Simply transforming text versions of disease-specific education to more visually oriented media (i.e., CD-ROM), while associated with improvements in satisfaction, does not appear to increase knowledge among patients with limited health literacy (Kim et al., 2001). Focus groups of patients with limited health literacy have identified health system navigation (finding resources within the health system, such as knowing whom, for what, and when to call for assistance with a problem) as a particularly daunting aspect of chronic disease management (Baker et al., 1996).

Community and Environmental Factors

Data from the National Adult Literacy Survey (Kirsch, 1993) demonstrate regional variation in literacy rates that parallels neighborhood patterns of socioeconomic status, immigrant status, age, and race and ethnicity. Studies in health-care settings (Gazmararian et al., 1999b; Williams et al., 1995b) indicate that patients with limited health literacy comprise a large sector of patients in public hospitals and community clinics that predominantly serve socioeconomically disadvantaged populations, and in private health systems that serve the elderly or those with low incomes, such as Medicare and Medicaid managed care organizations. Little work has been done exploring the relationship between limited health literacy and neighborhood characteristics, particularly those of direct relevance to chronic disease management. Recent work from social epidemiology (Berkman and Kawachi, 2000) and literacy theory (Wallerstein and Bernstein, 1988) can inform how community factors can either assist or hamper disease management efforts for patients with limited health literacy. Communities that have high rates of limited health literacy may be less able to assert political power and advocate for the health and health-care needs of their community (Nutbeam, 2000). Residents of medically underserved areas experience greater difficulties accessing a regular source of health care, a problem that has been shown to be associated with preventable hospitalizations for chronic conditions (Bindman et al., 1995). Other environmental attributes of communities, such as the availability of goods and services that promote health, the quality of the air and recreational physical space, and occupational risks associated with neighborhood employment may each interact with limited health literacy to lead to worse health. In addition, recent studies examining disparities in quality of care demonstrate racial and ethnic differences in level of trust in the health-care system that may influence how these communities interact with the health-care system (IOM, 2003). Finally, the focus of health promotion messages and activities that take place at the community level may not be aligned with the needs of patients with limited health literacy (Nutbeam, 2000).

Shaping the Chronic Care Model for Patients with Limited Health Literacy

One of the underlying assumptions of the Chronic Care Model is that the reorganization of health care will lead to more productive interactions between informed, involved patients, and prepared, proactive practice teams, which will, in turn, lead to better outcomes (Figure B-1). In order for this assumption to hold for populations with limited health literacy, we need to think more critically about the ways in which we communicate across the levels described above to ensure that interactions indeed are productive. If we apply the Chronic Care Model without also attending to the unique challenges to chronic disease management posed by limited health literacy, we may improve care for many but run the risk of perpetuating disparities in outcomes for those with limited health literacy.

In order to engage in more productive interactions with patients who have limited health literacy, solutions must primarily affect the nature, quality, and extent of communication. Previous research indicates patients want practical, concise information focused on the identification of the problem, what specifically the patient needs to do, why it is in their best interest, and what outcomes they can expect (Davis et al., 2001, 2002a, b). Communication strategies commonly employed by health professionals are often only marginally effective for those with limited health literacy. At present, clinicians do not have the means to uncover how patients learn best, nor the tools to more effectively engage patients who do not appear to be maximally benefiting from clinical interactions. In order to support patients' acquisition of self-management skills and increase confidence to carry out self-management tasks, efforts should be made to develop tools to assess how patients learn in the clinical setting, and to expand the repertoire of options to match patients' learning style or preferences. Some principles derived from the field of adult education may be relevant to chronic disease communication (Brookfield, 1986; Roter et al., 2001; Wallerstein, 1992). Learners (patients) should be involved in developing health education messages, materials, and programs (Davis et al., 1998a, b; Rudd and Comings, 1994). Learning should be participatory; patients should be actively involved in setting the agenda or curriculum and, at times, even leading it so as to ensure relevance (relating and reflecting on experience), encourage ongoing involvement, promote the development of behavior change through critical thinking (thoughtful action), and support other learners to succeed. This involvement will help ensure the education is relevant, understandable, culturally sensitive, and empowering. Interactions should involve exploration and problem-based learning (Cooper et al., 2003). Patient education activities should be designed so as to engage patients in ways relevant to their lives and their conditions and that enhance problem-solving skills (Center for Literacy Studies, 2003). Such activities educational focus may lead to patient-generated goal-setting, an important intermediate objective in successful chronic disease care (Anderson, 1995; Anderson et al., 1995). Group medical visits, an innovation in which groups of patients who share a common condition regularly meet with a health provider, have the potential to operate via these principles. Results of a small trial with diabetes patients suggests that, when designed with the collaboration of an expert in adult education, such visits can dramatically improve outcomes (Trento et al., 2001, 2002).

As chronic disease education, monitoring, and clinical support move beyond the office walls to include e-health and other forms of telemedicine, it is critical that patients with limited health literacy are not left behind (Robert Wood Johnson Foundation and the National Cancer Institute, 2002). Individuals with limited health literacy must be involved in all stages of intervention design and testing. This participatory development method allows for input during the generative phase of an intervention, provides opportunities for feedback during multiple points of pilot testing, and can engender trust and participation during the evaluation phase (Houts et al., 1998; Jacobson et al., 1999). As an example, our recent work at San Francisco General Hospital involves the development of an automated telephone diabetes management system for patients with limited health literacy. The idea for a telephone-based intervention was generated, in part, from patients. The program was developed with the active involvement of adult learners and patients with limited health literacy, which significantly altered numerous aspects of the program. Patients wanted to hear that we are actively listening and care about their well-being. They preferred narrative instead of instruction-based health education. Patients recommended we reduce the speed with which messages are delivered and limit the amount of technical language in order to make the messages more understandable. We are currently evaluating the effect of this system on diabetes-related outcomes.

If all patients with chronic diseases are to benefit from emerging technologies, particularly interventions that involve the Internet, research must explore how to best design such programs for patients with limited health literacy (Robert Wood Johnson Foundation and the National Cancer Institute, 2002). Such research will also require professional collaboration between disciplines such as computer science, health communication, education, economics, marketing, sociology, and library and information science.

If we are to redesign the health-care delivery system and better support patients in their self-management, it is important to recognize the needs that patients with limited health literacy have expressed with regards to system navigation. We must better understand the elements of successful system navigation and apply this understanding to support patients' navigation and self-advocacy skills, and better equip patients to get what they need from a complex system. We need to partner with patients with limited health literacy to identify those aspects of the system that represent bottlenecks and to design solutions that lower such barriers.

A crucial component to reducing the burden of limited health literacy lies with the providers of health care. In order to boost provider preparedness, we need to prime the workforce to more effectively care for patients who have chronic diseases and limited health literacy. Training of all health professionals that focuses on communication strategies to enhance clinician self-awareness (Frankel and Stein, 2001), mutual learning, partnership-building, collaborative goal-setting, and behavior change for chronic disease patients is essential (Wagner, 2003; Youmans and Schillinger, 2003). Such training should be expanded to include all members of the multidisciplinary health team, including lay health educators, both as learners and teachers. These efforts must be informed by new health communication research that involves patients with limited health literacy, a segment often under-represented in clinical research.

Community efforts should focus on developing relationships that foster trust, providing resources to measure and meet community needs, and ultimately preparing members of a community to effectively advocate for the needs of their community (Figueroa et al., 2002). Public health messages should take into account the health literacy skills of the population to whom the message is being targeted, involve the population from the beginning, and make use of appropriate channels to convey these messages (Bird et al., 1998).

Measuring Progress

In order to promote progress in chronic care delivery for patients with limited health literacy, quality-of-care measures must be designed to capture health literacy-related performance. If incentives are aligned to improve quality, such measures of health-care quality can, in turn, lead to the creation of standards of care and improve practice. There are several possible approaches to measuring the extent to which health systems are meeting the needs of patients with limited health literacy. An indirect approach, advocated by those involved in initiatives to reduce racial and ethnic disparities in quality of care (IOM, 2003; Sehgal, 2003) is to use existing measures of quality, such as Medicaid Health Plan Employer Data and Information Set indicators (that currently do not include any health literacy-specific indicators), and stratify a system's performance by race or ethnicity, or, in this case, health literacy level. Such an approach would enable a comparison of performance in process or outcome measures among those with inadequate health literacy in comparison to those with adequate health literacy. A health system can be considered improving if overall performance is improving and if the extent of health literacy-related variation in performance is narrowing over time. The main challenge to this strategy is the complexity involved in measuring health literacy. Current instruments take between 3 and 7 minutes and require in-person administration (Baker et al., 1999). Education level is not a useful proxy for health literacy, as there is only a modest correlation between education and health literacy. There also are interactions between education and other demographic characteristics (e.g., ethnicity, age, primary language) on health literacy (Beers et al., 2003; Guerra and Shea, 2003). A recent study suggests that a single questionnaire item may have reasonable sensitivity and specificity in detecting inadequate health literacy and appears to perform well if the prevalence of inadequate health literacy in the population is high enough (Chew and Bradley, 2003). In order for a strategy of reducing health literacy-related disparities by measuring health literacy-related quality is to succeed, research to develop a rapid and reliable measure of health literacy is needed.

A second approach is to develop novel measures of quality that may be less disease-specific, yet have particular relevance to patients with limited health literacy across chronic conditions. To our knowledge, relatively little work has been done in this regard. For example, the National Center for Quality Assurance (NCQA) for managed care organizations has created standards regarding the readability of the patient appeal of denial of services form (NCQA, 2003). While arguably of importance, the approach of assessing quality by measuring document readability is obviously narrow in scope, and does not capture a more comprehensive view of the patient experience. Other possibilities include measuring patients' reports of their experiences of communication (Schillinger et al., 2004), rates of discordance between patients' and providers' reports of medication regimens (Schillinger et al., 2003a), the extent to which home monitoring and support for chronic disease is available (Norris et al., 2002b), the range of learning options and media available to patients, the ease with which one can navigate a health system, or capturing the degree to which a health system has a family and community orientation (Starfield, 1998). In order for significant progress to be made, it is essential that research is done to develop appropriate quality indicators for health literacy-related performance.

CONCLUSIONS

Despite wide variation in literacy levels, our society places high literacy demands on its members. It is apparent that attempts to reduce health literacy-related disparities must revolve around either directly addressing the problem of basic literacy and/or creating a health-care system in which the gap between the literacy demands of the system and the literacy skills of the patients it serves is significantly narrowed. Modern chronic disease care requires that patients play an active role in their care, and that clinicians and the health systems in which they work take on the challenge of partnering with patients to promote successful outcomes. Meeting these goals is often most challenging for those patients who have the greatest need. When considered as a barrier to successful health communication as well as a marker for problems with navigation and self-advocacy, it becomes clear that the concerns related to limited health literacy are inescapably linked to the challenges of chronic disease management. In order to ensure that the Chronic Care Model and increasingly sophisticated chronic disease management programs can benefit patients with limited health literacy, attention must be paid to tailor design and implementation with the involvement of patients with limited health literacy, and to expand the reach of such programs. By promoting meaningful, collaborative communication between patients and the providers and systems that serve them, such a reorganization is likely to benefit all patients with chronic diseases.

REFERENCES

American Diabetes Association. 1998. Economic consequences of diabetes mellitus in the U.S. in 1997. *Diabetes Care*. 21(2): 296–309.

American Medical Association. 1999. Health literacy: Report of the Council on Scientific Affairs. Ad Hoc Committee on Health Literacy for the Council on Scientific Affairs, American Medical Association. *Journal of the American Medical Association*. 281(6): 552–557.

Anderson RM. 1995. Patient empowerment and the traditional medical model. A case of irreconcilable differences. *Diabetes Care*. 18(3): 412–415.

Anderson RM, Funnell MM, Butler PM, Arnold MS, Fitzgerald JT, Feste CC. 1995. Patient empowerment. Results of a randomized controlled trial. *Diabetes Care*. 18(7): 943–949.

Baker DW, Parker RM, Williams MV, Pitkin K, Parikh NS, Coates W, Imara M. 1996. The health care experience of patients with low literacy. *Archives of Family Medicine*. 5(6): 329–334.

Baker DW, Parker RM, Williams MV, Clark WS, Nurss J. 1997. The relationship of patient reading ability to self-reported health and use of health services. *American Journal of Public Health*. 87(6): 1027–1030.

Baker DW, Parker RM, Williams MV, Clark WS. 1998. Health literacy and the risk of hospital admission. *Journal of General Internal Medicine*. 13(12): 791–798.

Baker DW, Williams MV, Parker RM, Gazmararian JA, Nurss J. 1999. Development of a brief test to measure functional health literacy. *Patient Education and Counseling*. 38: 33–42.

Beers BB, McDonald VJ, Quistberg DA, Ravenell KL, Asch DA, Shea JA. 2003. Disparities in health literacy between African American and non-African American primary care patients. *Journal of General Internal Medicine*. 18(S1): 169.

Berkman LF, Kawachi, IO. 2000. *Social Epidemiology*. Oxford: Oxford University Press.

Berland GK, Elliott MN, Morales LS, Algazy JI, Kravitz RL, Broder MS, Kanouse DE, Munoz JA, Puyol JA, Lara M, Watkins KE, Yang H, McGlynn EA. 2001. Health information on the Internet: Accessibility, quality, and readability in English and Spanish. *Journal of the American Medical Association*. 285(20): 2612–2621.

Bertakis KD. 1977. The communication of information from physician to patient: A method for increasing patient retention and satisfaction. *Journal of Family Practice* 5(2): 217–222.

Bindman AB, Grumbach K, Osmond D, Komaromy M, Vranizan K, Lurie N, Billings J, Stewart A. 1995. Preventable hospitalizations and access to health care. *Journal of the American Medical Association.* 274(4): 305–311.

Bird JA, McPhee SJ, Ha NT, Le B, Davis T, Jenkins CN. 1998. Opening pathways to cancer screening for Vietnamese-American women: Lay health workers hold a key. *Preventive Medicine.* 27(6): 821–829.

Bodenheimer T. 1999. Disease management—Promises and pitfalls. *New England Journal of Medicine.* 340(15): 1202–1205.

Brookfield, S. 1986. *Understanding and Facilitating Adult Learning.* 1st edition. San Francisco, CA: Jossey-Bass.

Casalino L, Gillies RR, Shortell SM, Schmittdiel JA, Bodenheimer T, Robinson JC, Rundall T, Oswald N, Schauffler H, Wang MC. 2003. External incentives, information technology, and organized processes to improve health care quality for patients with chronic diseases. *Journal of the American Medical Association.* 289(4): 434–441.

CDC (Centers for Disease Control and Prevention). 2000. *National Diabetes Fact Sheet.* Atlanta, GA: Centers for Disease Control and Prevention.

Cegala DJ. 1997. A study of doctors' and patients' communication during a primary care consultation: Implications for communication training. *Journal of Health Communication.* 2(3): 169–194.

Center for Literacy Studies. 2003. *Equipped for the Future: EFF Center for Training and Technical Assistance.* University of Tennessee [Online]. Available: http:www.nifl.gov/lincs/collections/eff/eff.html [accessed: September, 2003].

Chew LD, Bradley KA. 2003. Brief questions to detect inadequate health literacy among VA patients. Abstract. *Journal of General Internal Medicine.* 18(Supplement 1): 170.

Chow KM. 2003. Information recall by patients. *Journal of the Royal Society of Medicine.* 96(7): 370.

Cole, SA, Bird J. 2000. *The Medical Interview: The Three-Function Approach.* 2nd edition. St. Louis: Mosby.

Cooper LA, Roter DL. 2003. Patient-provider communication: The effect of race and ethnicity on process and outcomes in health care. In: *Unequal Treatment: Confronting Racial and Ethnic Disparities in Health Care.* Smedley BD, Stith AY, Nelson AR, Editors. Washington, DC: The National Academies Press. Pp. 336–354.

Cooper HC, Booth K, Gill G. 2003. Patients' perspectives on diabetes health care education. *Health Education Research.* 18(2): 191–206.

Crane JA. 1997. Patient comprehension of doctor-patient communication on discharge from the emergency department. *Journal of Emergency Medicine.* 15(1): 1–7.

Davis TC, Crouch MA, Long SW, Jackson RH, Bates P, George RB, Bairnsfather LE. 1991. Rapid assessment of literacy levels of adult primary care patients. *Family Medicine.* 23(6): 433–435.

Davis TC, Berkel HJ, Arnold CL, Nandy I, Jackson RH, Murphy PW. 1998a. Intervention to increase mammography utilization in a public hospital. *Journal of General Internal Medicine* 13(4): 230–233.

Davis TC, Fredrickson DD, Arnold C, Murphy PW, Herbst M, Bocchini JA. 1998b. A polio immunization pamphlet with increased appeal and simplified language does not improve comprehension to an acceptable level. *Patient Education and Counseling.* 33(1): 25–37.

Davis TC, Fredrickson DD, Arnold CL, Cross JT, Humiston SG, Green KW, Bocchini JA Jr. 2001. Childhood vaccine risk/benefit communication in private practice office settings: A national survey. *Pediatrics.* 107(2): E17.

Davis TC, Fredrickson DD, Bocchini C, Arnold CL, Green KW, Humiston SG, Wilder E, Bocchini JA Jr. 2002a. Improving vaccine risk/benefit communication with an immunization education package: A pilot study. *Ambulatory Pediatrics.* 2(3): 193–200.

Davis TC, Williams MV, Marin E, Parker RM, Glass J. 2002b. Health literacy and cancer communication. *Ca: A Cancer Journal for Clinicians.* 52(3): 134–149.

Diabetes Control and Complications Trial Research Group. 1993. The effect of intensive treatment of diabetes on the development and progression of long-term complications in insulin-dependent diabetes mellitus. *New England Journal of Medicine.* 329(14): 977–986.

Diabetes Control and Complications Trial Research Group. 1996. Lifetime benefits and costs of intensive therapy as practiced in the diabetes control and complications trial. *Journal of the American Medical Association.* 276(17): 1409–1415.

Doak CC, Doak LG, Friedell GH, Meade CD. 1998. Improving comprehension for cancer patients with low literacy skills: Strategies for clinicians. [Review] [50 refs]. *Ca: A Cancer Journal for Clinicians.* 48(3): 151–162.

Figueroa ME, Kincaid DL, Rani M, Lewis G. 2002. *Communication for Social Change Working Paper Series.* Communication for Social Change: An Integrated Model for Measuring the Process and Its Outcomes. New York: The Rockefeller Foundation and Johns Hopkins University Center for Communication Programs.

Fiscella K, Franks P, Gold MR, Clancy CM. 2000. Inequality in quality: Addressing socioeconomic, racial, and ethnic disparities in health care. *Journal of the American Medical Association.* 283(19): 2579–2584.

Fox S, Fallows D. 2003 (July 16). Internet Health Resources: health searches and email have become more commonplace, but there is room for improvement in searches and overall Internet access. Washington, DC: Pew Internet & American Life Project.

Frankel RM, Stein T. 2001. Getting the most out of the clinical encounter: The four habits model. *Journal of Medical Practice Management.* 16(4): 184–191.

Gazmararian JA, Baker DW, Williams MV, Parker RM, Scott TL, Green DC, Fehrenbach SN, Ren J, Koplan JP. 1999a. Health literacy among Medicare enrollees in a managed care organization. *Journal of the American Medical Association.* 281(6): 545–551.

Gazmararian JA, Baker DW, Williams MV, Parker RM, Scott T, Greemn DCFSN, Ren J, Koplan JP. 1999b. Health literacy among Medicare enrollees in a managed care organization. *Journal of the American Medical Association.* 281(6): 545–551.

Guerra CE, Shea JA. 2003. Functional health literacy, comorbidity and health status. *Journal of General Internal Medicine.* 18(Supplement 1): 174.

HHS (U.S. Department of Health and Human Services). 2000. *Healthy People 2010: Understanding and Improving Health.* Washington, DC: U.S. Department of Health and Human Services.

Houts PS, Bachrach R, Witmer JT, Tringali CA, Bucher JA, Localio RA. 1998. Using pictographs to enhance recall of spoken medical instructions. *Patient Education and Counseling.* 35(2): 83–88.

Institute for Health and Aging. 1996. *Chronic Care in America: A 21st Century Challenge.* Princeton, NJ: The Robert Wood Johnson Foundation.

IOM (Institute of Medicine). 2001. *Crossing the Quality Chasm: A New Health System for the 21st Century.* Washington, DC: National Academy Press.

IOM. 2003. *Unequal Treatment: Confronting Racial and Ethnic Disparities in Health Care.* Washington, DC: The National Academies Press.

Jacobson TA, Thomas DM, Morton FJ, Offutt G, Shevlin J, Ray S. 1999. Use of a low-literacy patient education tool to enhance pneumococcal vaccination rates: A randomized controlled trial. *Journal of the American Medical Association.* 282(7): 646–650.

Kalichman SC, Rompa D. 2000. Functional health literacy is associated with health status and health-related knowledge in people living with HIV-AIDS. *Journal of Acquired Immune Deficiency Syndromes & Human Retrovirology.* 25(4): 337–344.

Kalichman SCP, Ramachandran BB, Catz SP. 1999. Adherence to combination antiretroviral therapies in HIV patients of low health literacy. *Journal of General Internal Medicine.* 14(5): 267–273.

Kim SP, Knight SJ, Tomori C, Colella KM, Schoor RA, Shih L, Kuzel TM, Nadler RB, Bennett CL. 2001. Health literacy and shared decision making for prostate cancer patients with low socioeconomic status. *Cancer Investigation.* 19(7): 684–691.

Kirsch IS (Educational Testing Service (ETS)). 1993. *Adult Literacy in America: A First Look at the Results of the National Adult Literacy Survey.* Washington, DC: U.S. Government Printing Office.

Kusec S, Brborovic O, Schillinger D. 2003. Diabetes websites accredited by the Health on the Net Foundation Code of Conduct: Readable or not? Studies in health technology and informatics. Vol. 95. In: *The New Navigators: From Professionals to Patients.* Baud R, Fieschi M, Le Beux P, Ruch P, Editors. Amsterdam, NE: IOS Press.

Lorig KR, Sobel DS, Stewart AL, Brown BW Jr, Bandura A, Ritter P, Gonzalez VM, Laurent DD, Holman HR. 1999. Evidence suggesting that a chronic disease self-management program can improve health status while reducing hospitalization: A randomized trial. *Medical Care.* 37(1): 5–14.

McCulloch DK, Price MJD, Hindmarsh M, Wagner EH. 2000. Improvement in diabetes care using an integrated population-based approach in a primary care setting. *Disease Management.* 3(2): 75–82.

NCQA (National Committee for Quality Assurance). 2003. *Measuring the Quality of America's Health Care.* [Online]. Available: http://www.ncqa.org [accessed: July, 2003].

Norris SL, Nichols PJ, Caspersen CJ, Glasgow RE, Engelgau MM, Jack L, Isham G, Snyder SR, Carande-Kulis VG, Garfield S, Briss P, McCulloch D. 2002a. The effectiveness of disease and case management for people with diabetes. A systematic review. *American Journal of Preventive Medicine.* 22(4 Supplement): 15–38.

Norris SL, Nichols PJ, Caspersen CJ, Glasgow RE, Engelgau MM, Jack L, Snyder SR, Carande-Kulis VG, Isham G, Garfield S, Briss P, McCulloch D. 2002b. Increasing diabetes self-management education in community settings. A systematic review. *American Journal of Preventive Medicine.* 22(4 Supplement): 39–66.

Nurss JR, Parker RM, Williams MV, Baker DW. 1995. *TOFHLA: Test of Functional Health Literacy in Adults.* Snow Camp, NC: Peppercorn Books & Press.

Nutbeam D. 2000. Health literacy as a public health goal: A challenge for contemporary health education and communication strategies into the 21st century. *Health Promotion International.* 15(3): 259–267.

Piette JD. 1999. Satisfaction with care among patients with diabetes in two public health care systems. *Medical Care.* 37(6): 538–546.

Piette JD. 2000. Interactive voice response systems in the diagnosis and management of chronic disease. *American Journal of Managed Care.* 6(7): 817–827.

Robert Wood Johnson Foundation. 2002. *Annual Report 2001.* Princeton, NJ: The Robert Wood Johnson Foundation.

Robert Wood Johnson Foundation and the National Cancer Institute. 2002. *A Research Dialogue: Online Behavior Change and Disease Management Research.* [Online]. Available: http://www.rwjf.org/publications/publicationsPdfs/onlineBehaviorChange.pdf [accessed: November 10, 2003].

Rost K, Roter D. 1987. Predictors of recall of medication regimens and recommendations for lifestyle change in elderly patients. *Gerontologist.* 27(4): 510–515.

Roter DL. 2000. The outpatient medical encounter and elderly patients. *Clinics in Geriatric Medicine.* 16(1): 95–107.

Roter DL, Hall JA. 1992. Doctors Talking with Patients/Patients Talking with Doctors: Improving Communication in Medical Visits. Westport, CT: Auburn House.

Roter DL, Stewart M, Putnam SM, Lipkin M Jr, Stiles W, Inui TS. 1997. Communication patterns of primary care physicians. *Journal of the American Medical Association.* 277(4): 350–356.

Roter DL, Rudd RE, Comings J. 1998. Patient literacy. A barrier to quality of care. *Journal of General Internal Medicine.* 13(12): 850–851.

Roter DL, Stashefsky-Margalit R, Rudd R. 2001. Current perspectives on patient education in the US. *Patient Education and Counseling.* 44(1): 79–86.

Rothman R, Pignone M, Malone R, Bryant B, Crigler B. 2003. A primary care-based, pharmacist led, disease management program improves outcomes for patients with diabetes: A randomized controlled trial *Journal of General Internal Medicine.* 18(Supplement 1): 155.

Rudd RE, Comings JP. 1994. Learner developed materials: An empowering product. *Health Education Quarterly.* 21(3): 313–327.

Schillinger D, Grumbach K, Piette J, Wang F, Osmond D, Daher C, Palacios J, Sullivan GaD, Bindman AB. 2002. Association of health literacy with diabetes outcomes. *Journal of the American Medical Association.* 288(4): 475–482.

Schillinger D, Machtinger E, Win K, Wang F, Chan L-L, Rodriguez ME. 2003a. Are pictures worth a thousand words? Communication regarding medications in a public hospital anticoagulation clinic *Journal of General Internal Medicine* 18(Supplement 1): 187.

Schillinger D, Piette J, Grumbach K, Wang F, Wilson C, Daher C, Leong-Grotz K, Castro C, Bindman AB. 2003b. Closing the loop: Physician communication with diabetic patients who have low health literacy. *Archives of Internal Medicine.* 163(1): 83–90.

Schillinger D, Bindman A, Stewart A, Wang F, Piette J. 2004. Functional health literacy and the quality of physician-patient communication among diabetes patients. *Patient Education and Counseling.* 52(3): 315–323.

Sehgal AR. 2003. Impact of quality improvement efforts on race and sex disparities in hemodialysis. *Journal of the American Medical Association.* 289(8): 996–1000.

Starfield B. 1998. *Primary Care: Balancing Health Needs, Services, and Technology.* New York: Oxford University Press.

Street RL Jr. 1991. Information-giving in medical consultations: The influence of patients' communicative styles and personal characteristics. *Social Science and Medicine.* 32(5): 541–548.

Trento M, Passera P, Tomalino M, Bajardi M, Pomero F, Allione A, Vaccari P, Molinatti GM, Porta M. 2001. Group visits improve metabolic control in type 2 diabetes: A 2-year follow-up. *Diabetes Care.* 24(6): 995–1000.

Trento M, Passera P, Bajardi M, Tomalino M, Grassi G, Borgo E, Donnola C, Cavallo F, Bondonio P, Porta M. 2002. Lifestyle intervention by group care prevents deterioration of Type II diabetes: A 4-year randomized controlled clinical trial. *Diabetologia.* 45(9): 1231–1239.

United Kingdom Prospective Diabetes Study Group. 1998. Intensive blood-glucose control with sulphonylureas or insulin compared with conventional treatment and risk of complications in patients with type 2 diabetes (UKPDS 33). *Lancet.* 352(9131): 837–853.

Vinicor F, Burton B, Foster B, Eastman R. 2000. Healthy people 2010: Diabetes. *Diabetes Care.* 23(6): 853–855.

Von Korff M, Gruman J, Schaefer J, Curry SJ, Wagner EH. 1997. Collaborative management of chronic illness. *Annals of Internal Medicine.* 127(12): 1097–1102.

Wagner EH. 1995. Population-based management of diabetes care. *Patient Education and Counseling.* 26(1–3): 225–230.

Wagner EH. 1998. Chronic disease management: What will it take to improve care for chronic illness? *Effective Clinical Practice.* 1(1): 2–4.

Wagner, EH. 2003. *The Chronic Care Model: Improving Chronic Illness Care.* [Online]. Available: http://www.improvingchroniccare.org/change/model/components.html [accessed: March, 2003].

Wallerstein N. 1992. Powerlessness, empowerment, and health: Implications for health promotion programs. *American Journal of Health Promotion.* 6(3): 197–205.

Wallerstein N, Bernstein E. 1988. Empowerment education: Freire's ideas adapted to health education. *Health Education Quarterly.* 15(4): 379–394.

Weiss BD, Hart G, McGee DL, D'Estelle S. 1992. Health status of illiterate adults: Relation between literacy and health status among persons with low literacy skills. *Journal of the American Board of Family Practice.* 5(3): 257–264.

Williams MV, Parker RM, Baker DW, Coates W, Nurss J. 1995a. The impact of inadequate functional health literacy on patients' understanding of diagnosis, prescribed medications, and compliance. *Academic Emergency Medicine.* 2: 386.

Williams MV, Parker RM, Baker DW, Parikh NS, Pitkin K, Coates WC, Nurss JR. 1995b. Inadequate functional health literacy among patients at two public hospitals. *Journal of the American Medical Association.* 274(21): 1677–1682.

Williams MV, Baker DW, Honig EG, Lee TM, Nowlan A. 1998a. Inadequate literacy is a barrier to asthma knowledge and self-care. *Chest.* 114(4): 1008–1015.

Williams MV, Baker DW, Parker RM, Nurss JR. 1998b. Relationship of functional health literacy to patients' knowledge of their chronic disease. A study of patients with hypertension and diabetes. *Archives of Internal Medicine.* 158(2): 166–172.

Williams MV, Davis T, Parker RM, Weiss BD. 2002. The role of health literacy in patient-physician communication. *Family Medicine.* 34(5): 383–389.

Win K, Schillinger D. 2003. Understanding of warfarin therapy and stroke among ethnically diverse anticoagulation patients at a public hospital. *Journal of General Internal Medicine.* 18(Supplement 1): 278.

Youmans S, Schillinger D. 2003. Functional health literacy and medication management: The role of the pharmacist. *Annals of Pharmacotherapy.* 37(11): 1726–1729.

Zarcadoolas C, Blanco M, Boyer JF, Pleasant A. 2002. Unweaving the Web: An exploratory study of low-literate adults' navigation skills on the World Wide Web. *Journal of Health Communication.* 7(4): 309–324.

Outside the Clinician–Patient Relationship:
A Call to Action for Health Literacy

Barry D. Weiss, M.D.

Many governmental, corporate, and nonprofit businesses, organizations, and agencies have, or should have, an interest in the health literacy problem—because limited health literacy is prevalent in the groups for which these entities are responsible. These entities can be broadly categorized as insurers, employers, and advocacy groups.

Insurers should have an interest in the health literacy problem because they pay for the medical care provided to individuals with limited literacy skills, and these individuals have higher illness rates and higher health-care costs than the population in general. Employers should care about literacy because they pay for the health insurance of their workers who have limited literacy skills, and they also lose worker productivity as a result of their employee's limited literacy. Advocacy groups should care about the literacy problem because limited literacy skills often prevent their constituents from achieving full potential in society. Methods by which these and other organizations and systems might help improve America's health literacy issue are shown in Table B-5, below.

Insurers

Several entities provide medical insurance coverage groups in which low literacy is most prevalent. They include the publicly funded Medicare and Medicaid programs and the military's Tricare program.

Medicare

The Medicare program is a federally funded program that provides health insurance benefits to most elderly U.S. citizens. Medicare's costs are heavily influenced by limited health literacy because of the high rate of limited literacy skills among elderly individuals. According to the Centers for Medicare and Medicaid Services, around 35 million persons over 65 years old currently receive Medicare benefits, and the number of beneficiaries increases annually (Figure B-3).

Federal expenditures for the Medicare program now exceed $240 billion per year for medical benefits, administrative costs, and program integrity costs, representing some 20 percent of all health-care spending in the country. These costs will all increase as the number of beneficiaries continues to grow (Figure B-4) (CMS, 2002).

TABLE B-5   How Organizations and Systems Might Act to Improve America's Health Literacy

Insurers

- Provide insurance premium discounts and/or co-payment waivers to non-high school graduates who enroll in and successfully complete graduate equivalency diploma (GED) programs.
- Medicaid and Medicare could provide health education on common health problems to their enrollees at community-based courses and seminars around the nation.
- Tricare could sponsor health education seminars around the nation for military personnel and their dependents.
- Medicare, Medicaid, and Tricare insurance plans could all partner with community-based literacy enhancement programs, such as those operated by ProLiteracy, to provide literacy enhancement education to enrollees in those insurance plans.

Employers

- Partner with public school systems to enhance general literacy and biological science and health education in elementary and secondary schools.
- Partner with community-based literacy enhancement programs (e.g., ProLiteracy) to expand availability of such programs, many of which are currently oversubscribed and cannot meet community needs.
- Expand workplace literacy education programs to include an emphasis on health literacy.
- Fast food restaurants could provide education to employees regarding modes of transmission of infectious disease, thus improving both employees' health literacy and sanitation in restaurants.

Advocacy Organizations

- Advocacy organizations for the elderly could provide health education courses and classes on common health problems of older persons, specifically designed for seniors with limited literacy skills.
- Professional advocacy organization could create a nationwide corps of volunteer physicians and other health professionals to teach health education and prevention topics in elementary and secondary schools across the nation.
- Professional health advocacy organizations could establish a well-publicized national health literacy bee, analogous to current national spelling or geography bees, in which children and adolescents would compete to demonstrate their knowledge of health information.

Governmental and Social Service Agencies

- Public housing facilities for the poor could provide health education videotapes for residents to view in their homes.
- Head Start and similar daycare programs could provide pediatric health education information to parents of enrolled children.
- Homeless shelters could provide health education.
- Homeless shelters could link with community-based literacy programs to facilitate entry of clients into those literacy programs.

TABLE B-5 Continued

- Provide health information—perhaps via live speakers and/or video presentations—to individuals visiting agencies at which waiting times are typically extensive—e.g., motor vehicle department, welfare offices, post offices, etc.
- Prison systems could expand current inmate education programs to include greater emphasis on health topics.

Others

- Assisted living centers for the elderly could provide health education videotapes for residents to view in their homes.
- Health education messages could be displayed on the inside or bathroom stall doors in all public restrooms.
- Health messages, perhaps in quiz form, could be displayed on movie theater screens for the audience to view while waiting for the movie to begin.
- Sports celebrities could appear on national media to promote important health issues.
- Cell phone display screens could provide a "health tip of the day."

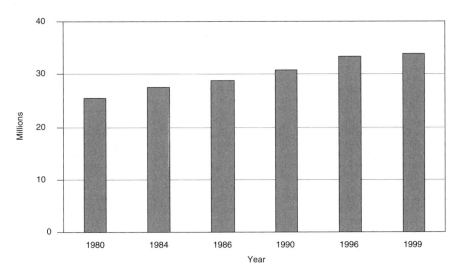

FIGURE B-3 Number of Medicare enrollees.
SOURCE: Number of Medicare Enrollees, by Age of Enrollee: Selected Calendar Years July 1, 1980–1999. Center for Medicare & Medicaid Services, Office of Information Services (http://hcms.hhs.gov/review/supp/table7b.pdf).

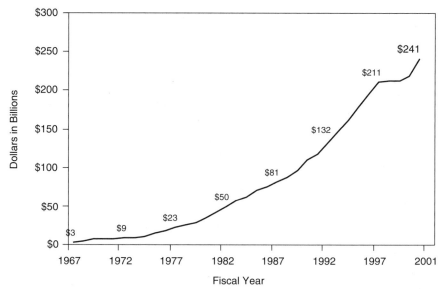

FIGURE B-4 Federal spending for Medicare. Note that overall spending includes benefit dollars, administrative costs, and program integrity costs (federal spending only).
SOURCE: Medicare Program Spending. Centers for Medicare and Medicaid Services, Office of the Actuary, June 2002 (http://www.cms.hhs.gov/charts/default.asp).

By combining Medicare expenditure figures with results from the National Adult Literacy Survey (NALS), which indicate that 80 percent of persons over 65 have limited literacy skills, one can estimate that about 80 percent of Medicare beneficiaries—32 million individuals—have limited literacy skills. Thus, most of the $240 billion annual Medicare expenditures are related to providing benefits for persons with limited literacy. Addressing the health literacy of Medicaid enrollees (Table B-5) can potentially result in substantial cost savings for the Medicare program.

Medicaid

The Medicaid program, funded by state and federal tax dollars, provides medical insurance benefits for about 45 million persons, most of whom are poor (CMS, 2000). Total expenditures by the Medicaid system were $175 billion per year in 1998, accounting for about 15 percent of all health-care spending in the United States (Health Care Financing Administration, 2000). The cost of the Medicaid program is expected to grow to $444 billion by 2010 (Figure B-5).

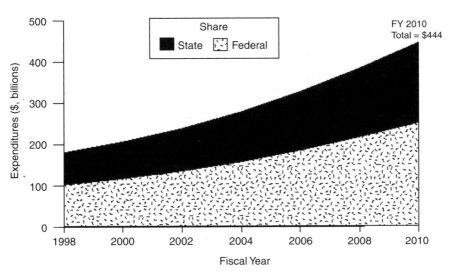

FIGURE B-5   Predicted Medicaid expenditures.
SOURCE: Health Care Financing Administration. *A Profile of Medicaid: Chartbook 2000*, Section III. Medicaid Expenditures. Pp. 27–51 (http://www.cms.hhs.gov/charts/medicaid/2Tchartbk.pdf).

The rate of limited literacy is high among Medicaid enrollees. A study of a random sample of Medicaid enrollees in Arizona (Weiss et al., 1994) found that the mean literacy skills of the enrollees were at just over grade-level 5. More than a quarter of subjects had reading skills at or below the fourth-grade level, in contrast to the eighth-grade average reading level of U.S. adults. Subjects in the study who indicated that their preferred language for reading was Spanish had their literacy skills assessed in Spanish, and their average reading level was at grade level 3.1.

The limited literacy skills of Medicaid enrollees are associated with high health-care costs. Indeed, in the Arizona study Medicaid recipients with the highest reading levels had average annual health-care costs of $2,969, similar to the $2,400 average cost of health care for all U.S. citizens at the time of the study. In contrast, those with reading levels at or below grade-level 3 had annual health-care costs averaging $10,688 (Weiss and Palmer, 2004). These results are remarkable, given that the subjects had relatively homogenous sociodemographic characteristics (all poor and un-employed or employed at very low-paying jobs), and the statistical relationship between literacy and costs remained strong even after a multivariable analysis that accounted for education, gender, ethnic group, and preferred language. Thus, to the extent that interventions to improve health literacy (Table B-5) can reduce health-care costs, such interventions can potentially result in substantial cost savings for Medicaid programs.

Tricare

The Tricare program provides health insurance benefits for the nation's military personnel (active- and non-active-duty) and their dependents. The program covers direct medical care, prescriptions, dental care, and a variety of other health-related benefits.

Tricare is an expensive program. Spending by the federal government for direct medical and administrative costs totaled $8.3 billion in 1998 for some 4 million Tricare enrollees (Stoloff et al., 2000).

As noted earlier, many military recruits have limited literacy skills. Given the association between limited literacy and higher health-care costs, and given the cost of the Tricare system, significant cost savings might accrue to the U.S. military if the health literacy skills of the military recruits were improved. Thus, the military is an entity with large potential gain from improvement in its members' health literacy.

As mentioned, the military currently engages in literacy-skill enhancement for its recruits to enable them to function adequately in the roles as soldiers. Incorporating health knowledge within literacy training (Table B-5) might provide further benefit by reducing excess costs related to limited health literacy.

Employers

Business leaders have long recognized the need for literacy enhancement in the workforce, as workers' limited literacy skills often interfere with productivity and safety (Rockefeller Foundation Conference Proceedings, 1989). This concern is of particular importance for businesses that employ large numbers of routine service providers and production workers, because these groups have an over-representation of undereducated individuals (Reich, 1992). Some large employers already offer literacy training to their employees to address concerns about workplace literacy (Academy of Human Resource Development, 2000; Askov and Van Horn, 1993; National Institute for Literacy, 1994).

Businesses should also have an interest in health literacy because of its relationship to health-care costs. Government agencies have reported that nearly two-thirds of Americans under age 65 obtain health insurance through their workplace (Monheit and Vistnes, 1997), with more than 150 million workers and dependents in the United States, and an additional 5 million retirees, receiving job-based health insurance benefits (Gabel et al., 2000). On average, health benefits currently cost employers about $1.29 per hour per employee (U.S. Department of Labor, 2002).

The result of these costs, based on recent data from the Agency for Healthcare Research and Quality (AHRQ), is that each year private employers in the United States pay in the range of $350 billion to cover the cost of hospitalizations and physicians' services for their employees and families (Table B-6) (AHRQ, 2000). Public employers, including federal, state, and local governments, pay approximately $60 billion dollars per year. These costs rise annually—an 8 percent increase in 2000 and an 11 percent increase in 2001—with similar increases anticipated in the future (Mercer, 2003). Health insurance premiums paid by employers increase at a faster rate than wages or overall inflation (Gabel et al., 2001). Indeed, the Health Care Financing Administration has estimated that by 2008, health-care spending in the United States will reach $2.2 trillion (CMS, 2003).

To the extent that improving literacy skills will reduce health-care costs, employers would benefit substantially from initiatives that improve worker literacy. This is especially true for employers with a workforce that includes large numbers of routine service and production workers, as these groups have high rates of limited literacy. Partners in such initiatives could

TABLE B-6 National Totals for Enrollees and Cost of Hospitalization and Physician Service Health Plans for the Private Sector, United States, 2000

Enrollee Category	Total (in thousands of persons)
Total Enrollees	71,253
Active enrollees	64,284
Enrollees through COBRA	2,766
Retired enrollees	4,203
Costs	Total (in millions of dollars)
Total Costs	349,612
Employer contribution single coverage	69,066
Employer contribution family coverage	191,916
Employee contribution single coverage	18,251
Employee contribution family coverage	70,379

SOURCE: Agency for Healthcare Research and Quality, Center for Cost and Financing Studies. *2000 Medical Expenditure Panel Survey—Insurance Component* (http://meps.ahrq.gov/ MEPSDATA/ic/2000/Tables_IV/TableIVA1.htm).

include not only employers, but also community-based literacy programs and local governments seeking to attract employers that would be drawn to communities with a more literate workforce.

An additional approach to improving workforce literacy, including health literacy, could focus on science education in secondary schools and universities, where most students currently are taught basic science facts, rather than applied health sciences—and many students study little or no science at all. Indeed, data from the National Center for Education Statistics indicate that only 75 percent of U.S. high school students take more than one science course. While biology is the most popular science course offered in high school (i.e., most students select biology as their one science course), only about 1 in 6 takes an advanced course in biology (National Center for Education Statistics, 2001). The result is that many, if not most, students, even some destined for a career in the health sciences, graduate from high schools without a substantive understanding of the anatomy, physiology, and etiology of common diseases like atherosclerosis, diabetes, and cancer. Incorporating an applied "health literacy approach" into science education in schools and universities could have a major benefit for improving the health literacy of the nation's workforce and for reducing health-care expenditures for employers (Table B-5).

Advocacy Organizations

There are many national-level organizations with missions dedicated to improving opportunities and quality of life for their constituents. Of note, some of these organizations advocate on behalf of the groups with the highest rates of limited literacy—the elderly, Hispanics, and African Americans—and these organizations could implement programs to improve their constituents' health literacy (Table B-5). Although not discussed here, there are also advocacy groups on both local and national levels that represent the other high-risk groups, such as other ethnic minority groups, immigrants, the homeless, the poor, and prisoners.

Advocates for the Elderly

The most well known, and perhaps the most important, senior citizens' advocacy group is the American Association of Retired Persons (now known only by the acronym AARP)—which represents over 35 million older Americans (AARP, 2002). In addition to general advocacy on behalf of the nation's elderly, AARP places particular emphasis on health and the cost of health care for senior citizens.

Given the very high rate of limited literacy among older individuals, and relationship of those limited literacy skills to health status, health-care costs, employment opportunities, and quality of life, a focus on literacy—including health literacy—would advance AARP's mission and improve quality of life for its constituents. Other senior citizens' advocacy groups share similar goals.

Advocates for Hispanics

There are many advocacy organizations for Hispanics, but two stand out as particularly respected and influential: the National Council of La Raza and the Mexican American Legal Defense and Educational Fund. In addition, the National Hispanic Medical Association has particular interest in health-related issues, which could include health literacy.

National Council of La Raza

The National Council of La Raza is a private, nonprofit organization established in 1968. It has 270 formal affiliates in 40 states, and a much broader network of 20,000 groups and individuals nationwide. Its mission is to "improve life opportunities for Hispanic Americans" (National Council of La Raza, 2003). Life opportunities are diminished when individuals have limited literacy skills, and the literacy skills of Hispanics are currently the lowest of any major ethnic group in the United States (Table B-7). Enhancing literacy skills, including health literacy skills, as an area of emphasis for the National Council of La Raza and similar organizations has the potential to improve economic opportunities and health care for Hispanic Americans.

Mexican American Legal Defense and Educational Fund

The Mexican American Legal Defense and Educational Fund is a national nonprofit organization whose mission includes assuring that "there are no obstacles preventing [the Latino] community from realizing its dreams . . ." (Mexican American Legal Defense and Educational Fund, 2003). Limited literacy is one such obstacle, and the Mexican American Legal Defense and Educational Fund could participate in efforts to enhance literacy and health literacy skills of Hispanics.

National Hispanic Medical Association

The National Hispanic Medical Association is an organization that represents Hispanic medical providers. The organization expresses a commitment to providing policy makers and health-care providers with expert medical information, and to supporting and strengthening delivery of health

TABLE B-7 Percentage of Adult Population Groups with Literacy Skills at NALS Levels 1 or 2

	Percent	
Group	Level 1	Level 2
All NALS Respondents	22	28
Age		
16–54 years	15	28
55–64 years	28	33
65 years and older	49	32
Highest Education Level Completed		
0–8 years	77	19
9–12 years (no high school graduation)	44	37
High school diploma/GED (no college study)	18	37
Racial/Ethnic Group		
White	15	26
American Indian/Alaska Native	26	38
Asian Pacific Islander	35	25
Black	41	36
Hispanic (all groups)	52	26
Immigrants to U.S. (various countries of origin)		
0–8 years of education prior to arrival in U.S.	60	31
9 + years of education prior to arrival in U.S.	44	27

SOURCE: Unadjusted averages of prose and document literacy scores on the NALS as reported on Tables 1.1A, 1.1B, 1.2A, and 1.2B in Kirsch I, Jungeblut A, Jenkins L, Kolstad A. *Adult Literacy in America: A First Look at the Results of the National Adult Literacy Survey.* Washington, DC: National Center for Education Statistics, U.S. Department of Education; September, 1993, and on Table B3.13 in U.S. Department of Education. National Center for Education Statistics. *English Literacy and Language Minorities in the United States*, NCES 2001–464, by Greenberg E, Macías RF, Rhodes D, Chan T. Washington, DC: 2001.

services to Hispanic communities across the nation (National Hispanic Medical Association, 1997). Aiding in the improvement of health literacy for Hispanics would go hand in hand with these goals, and it would seem logical for the National Hispanic Medical Association to participate in health literacy efforts.

Advocates for African-Americans

African-Americans are also represented by a number of advocacy organizations. Two of the most respected organizations are the National Association for the Advancement of Colored People (NAACP) and the National Urban League. The National Medical Association, the organization that represents African-American physicians, also has a specific interest in the health status of African-American citizens.

NAACP

NAACP is the nation's oldest and largest civil rights organization. NAACP has a specific health division, with goals that include "developing national health advocacy and education initiatives that promote equity in health status," "sponsoring collaborative initiatives with other national and local health groups," and "expanding outreach on health advocacy and awareness in communications" (NAACP, 2003). Assuring adequate health literacy as a component of initiatives meets all of those goals, and NAACP may thus be an effective advocate for enhancing health literacy among African Americans.

National Urban League

The National Urban League has affiliates in more than 100 cities in 24 states. While the organization's goal is broadly aimed at enabling "African Americans to secure economic self-reliance, parity and power and civil rights," its mission also includes a specific goal of "ensuring that our children are well educated" (National Urban League, 2002). Efforts to improve literacy in general, and health literacy in particular, would fall within the mission of the National Urban League.

National Medical Association

The National Medical Association represents the interests of more than 25,000 African-American physician and their patients. One of the organization's key missions is "to improve the status of health and quality and availability of health care to African-American and underserved populations" (National Medical Association, 2003). This mission would be enhanced by efforts to improve health literacy.

Other Organizations and Systems

There are many other organizations and systems that provide services to groups with high rates of limited literacy. Among these are prison systems and social service agencies that work with undereducated individuals. Professional organizations that represent health-care providers (in addition to the National Medical Association and National Hispanic Medical Association) also have a role to play in improving health literacy (Table B-5).

Prison Systems

Inmates in most prisons already have access to literacy improvement programs. Given the large and growing size of the U.S. prison population, however, and the costs associated with providing health care to prisoners, incorporating health literacy content might enhance current literacy improvement programs.

Social Service Agencies

Social service agencies in virtually all U.S. communities interact with low-literate individuals every day, because clientele of these agencies include large numbers of unemployed persons with limited education. Some of these agencies, particularly adult education programs, focus on literacy enhancement as a core mission through adult basic education, GED programs, and "English as a Second Language" programs.

The majority of individuals with limited literacy, however, do not enter such education programs. Rather their interaction with social service agencies is often through county and state public assistance programs, unemployment agencies, childcare programs, and others. These social service agencies spend large sums of money providing services to their clientele, and those sums might be reduced if clientele had better literacy skills that permitted easier entry into the workforce. To the extent that clientele of these agencies have chronic health problems—and many do—costs might further be reduced if clientele had better health literacy.

Public assistance, unemployment, and childcare agencies could link with local adult education programs, or with national literacy programs such as ProLiteracy America (Proliteracy Worldwide, 2002), to facilitate easy referral into literacy training programs. In fact, literacy training programs could be located on site with, or in close geographic proximity to, a variety of social service agencies, including medical clinics whose clients might benefit from literacy enhancement. Such partnerships, some emphasizing health literacy, are currently in place in a number of communities (Community Health Partners, 2003; El Paso Community College/Community Education Program, 2001). More such partnerships should be encouraged.

Professional Associations

Finally, professional associations representing health-care providers have an interest in assuring and improving health and health care for individual patients. With evidence showing that limited literacy skills are associated with poorer health status, all professional associations representing health-care providers should have a *de facto* interest in improving health literacy.

Some professional associations, such as the American Medical Association, have already produced educational materials to enhance health providers' understanding of the health literacy problem and give them suggestions for how to more effectively communicate with patients (Weiss, 2003). The materials include educational monographs and videotapes, train-the-trainer programs, and outreach efforts to local medical societies. Other professional organizations, such as the American Academy of Neurology, the Virginia Medical Society, the Iowa Medical Society, and the Georgia Academy of Family Physicians have also developed programs, or are planning to do so.

Additional efforts from professional associations could include lobbying efforts aimed at securing support for health literacy content in adult basic education programs. Finally, professional organizations could improve the public's health literacy by working with school systems to develop and implement health education curricula for use in elementary and secondary schools.

CONCLUSION

The unique vocabulary and concepts of medicine make it difficult for many individuals to fully understand health information provided to them by clinicians. This lack of understanding translates into poor health literacy—i.e., a limited ability to read, understand, and use health information to make effective health-care decisions and follow recommendations for treatment. While limited health literacy occurs in all segments of society, it is a particular problem for individuals with limited reading skills (i.e., limited general literacy).

Limited literacy is more prevalent in certain groups. These groups include the elderly, racial and ethnic minorities, persons with limited education, immigrants, prisoners, the poor and homeless, and military recruits. In some of these groups, such as the elderly, certain ethnic minorities, and persons who did not complete school, the prevalence of limited literacy exceeds 80–90 percent.

Persons with limited general and health literacy, on average, have poorer health knowledge, poorer health status, and higher health-care costs than do persons with higher-level literacy skills. The relationship between limited literacy and poorer health and higher costs is strong and independent of other socioeconomic factors.

Based on results of the NALS, about half of U.S. adults have literacy skills that are inadequate to meet the demands of today's health system. Health-care systems could address this problem through processes and policies that enhance employee awareness of patients' health literacy skills, and by delivering information in ways that patients can understand.

A variety of public and private entities have a stake in the health literacy problem. These include health insurers, employers, and advocacy groups. Insurers have a stake in the problem because of the high cost of health care for persons with limited literacy. For example, because limited literacy skills are so common among the elderly, most of Medicare's $240 billion annual budget goes to providing care for persons with limited literacy.

Employers, especially those that employ large numbers of undereducated service and production workers, also have a stake in health literacy. Employers pay the high cost of their employee's health insurance benefits, and their businesses lose productivity due to higher rates of illness among employees with limited literacy.

REFERENCES

AARP. 2002. *AARP Facts.* [Online]. Available: http://www.aarp.org/what_is.html [accessed: August, 2003].

Academy of Human Resource Development. 2000. Workforce Development. Symposium 37 [concurrent Symposium Session at AHRD Annual Conference, March 8–12, 2000]. Raleigh-Durham, NC: Academy of Human Resource Development.

AHRQ (Agency for Healthcare Research and Quality, Center for Cost and Financing Studies). 2000. *Medical Expenditure Panel Survey—Insurance Component.* [Online]. Available: http://meps.ahrq.gov/MEPSDATA/ic/2000/Tables_IV/TableIVA1.htm [accessed August, 2003].

Askov EN, Van Horn B. 1993. Adult educators and workplace literacy: Designing customized basic skills instruction. *Adult Basic Education.* 3(2): 115–125.

CMS (Centers for Medicare and Medicaid Services). 2000. *Medicaid Eligables—Fiscal Year 2000 by Maintenance Assistance Status and Basis of Eligibility.* [Online]. Available: http://www.cms.hhs.gov/medicaid/msis/00total.pdf [accessed: August, 2003].

CMS. 2002. *Medicare Program Spending.* [Online]. Available: http://www.cms.hhs.gov/charts/series/sec3-a.ppt [accessed: August, 2003].

CMS. 2003. *Health Accounts: Estimates.* [Online]. Available: http://hcfa.gov/stats/NHE-proj/ [accessed: August, 2003].

Community Health Partners. 2003. *A Partnership for Health.* [Online]. Available: http://chphealth.org/ [accessed: August, 2003].

El Paso Community College/Community Education Program. 2001. *The El Paso Collaborative Health Literacy Curriculum.* [Online]. Available: http://www.worlded.org/us/health/docs/elpaso/index.htm [accessed: August, 2003].

Gabel J, Levitt L, Pickreign J, Whitmore H, Holve E, Hawkins S, Miller N. 2000. Job-based health insurance in 2000: Premiums rise sharply while coverage grows. *Health Affairs.* 19(5): 144–151.

Gabel J, Levitt L, Pickreign J, Whitmore H, Holve E, Rowland D, Dhont K, Hawkins S. 2001. Job-based health insurance in 2001: Inflation hits double digits, managed care retreats. *Health Affairs.* 20(5): 180–186.

Health Care Financing Administration. 2000. *A Profile of Medicaid: Chartbook 2000.* [Online]. Available: http://www.cms.hhs.gov/charts/medicaid/2Tchartbk.pdf [accessed: August, 2003].

Mercer, WM. 2000. *15th Annual Mercer/Foster Higgins National Survey of Employer-Sponsored Health Plans.* [Online]. Available: http://imercer.com/us/imercercommentary/BBfinal.pdf [accessed: August, 2003].

Mexican American Legal Defense and Education Fund. 2003. *Mission Statement.* [Online]. Available: http://www.maldef.org/about/mission.htm [accessed: August, 2003].

Monheit AC, Vistnes JP 1997. *MEPS Research Findings No. 2. Health Insurance Status of Workers and Their Families.* Rockville, MD: Agency for Health Care Policy and Research.

NAACP (National Association for the Advancement of Colored People). 2003. *NAACP Health Division Fact Sheet.* [Online]. Available: http://www.naacp.org/programs/health/FactSheet.shtml [accessed: August, 2003].

National Center for Education Statistics. 2001. *The 1998 High School Transcript Study Tabulations: Comparative Data on Credits Earned and Demographics for 1998, 1994, 1990, 1987, 1982 High School Graduates.* Washington, DC: U.S. Department of Education, Office of Educational Research and Improvement.

National Council of La Raza. 2003. *Mission Statement.* [Online]. Available: http://www.nclr.org/about/index.html [accessed: August, 2003].

National Hispanic Medical Association. 1997. *Home Page.* [Online]. Available: http://www.nhmamd.org [accessed: August, 2003].

National Institute for Literacy. 1994. *What Kind of Adult Literacy Policy Do We Need If We Are Serious About Enabling Every Adult to Become a High Skills/High Wage Worker in the Global Economy?* Washington, DC: National Institute for Literacy.

National Medical Association. 2003. *National Medical Association Overview.* [Online]. Available: http://www.nmanet.org [accessed: August, 2003].

National Urban League. 2002. *Mission Statement.* [Online]. Available: http://www.nul.org/about/mission.htm [accessed: August, 2003].

Proliteracy Worldwide. 2002. *Proliteracy America.* [Online]. Available: http://www.proliteracy.org/proliteracy_america/index.asp [accessed: August, 2003].

Reich RB. 1992. *The Work of Nations: Preparing Ourselves for 21st Century Capitalism.* New York: Vintage Press.

Rockefeller Foundation Conference Proceedings. 1989. *Literacy and the Marketplace.* New York: The Rockefeller Foundation.

Stoloff, PH, Lurie, PM, Goldmerg, L, Almendarez, M 2000. *Evaluation of the TRICARE Program: FY 2000 Report to Congress.* [Online]. Available: http://www.defenselink.mil/pubs/tricare02202001.pdf [accessed: August, 2003].

U.S. Department of Labor. Bureau of Labor Statistics. 20002. *Cost of Health Benefits in Private Industry, March 2002.* [Online]. Available: http://www.bls.gov/opub/ted/2002/jul/wk3/art01.htm [accessed: August, 2003].

Weiss BD. 2003. *Health Literacy: A Manual for Clinicians.* Chicago, IL: American Medical Association Foundation.

Weiss BD, Palmer R. 2004. Relationship between health care costs and very low literacy skills in a medically needy and indigent Medicaid population. *Journal of the American Board of Family Practice.* 17(1): 44–47.

Weiss BD, Blanchard JS, McGee DL, Hart G, Warren B, Burgoon M, Smith KJ. 1994. Illiteracy among Medicaid recipients and its relationship to health care costs. *Journal of Health Care for the Poor & Underserved.* 5(2): 99–111.

C

Sample Material from Selected Assessments of Literacy and Health Literacy

his appendix presents background and sample items from some of the measures that have been discussed in this report. For more information about the development and use of these measures, please see Chapter 2.

CONTENTS

RAPID ESTIMATE OF ADULT LITERACY IN MEDICINE (REALM)©

TABLE C-1　REALM

Patient Name/
Subject # _____　　Date of
　　　　　　　　　　　　　　Birth _____　　Reading
　　　　　　　　　　　　　　　　　　　　　　Level _____

Date _____ Clinic _____　Examiner _____　Grade
　　　　　　　　　　　　　　　　　　　　　　Completed _____

List 1	List 2	List 3
Fat	Fatigue	Allergic
Flu	Pelvic	Menstrual
Pill	Jaundice	Testicle
Dose	Infection	Colitis
Eye	Exercise	Emergency
Stress	Behavior	Medication
Smear	Prescription	Occupation
Nerves	Notify	Sexually
Germs	Gallbladder	Alcoholism
Meals	Calories	Irritation
Disease	Depression	Constipation
Cancer	Miscarriage	Gonorrhea
Caffeine	Pregnancy	Inflammatory
Attack	Arthritis	Diabetes
Kidney	Nutrition	Hepatitis
Hormones	Menopause	Antibiotics
Herpes	Appendix	Diagnosis
Seizure	Abnormal	Potassium
Bowel	Syphilis	Anemia
Asthma	Hemorrhoids	Obesity
Rectal	Nausea	Osteoporosis
Incest	Directed	Impetigo

SCORE

List 1 _____
List 2 _____
List 3 _____

Raw Score _____

Directions:

1. Give the patient a laminated copy of the REALM and score answers on an unlaminated copy that is attached to a clipboard. Hold the clipboard at an angle so that the patient is not distracted by your scoring procedure. Say:

> "I want to hear you read as many words as you can from this list. Begin with the first word on List 1 and read aloud. When you come to a word you cannot read, do the best you can or say "blank" and go on to the next word."

2. If the patient takes more than five seconds on a word, say "blank" and point to the next word, if necessary, to move the patient along. If the patient begins to miss every word, have him or her pronounce only known words.

3. Count as an error any word not attempted or mispronounced. Score by marking a plus (+) after each correct word, a check (✓) after each mispronounced word, and a minus (–) after words not attempted. Count as correct any self-corrected word.

4. Count the number of correct words for each list and record the numbers in the "SCORE' box. Total the numbers and match the total score with its grade equivalent in the table below (Table C-2).

TABLE C-2 Scores and Grade Equivalents for the REALM

	GRADE EQUIVALENT
Raw Score	Grade Range
0–18	3rd Grade and below • Will not be able to read most low literacy materials; will need repeated oral instructions, materials composed primarily of illustrations, or audio or videotapes
19–44	4th to 6th Grade • Will need low literacy materials; may not be able to read prescription labels
45–60	7th to 8th Grade • Will struggle with most patient education materials; will not be offended by low literacy materials
61–66	High School • Will be able to read most patient education materials

Excerpts taken from: Davis TC, Crouch MA, Long SW. 1993. *Rapid Estimate of Adult Literacy in Medicine: A Shortened Screening Instrument*. Louisiana State University. Reprinted with permission.

EXCERPTS FROM THE TEST OF FUNCTIONAL HEALTH LITERACY IN ADULTS

Numeracy

The numeracy section of the TOFHLA measures the patient's ability to understand and act on numerical directions given by a health-care provider or pharmacist. The test items reproduce real-life situations in receiving, following, and paying for medication plans. The numeracy section uses a series of prompts to which the patient responds. These prompts consist of prescription vials, an appointment slip, a chart describing eligibility for financial aid, and an example of results from a medical test. The patient is handed the prompt for each question, the administrator reads each question, and the responses are recorded.

Sample Items

At the beginning of this section, the following introduction is read: "These are directions you or someone else might be given at the hospital. Please read each direction to yourself. Then I will ask you some questions about what it means." For the first few questions in this section the patient is given Prompt 1, a prescription bottle that has the label shown in Figure C-1 below taped to it.

GARFIELD IM   16 Apr 93
FF941858 Dr. Lubin, Michael

PENICILLIN VK
250MG 40/0
Take one tablet by mouth four
times a day 02 (4 of 40)

FIGURE C-1   Prompt 1 for TOFHLA. Prescription label that should taped onto an actual prescription bottle that can be handed to the patient to read.

Questions for Prompt 1:

If you take your first tablet at 7:00 am, when should you take the next one?

And the next one after that?

What about the last one for the day, when should you take that one?

At the end of the numeracy section, the patient is given Prompt 10, a laminated card with information shown in Figure C-2 below.

You can get care at no cost if after deductions your monthly income and other resources are less than:

$581 for a family of one $1,196 for a family of four
$786 for a family of two $1,401 for a family of five
$991 for a family of three $1,606 for a family of six.

FIGURE C-2   Prompt 10 for TOFHLA. Laminated card with financial information about clinic services.

Question for Prompt 10:

Let's say that after deductions, your monthly income and other resources are $1,129. And, let's say you have 3 children. Would you have to pay for your care at that clinic?

Reading Comprehension

The reading comprehension section of the TOFHLA measures a patient's ability to read passages using real materials from the health-care setting using a modified Cloze procedure. Passages included come from instructions for preparation for an upper GI series, the patient rights and responsibilities section of a Medicaid application form, and standard hospital informed consent language.

Sample Items

At the beginning of the reading comprehension section of the TOFHLA, the following instructions are read:

Here are some other medical instructions that you or anybody might see around the hospital. These instructions are in sentences that have some of the words missing. Where a word is missing, a blank line is drawn, and 4 possible words that could go in the blank appear just below it. I want you to figure out which of those 4 words should go in the blank, which word makes the sentence make sense. When you think you know which one it is, circle the letter in front of that word, and go on to the next one. When you finish the page, turn the page, and keep going until you finish all the pages.

The reading comprehension section consists of three passages; one of these passages is shown on the next page.

PASSAGE B: Medicaid Rights and Responsibilities

I agree to give correct information to _____ if I can receive Medicaid.
                    a. hair
                    b. salt
                    c. see
                    d. ache

I _____ to provide the county information to _____ any
  a. agree   a. hide
  b. probe   b. risk
  c. send   c. discharge
  d. gain   d. prove

statements given in this _____ and hereby give permission to
                a. emphysema
                b. application
                c. gallbladder
                d. relationship

the _____ to get such proof. I _____ that for
    a. inflammation   a. investigate
    b. religion   b. entertain
    c. iron   c. understand
    d. county   d. establish

Medicaid I must report any _____ in my circumstances
                  a. changes
                  b. hormones
                  c. antacids
                  d. charges

within _____ (10) days of becoming _____ of the change.
    a. three   a. award
    b. one   b. aware
    c. five   c. away
    d. ten   d. await

I understand _____ if I DO NOT like the _____ made on my
    a. thus   a. marital
    b. this   b. occupation
    c. that   c. adult
    d. than   d. decision

case, I have the _____ to a fair hearing. I can _____ a
    a. bright   a. request
    b. left   b. refuse
    c. wrong   c. fail
    d. right   d. mend

hearing by writing or _____ the county where I applied.
              a. counting
              b. reading
              c. calling
              d. smelling

If you _____ AFDC for any family _____, you will have to
      a. wash   a. member,
      b. want   b. history,
      c. cover   c. weight,
      d. tape   d. seatbelt,

_____ a different application form. _____, we will use
    a. relax   a. Since,
    b. break   b. Whether,
    c. inhale   c. However,
    d. sign   d. Because,

the _____ on this form to determine your _____.
      a. lung   a. hypoglycemia.
      b. date   b. eligibility.
      c. meal   c. osteoporosis.
      d. pelvic   d. schizophrenia.

Excerpts taken from: Nurss JR, Parker RM, Williams MV, Baker DW. 2001. *Test of Functional Health Literacy in Adults.* Available from Peppercorn Books and Press, Inc. Reprinted with permission.

EXCERPTS FROM THE NATIONAL ADULT LITERACY SURVEY

Prose Literacy and Sample Items

Prose refers to any written text such as editorials, news stories, poems, and fiction, and can be broken down into two types: expository prose and narrative prose. Expository prose consists of printed information that defines, describes, or informs, such as newspaper stories or written instructions. Narrative prose tells a story. Prose varies in its length, density, and structure (e.g., use of section headings or topic sentences for paragraphs). Prose literacy tasks include locating all the information requested, integrating information from various parts of a passage of text, and writing new information related to the text.

Prose Literacy Levels

Adults included in level 1 were those who could succeed at level 1 tasks, but not at level 2 tasks, as well as those who could not succeed at level 1 tasks and those who were not literate enough in English to take the test at all. Adults in levels 2 through 4 were able to succeed at tasks at their proficiency level, but not at tasks for the next more difficult level. Adults in level 5 are able to succeed at level 5 tasks.

Prose Level 1. Level 1 prose literacy tasks required a person to read a short passage of text and locate a single piece of information that is identical to or synonymous with the information given in the question. If plausible but incorrect information was present in the text, it tended not to be located near the correct information.

Sample Prose Item (Level 1): Swimmer Article: Locate Fact with No Distractor

Task: Use the article "Swimmer completes Manhattan marathon" (See Figure C-3) to answer the following question.

Underline the sentence that tells what Ms. Chanin ate during the swim.

The answer is correct if respondent underlines, circles, or puts a mark next to the sentence beginning A Spokesman for the Swimmer, or underlines, circles, or puts a mark next to any part of the sentence that just lists the foods.

This level 1 task asks respondents to read a newspaper article about a marathon swimmer and to underline the sentence that tells what she ate

Swimmer completes Manhattan marathon

The Associated Press
NEW YORK—University of Maryland Senior Stacy Chanin on Wednesday became the first person to swim three 28-mile laps around Manhattan.

Chanin, 23, of Virginia, climbed out of the East River at 96th Street at 9:30 p.m. She began the swim at noon on Tuesday.

A spokesman for the swimmer, Roy Brunett, said Chanin had kept up her strength with "banana and honey" sandwiches, hot chocolate, lots of water and granola bars."

Chanin has twice circled Manhattan before and trained for the new feat by swimming about 28.4 miles a week. The Yonkers native has competed as a swimmer since she was 15 and hoped to persuade Olympic authorities to add a long-distance swimming event.

The Leukemia Society of America solicited pledges for each mile she swam.

In July 1983, Julie Ridge became the first person to swim around Manhattan twice. With her three laps, Chanin came up just short of Diane Nyad's distance record, set on a Florida-to-Cuba swim.

Reduced from original copy

FIGURE C-3   Article "Swimmer completes Manhattan marathon" used in NALS.

during a swim. Only one reference to food is contained in the passage, and it does not use the word "ate." Rather, the article says the swimmer "kept up her strength with banana and honey sandwiches, hot chocolate, lots of water and granola bars." The reader must match the word "ate" in the directive with the only reference to foods in the article.

Prose Level 2. Prose literacy tasks at level 2 required a person to locate a single piece of information in the text, compare and contrast easily identifiable information based on criteria provided in the question, or integrate two or more pieces of information, when distractors were present or when low level inferences were required.

Sample Prose Item (Level 2): Swimmer Article: Locate Fact with Distractor

Task: Use the article "Swimmer completes Manhattan marathon" (see Figure C-3 above) to answer the following question.

At what age did Chanin begin swimming competitively?

Acceptable responses are underlining or circling age or the sentence containing the age in the article.

This level 2 task requires the reader to locate information in the text. The reader is asked to identify the age at which the marathon swimmer began to swim competitively. The article first provides the swimmer's current age of 23, which is a plausible but incorrect answer. The correct information, age 15, is found toward the end of the article.

Prose Level 3. Prose literacy tasks at level 3 required a person to match literal or synonymous information in the text with that requested in the question, to integrate multiple pieces of information from dense or lengthy text, or to generate a response based on information that could be easily identified in the text. Distracting information was present, but was not located near the correct information.

Sample Prose Item (Level 3): Discrimination Article

Task: Refer to the article below (Figure C-4) to answer this question.

> List two things that Chen became involved in or has done to help resolve conflicts due to discrimination.

The answer is correct if the respondent lists any two of the following:

- worked for EEO Commission or was litigator on behalf of plaintiffs who experienced discrimination
- served on Philadelphia Commission on Human Relations or worked with community leaders (to resolve racial and ethnic tensions)
- contributed free legal counsel (to a variety of activist groups)
- called for a meeting of community leaders to help resolve conflict over desecration of Korean street signs
- involved in Hispanic, Jewish, and black issues
- involved in Ethnic Affairs Committee of Anti-Defamation League of B'nai B'rith or just B'nai B'rith

This level 3 item requires the reader to read a magazine article about an Asian-American woman and to provide two facts that support an inference made from the text. The question directs the reader to identify what Ida Chen did to help resolve conflicts due to discrimination.

Prose Level 4. Prose literacy tasks at level 4 required a person to search through text and match multiple features, and to integrate or synthesize multiple pieces of information from complex or lengthy passages. More complex inferences were required, and conditional information had to be taken into consideration for these tasks.

IDA CHEN is the first Asian-American woman to become a judge of the Commonwealth of Pennsylvania.

She understands discrimination because she has experienced it herself.

Soft-spoken and eminently dignified, Judge Ida Chen prefers hearing about a new acquaintance rather than talking about herself. She wants to know about career plans, hopes, dreams, fears. She gives unsolicited advice as well as encouragement. She instills confidence.

Her father once hoped that she would become a professor. And she would have also made an outstanding social worker or guidance counselor. The truth is that Chen wears the caps of all these professions as a Family Court judge of the Court of Common Pleas of Philadelphia County, as a participant in public advocacy for minorities, and as a particularly sensitive, caring person.

She understands discrimination because she has experienced it herself. As an elementary school student, Chen tried to join the local Brownie troop. "You can't be a member," she was told. "Only American girls are in the Brownies."

Originally intent upon a career as a journalist, she selected Temple University because of its outstanding journalism department and affordable tuition. Independence being a personal need, she paid for her tuition by working for Temple's Department of Criminal Justice. There she had her first encounter with the legal world and it turned her career plans in a new direction — law school.

Through meticulous planning, Chen was able to earn her undergraduate degree in two and a half years and she continued to work three jobs. But when she began her first semester as a Temple law student in the fall of 1973, she was barely able to stay awake. Her teacher Lynne Abraham, now a Common Pleas Court judge herself, couldn't help but notice Chen yawning in the back of the class, and when she determined that this student was not a party animal but a workhorse, she arranged a teaching assistant's job for Chen on campus.

After graduating from Temple Law School in 1976, Chen worked for the U.S. Equal Employment Opportunity Commission where she was a litigator on behalf of plaintiffs who experienced discrimination in the workplace, and then moved on to become the first Asian-American to serve on the Philadelphia Commission on Human Relations.

Appointed by Mayor Wilson Goode, Chen worked with community leaders to resolve racial and ethnic tensions and also made time to contribute free legal counsel to a variety of activist groups.

The "Help Wanted" section of the newspaper contained an entry that aroused Chen's curiosity — an ad for a judge's position. Her application resulted in her selection by a state judicial committee to fill a seat in the state court. And in July of 1988, she officially became a judge of the Court of Common Pleas. Running as both a Republican and Democratic candidate, her position was secured when she won her seat on the bench at last November's election.

At Family Court, Chen presides over criminal and civil cases which include adult sex crimes, domestic violence, juvenile delinquency, custody, divorce and support. Not a pretty picture.

Chen recalls her first day as judge, hearing a juvenile dependency case — "It was a horrifying experience. I broke down because the cases were so depressing," she remembers.

Outside of the courtroom, Chen has made a name for herself in resolving interracial conflicts, while glorying in her Chinese-American identity. In a 1986 incident involving the desecration of Korean street signs in a Philadelphia neighborhood, Chen called for a meeting with the leaders of that community to help resolve the conflict.

Chen's interest in community advocacy is not limited to Asian communities. She has been involved in Hispanic, Jewish and Black issues, and because of her participation in the Ethnic Affairs Committee of the Anti-Defamation League of B'nai B'rith, Chen was one of 10 women nationwide selected to take part in a mission to Israel.

With her recently won mandate to judicate in the affairs of Pennsylvania's citizens, Chen has pledged to work tirelessly to defend the rights of its people and contribute to the improvement of human welfare. She would have made a fabulous Brownie.

— Jessica Schultz

FIGURE C-4   Discrimination article used in NALS.

Sample Prose Item (Level 4): Korean Jet Article

Task: This question directs the reader to state what argument Tom Wicker is making in the editorial below (Figure C-5).

In this level 4 item, the answer is correct if the argument is identified and respondents make a statement about the author's main point. Answers were marked incorrect if the argument was not identified, respondents wrote what the article was about, or listed evidence without stating the argument. Answers that used the prompt as a basis for personal digression were also marked incorrect. The item is reflective of other tasks at this level of difficulty, which often have repetitive statements that are elaborated in the text so that the propositions supporting the theme, though repetitive, are widely separated in the text.

Prose Level 5. Prose literacy tasks at level 5 required a person to search through text and match multiple features contained in dense text with a number of plausible distractors, to compare and contrast complex information, or to generate new information making high-level inferences or using specialized background knowledge.

Document Literacy and Sample Items

Documents are short forms or graphically displayed information found in everyday life, including job applications, payroll forms, transportation schedules, maps, tables, and graphs. Document literacy tasks included locating a particular intersection on a street map, using a schedule to choose the appropriate bus, or entering information on an application form.

Document Literacy Levels

Adults included in level 1 were those who could succeed at level 1 tasks, but not at level 2 tasks, as well as those who could not succeed at level 1 tasks and those who were not literate enough in English to take the test at all. Adults in levels 2 through 4 were able to succeed at tasks at their proficiency level, but not at tasks for the next more difficult level. Adults in level 5 are able to succeed at level 5 tasks.

Document Level 1. Document literacy tasks at level 1 required a person to locate information based on a literal match to the question or to enter information from personal knowledge into a document. Little, if any, distracting information was present.

Did U.S. know Korean

THE COMPLICITY with government into which the press has sunk since Vietnam and Watergate has seldom been more visible than on the first anniversary of Soviet destruction of Korean Air Lines Flight 007.

On Sept. 1, headlines, of course, reported the Reagan administration's statements that the event had boosted, during the year, U.S. standing in the world relative to that of the U.S.S.R.

But the press effectively ignored an authoritative article in The Nation (for Aug. 18-25) establishing to a reasonable certainty that numerous U.S. government agencies knew or should have known, almost from the moment Flight 007 left Anchorage, Alaska, that it was off course and headed for intrusion into Soviet air space, above some of the most sensitive Soviet military installations.

Yet no agency, military or civilian, warned Flight 007 or tried to guide it out of danger; neither did the Japanese. As

late as Aug. 28, in a briefing, a State Department spokesman claimed "no agency of the U.S. government even knew the plane was off course and was in difficulty until after it was shot down."

If that's true, the author of The Nation's article—David Pearson, an authority on the Defense Department's World Wide Military Command and Control System, who spent a year researching his lengthy article—concludes, "the elaborate and complex system of intelligence, warnings and security that the U.S. has built up over decades suffered an unprecedented and mind-boggling breakdown."

But Pearson shows in excruciating detail why it's most unlikely there was any such "simultaneous failure of independent intelligence systems" of the Navy, Army, Air Force, National Security Agency, Central Intelligence Agency "or the Japanese self-defense agency"—all of which, he shows, had ability to track Flight 007 at various stages

Tom Wicker

across the Pacific.

What's the alternative to the staggering idea of such a breakdown? That all these agencies deliberately chose not to guide the airliner back on a safe course, because its projected overflight of the Kamchatka Peninsula and Sakhalin Island would activate Soviet radar and air defenses and thus yield a "bonanza" of intelligence information to watching and listening U.S. electronic devices. Despite all administration protests to the contrary, the evidence Pearson presents raises this alternative at least to the high probability level.

But Pearson does not assert as a fact that the United States, South Korea or both deliberately planned an intelligence mission for Flight

jet was astray?

007; he concedes the possibility that it simply "blundered" into sensitive Soviet air space, and that electronic onlookers for the United States decided on the spot to take intelligence advantage of the error—never dreaming the Russians would shoot down an unarmed airliner.

But if the disaster happened that way, Pearson notes, two experienced pilots (nearly 20,000 flying hours between them) not only made an error in setting the automatic pilot but "sat in their cockpit for five hours, facing the autopilot selector switch directly in front of them at eye level, yet failed to see that it was set improperly." Nor in all that time could they have used the available radar and other systems to check course and position.

Pearson also presents substantial evidence that Soviet radar detection and communications systems over Kamchatka and Sakhalin were being jammed that night, which would help account for their documented difficulty in

catching up to Flight 007. He reconstructs electronic evidence too, to show that the airliner changed course slightly after passing near a U.S. RC-135 reconnaissance plane; otherwise it would have crossed Sakhalin far north of the point where a Soviet fighter finally shot it down.

The jamming and course change, as detailed by Pearson, strongly suggest what he obviously fears: "that KAL 007's intrusion into Soviet air space, far from being accidental, was well orchestrated," with the Reagan administration, at some level, doing the orchestrating. Even if not, the deliberate silence—or shocking failure—of so many U.S. detection systems argue that President Reagan and the security establishment have greater responsibility for Flight 007's fate than they admit—or that a complaisant press has been willing to seek.

Copyright ©1984 by The New York Times Company. Reprinted by permission.

FIGURE C-5 Korean jet article used in NALS.

1.   You have gone to an employment center for help in finding a job. You know that this center handles many different kinds of jobs. Also, several of your friends who have applied here have found jobs that appeal to you.

The agent has taken your name and address and given you the rest of the form to fill out. Complete the form so the employment center can help you get a job.

Birth date_____   Age_____   Sex: Male_____   Female_____

Height_____   Weight_____   Health_____

Last grade completed in school_____

Kind of work wanted:

   Part-time_____   Summer_____

   Full-time_____   Year-round_____

FIGURE C-6   Job application used in NALS.

Sample Document Item (Level 1): Job Application (Figure C-6)

Task:

The answer is correct if the respondent satisfactorily completes the form portion (birth date, age, sex, height, weight, health, grade).

In this task, readers were asked to complete a section of a job application by providing several pieces of information. Here, respondents had to conduct a series of one-feature matches.

Sample Document Item (Level 1): Net Pay

Task: Here is a wage and tax statement that comes with a paycheck (Figure C-7). What is the current net pay?

The correct answer to this item is: 459.88.

This level 1 question asks, "what is the current net pay?" Since the term appears only once on the pay stub and there is only one number in the column, this task requires only a one-feature match and receives a difficulty value that lies within the level 1 range on the document scale.

Document Level 2. Document literacy tasks at level 2 required the reader to match a piece of information either when several distractors were present

	HOURS			PERIOD ENDING 03/15/00	REGULAR	OVERTIME	GROSS	DEF. ANN	NET PAY
REGULAR	2ND SHIFT	OVERTIME	TOTAL	CURRENT	625,00		625,00		459,88
5,00			5,00	YEAR-TO-DATE			4268,85		

	FED. WH	STATE WH	CITY WH	FICA		CR UNION		UNITED FD	PERS INS	MISC.	MISC CODE
		TAX DEDUCTIONS						OTHER DEDUCTIONS			
CURRENT	108,94	13,75		38,31							
YEAR-TO-DATE	734,98	82,50		261,67							

NON-NEGOTIABLE

		OTHER DEDUCTIONS				
CODE	TYPE	AMOUNT	CODE	TYPE	AMOUNT	
07	DEN	4,12				

Reduced from original copy

FIGURE C-7 Wage and tax statement used in NALS.

or when low-level inferences were required. Tasks at this level also asked the reader to cycle through information in a document or to integrate information from various parts of a document.

Sample Level 2 Item

Task: You are a marketing manager for a small manufacturing firm. This graph (Figure C-8) shows your company's sales over the last three years. Given the seasonal pattern shown on the graph, predict the sales for Spring 1985 (in thousands) by putting an "x" on the graph.

The answer is correct if the respondent puts an "x" or other mark on the graph at any point above the point for Winter, 1984, in the area under 1985.

This level 2 task asks respondents to study a line graph showing a company's seasonal sales over a three-year period, then predict the level of sales for the following year, based on the seasonal trends shown in the graph. It requires readers to integrate information from different parts of the document by looking for similarities or differences.

Document Level 3. Document literacy tasks at level 3 required a person to integrate multiple pieces of information from one or more documents. Other tasks asked readers to cycle through complex tables or graphs and locate particular features. The displays contained information that was irrelevant or inappropriate to the task.

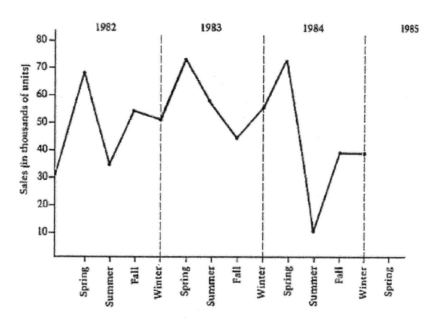

FIGURE C-8   Sales graph used in NALS.

Sample Level 3 Item: Energy Chart (Figure C-9)

Question: In the year 2000, which energy source is predicted to supply a
larger percentage of total power than it did in 1971?
  A   Coal
  B   Petroleum
  C   Natural Gas
  D   Nuclear Power
  E   Hydropower
  F   I don't know
  The correct answer to this item is: *D. Nuclear power.*
  This level 3 task directs the reader to a stacked bar graph depicting
estimated power consumption by source for four different years. The reader
is asked to select an energy source that will provide a larger percentage of
total power in the year 2000 than it did in 1971. To succeed on this task,
the reader must first identify the correct years and then compare each of the
five pairs of energy sources given.

Document Level 4. Document literacy tasks at level 4 required a person to
perform multiple-feature matches, cycle through documents, and integrate

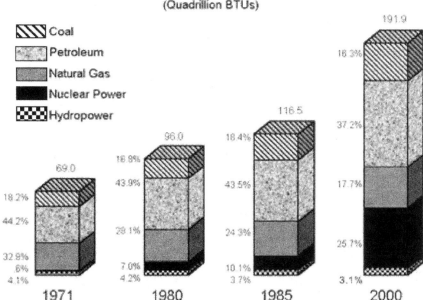

FIGURE C-9 Energy chart used in NALS.
SOURCE: U.S. Department of Interior United States Energy through the year 2000.
BTU: Quantity of heat required to raise temperature of one pound of water one degree Fahrenheit.
Copyright 1973 Congressional Quarterly Inc.

information, all of which required high-level inferences. Many of these tasks required readers to provide numerous responses but did not designate how many responses were needed. Conditional information was also present in the tasks at this level and had to be taken into account by the reader.

Sample Level 4 Item: Bus Schedule (Figure C-10)

On Saturday afternoon, if you miss the 2:35 bus leaving Hancock and Buena Ventura going to Flintridge and Academy, how long will you have to wait for the next bus?

The correct answer to this item is: *C. Until 3:35 p.m.*

This level 4 task combines many of the variables that contribute to difficulty in level 5. These include multiple feature matching, complex dis-

A   Until 2:57 p.m.
B   Until 3:05 p.m.
C   Until 3.35 p.m.
D   Until 3:57 p.m.
E   I don't know.

FIGURE C-10   Bus schedule used in NALS.

plays involving nested information, numerous distracters, and conditional information that must be taken into account in order to arrive at a correct response. Using the bus schedule, readers are asked to select the time of the next bus on a Saturday afternoon, if they miss the 2:35 bus leaving Hancock and Buena Ventura going to Flintridge and Academy. Several departure times are given, from which respondents must choose the correct one.

Document Level 5. Document literacy tasks at level 5 required a person to search through complex displays that contained multiple distractors, to make high-level text-based inferences, and to use specialized knowledge. Tasks required readers to integrate information, compare and contrast data points, and to summarize the results.

Quantitative Literacy and Sample Items

Quantitative information may be displayed visually in graphs or charts or in numerical form using whole numbers, fractions, decimals, percentages, or time units (hours and minutes). These quantities appeared in both prose and document form. Quantitative literacy refers to locating quantities, integrating information from various parts of a document, determining the necessary arithmetic operation, and performing that operation. Quantitative literacy tasks included balancing a checkbook, completing an order form, and determining the amount of interest paid on a loan.

Quantitative Literacy Levels

Adults included in level 1 were those who could succeed at level 1 tasks, but not at level 2 tasks, as well as those who could not succeed at level 1 tasks and those who were not literate enough in English to take the test at all. Adults in levels 2 through 4 were able to succeed at tasks at their proficiency level, but not at tasks for the next more difficult level. Adults in level 5 are able to succeed at level 5 tasks.

Quantitative Level 1. Quantitative literacy tasks at level 1 required a person to perform single, relatively simple arithmetic operations, such as addition, when the question included the numbers to be used and the arithmetic operation to be performed.

Sample Quantitative Item (Level 1): Adding Deposits (Figure C-11)

Task: You wish to use the automatic teller machine at your bank to make a deposit. Figure the total amount of the two checks being deposited. Enter the amount on the form in the space next to TOTAL.

The correct answer to this item is $632.19.

This level 1 item is the least demanding task on the quantitative scale. It requires the reader to total two numbers on a bank deposit slip. In this task, both the numbers and the arithmetic operation are judged to be easily identified and the operation involves the simple addition of two decimal numbers that are set up in column format.

Quantitative Level 2. Quantitative literacy tasks at level 2 required a person to locate numbers by matching the required information with that given, infer the necessary arithmetic operation, or perform an arithmetic operation when the tasks specified the numbers and the operation to be performed. The quantities could be easily located in the text, and the operation could be determined from the format of the material.

Quantitative Level 3. Quantitative literacy tasks at level 3 required a person to locate numbers by matching the required information with that given, infer the necessary arithmetic operation and perform arithmetic operations

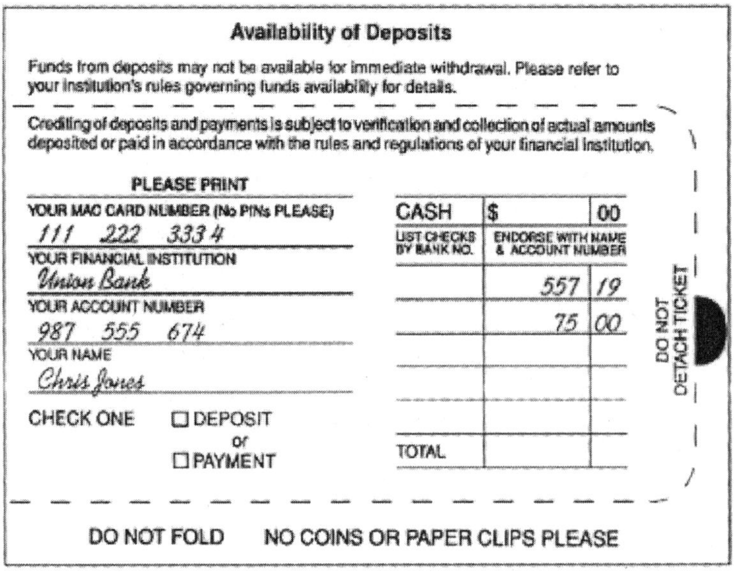

Availability of Deposits

Funds from deposits may not be available for immediate withdrawal. Please refer to your institution's rules governing funds availability for details.

Crediting of deposits and payments is subject to verification and collection of actual amounts deposited or paid in accordance with the rules and regulations of your financial institution.

PLEASE PRINT

YOUR MAC CARD NUMBER (No PINs PLEASE)
111 222 3334

YOUR FINANCIAL INSTITUTION
Union Bank

YOUR ACCOUNT NUMBER
987 555 674

YOUR NAME
Chris Jones

CHECK ONE ☐ DEPOSIT or ☐ PAYMENT

CASH	$	00
LIST CHECKS BY BANK NO.	ENDORSE WITH NAME & ACCOUNT NUMBER	
	557	19
	75	00
TOTAL		

DO NOT DETACH TICKET

DO NOT FOLD NO COINS OR PAPER CLIPS PLEASE

FIGURE C-11 Bank deposit slip used in NALS.

on two or more numbers, or to solve a problem, when the numbers must be located in the text or document. The required operation(s) could be determined from the arithmetic-relation terms used in the question.

Quantitative Level 4. Quantitative literacy tasks at level 4 required a person to perform two or more sequential arithmetic operations or a single arithmetic operation, when the quantities could be found in different displays, or when the operations had to be inferred from semantic information given or drawn from prior knowledge.

Sample Quantitative Item (Level 4): Unit Price (Figure C-12)

Task: Estimate the cost per ounce of the creamy peanut butter. Write your estimate on the line provided.

The correct answer to this item is: *Any figure from 9 (.09) to 10 (.10).*

This level 4 item task requires the reader to select from two unit price labels to estimate the cost per ounce of creamy peanut butter. To perform this task successfully, readers may have to draw some information from prior knowledge.

Level 4 tasks require either two sequential operations or the application

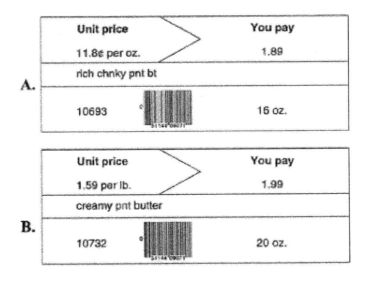

FIGURE C-12 Peanut butter label used in NALS.

of a single higher level operation, such as multiplication. In this example, readers are shown a menu and are required to compute the cost of a specified meal and use multiplication to determine a ten percent tip.

Quantitative Level 5. Quantitative literacy tasks at level 5 required a person to perform multiple arithmetic operations sequentially, when the features of the problem had to be extracted from text; or when background knowledge was required to determine the quantities or operations needed.

Sample Quantitative Item (Level 5): Interest Charges (Figure C-13)

Task: Use the ad for Home Equity Loans to answer this question.

You need to borrow $10,000. Explain to the interviewer how you would compute the total amount of interest charges you would pay under this loan plan. Please tell the interviewer when you are ready to begin.

The answer is correct if the speaker explains the two basic steps in computing the total interest charges, i.e., the monthly payment ($156.77) times the number of payments (120) equals the total loan payment; the total loan payment minus the amount of the loan ($10,000) equals the total interest charges.

One of the most difficult tasks on the quantitative scale, this item requires readers to look at an advertisement for a home equity loan and then, using the information given, explain how they would calculate the total amount of the interest charges associated with the loan.

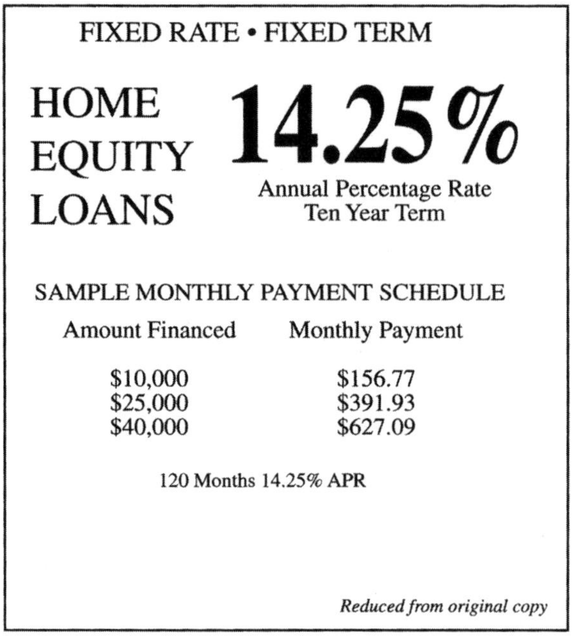

FIXED RATE • FIXED TERM

HOME
EQUITY **14.25%**
LOANS
Annual Percentage Rate
Ten Year Term

SAMPLE MONTHLY PAYMENT SCHEDULE

Amount Financed	Monthly Payment
$10,000	$156.77
$25,000	$391.93
$40,000	$627.09

120 Months 14.25% APR

Reduced from original copy

FIGURE C-13   Home equity loan advertisement used in NALS.

Excerpts taken from: National Center for Education and Statistics, U.S. Department of Education. *Defining Literacy and Sample Items.* [Online]. Available: http://nces.ed.gov/naal/defining/defining.asp [accessed: October, 2003].

D

Committee and Staff Biographies

David A. Kindig, M.D., Ph.D. (*Chair*), is Emeritus Professor of Population Health Sciences and Emeritus Vice Chancellor for Health Sciences at the University of Wisconsin-Madison. He is also Co-director of the Wisconsin Public Health and Health Policy Institute. He served as Vice Chancellor for Health Sciences at the University of Wisconsin-Madison (1980–1985), Director of Montefiore Hospital and Medical Center (1976–1980), Deputy Director of the Bureau of Health Manpower, U.S. Department of Health, Education and Welfare (1976), and medical director of the National Health Service Corps (1971–1973). He served as Chair of the federal Council of Graduate Medical Education (1995–1997), President of the Association for Health Services Research (1997–1998), ProPAC Commissioner (1991–1994) and Senior Advisor to Donna Shalala, Secretary of Health and Human Services (1993–1995). In 1996 he was elected to the Institute of Medicine (IOM), National Academy of Sciences. Dr. Kindig received a B.A. from Carleton College and M.D. and Ph.D. degrees from the University of Chicago School of Medicine. His research interests include population health status, supply and distribution of health professionals, equity in health services, and physician and nurse executives. His current work derives from his 1997 book "Purchasing Population Health: Paying for Results."

Dyanne D. Affonso, Ph.D., R.N., F.A.A.N., is Dean of the Faculty of Nursing at the University of Toronto. She is a leading educator who has advocated for curricula reforms in the health sciences to produce culturally competent health professionals. She is a researcher in women's health issues, community-based interventions, and reducing health disparities through studies on testing community prenatal care programs for ethnically diverse women, post-partum depression screening among culturally diverse women, and school-based violence prevention program for ethnically diverse children. She designed several DHSS-HRSA special projects to customize health-care services to immigrant and low-income families across the United States. She has participated in several National Institutes of Health (NIH) initiatives and review groups addressing the health needs of culturally diverse populations, specifically the National Cancer Institute's (NCI's) Special Population Networks and NCMH's Centers for Reducing Health Disparities. A member of the IOM since 1994, she received her Ph.D. in clinical psychology from the University of Arizona, a master's degree in nursing from the University of Washington, and a bachelor's degree in nursing from the University of Hawaii.

Eric H. Chudler, Ph.D., is a Research Associate Professor in the Department of Anesthesiology at the University of Washington in Seattle, WA. His current research interests include how Parkinson's disease affects the brain, how the brain processes pain signals, and how the nervous system reacts to nerve injury. Dr. Chudler creates neuroscience curricula, and provides information to teachers and students (grades K-12) who want to learn more about the nervous system. He also created the Neuroscience for Kids website, funded by the NIH. Dr. Chudler received his M.S. and Ph.D. degrees from the Department of Psychology at the University of Washington, and received his post-doctoral training from the NIH. He was also an Instructor in the Department of Neurosurgery at the Massachusetts General Hospital in Boston.

Marilyn H. Gaston, M.D., is a past Assistant Surgeon General of the United States and Director of the Bureau of Primary Health Care of the Health Resources and Services Administration. Her career has focused on improving the health of poor and minority families through the delivery of quality primary patient care through the provision of medical education, involvement in clinical research, and the administration of local and federal programs directed to services to the underserved. Dr. Gaston is internationally recognized for her leadership in sickle cell disease. Through her work at the NIH, changes in management of children with this illness have resulted significantly in decreasing the morbidity and mortality in young children. Elected to the IOM in 1996, she frequently speaks on improving access to quality care, elimination of health disparities, African-American women's health, sickle cell disease, and the health needs of youths.

Cathy D. Meade, Ph.D., R.N., F.A.A.N., is Professor in the Department of Interdisciplinary Oncology, Division of Cancer Prevention and Control at the University of South Florida College of Medicine, and Director of the Education Program at the H. Lee Moffitt Cancer Center & Research Institute. She also holds a joint appointment in the College of Nursing. She was one of the first investigators to conduct studies in the area of patient understanding identifying the mismatches between patients' reading levels and the reading levels of health information. She has extensive experience in the development of relevant cancer communications and has produced numerous printed and electronic materials and media for lay and professional audiences. Practical aspects of this work have been published widely to help professionals develop easy-to-understand educational materials and interventions. Her research interests center on crafting culturally, linguistically, and literacy-appropriate health communications, creating sustained community-based cancer education, outreach, and screening initiatives for underserved priority populations, examining understanding of the clinical trial and informed consent process, and developing innovative cancer education and training programs to increase the number of researchers from underrepresented groups. Dr. Meade has served as a member on NCI's work groups on Cancer and Literacy, and Informed Consent in Cancer Clinical Trials for increasing awareness of the impact of literacy in health care. Dr. Meade also provides leadership for numerous education and training initiatives that address the nexus of cancer, culture, and literacy.

Ruth Parker, M.D., is Associate Professor of Medicine, and Associate Director of Faculty Development for the Division of General Medicine at the Emory University School of Medicine. Her primary research interests are in medical education and health services of underserved populations. Dr. Parker has focused extensively on the health-care issues of underserved populations, particularly health literacy. She was principal investigator in the Robert Wood Johnson Literacy in Health Study, and worked with collaborators to develop the Test of Functional Health Literacy in Adults (TOFHLA), a measurement tool to quantify patients' ability to read and understand health information. She is widely published in health literacy, and co-edited the complete bibliography of medicine on health literacy for the National Library of Medicine. She is chair of the American Medical Association (AMA) Foundation steering committee for the national program on health literacy, a member of the ACP Foundation Health Communication Intiative Committee, and former chair of the AMA expert panel for the Council of Scientific Affairs.

Victoria Purcell-Gates, Ph.D., is a Professor of Literacy and Teacher Education at Michigan State University, where she teaches courses in literacy teaching and research. A former middle and high school teacher, Purcell-Gates had directed literacy centers for children needing help with reading and writing at both the University of Cincinnati and Harvard University. She studies literacy acquisition and development in the context of families, communities, and schools. As part of this, she studies the influence of culture, class, gender, and SES on literacy development and on access to literacy learning in schools. She has just concluded a longitudinal experimental study of text genre instruction in second- and third-grade science classes, sponsored by the National Science Foundation and IERI. Her latest book (*Print Literacy Development*), to be issued by Harvard University Press in 2004, is based on a multiyear study of relationships between adult literacy instructional factors and change in home literacy practices, sponsored by the National Center for the Study of Adult Literacy and Learning. Her teaching experience has been primarily with children and adults who have experienced difficulty learning to read and write in school.

Irving Rootman, Ph.D., is Professor and Michael Smith Foundation for Health Research Distinguished Scholar in the Faculty of Human and Social Development at the University of Victoria in British Columbia, Canada, and was Professor of Public Health Sciences and Director of the Centre for Health Promotion at the University of Toronto. He was Director of the Health and Welfare Canada Program Resources Division and Chief of Health Promotion Studies in the Health Promotion Directorate, and Chief of Epidemiological and Social Research in the Non-Medical Use of Drugs Directorate. He has acted as Senior Scientist, consultant, and technical advisor for the World Health Organization (WHO), and chaired the WHO-EURO Working Group on Health Promotion Evaluation. He has published widely in the field of health promotion, and co-authored a book entitled *People-Centred Health Promotion*. Dr. Rootman serves on the Health Promotion and Disease Prevention Board of the IOM and is a former member of the Canadian Minister of Health's Science Advisory Board.

Rima Rudd, Sc.D., is Senior Lecturer on Society, Human Development, and Health at the Harvard University School of Public Health. She is a public health educator and her work centers on health communication and on the design and evaluation of public health community-based programs. She teaches graduate courses on health literacy, innovative strategies in health education, and program planning and evaluation. Dr. Rudd's current research is focused on health disparities and on literacy-related barriers to health programs, services, and care. She works closely with the adult education, public health, and medical sectors. She is a research fellow of the

National Center for the Study of Adult Learning and Literacy and is Principal Investigator (PI) for the Health and Adult Literacy studies. Dr. Rudd also serves as PI for the Literacy in Arthritis Management: A Randomized Controlled Trial of a Novel Patient Education Intervention with the RB Brigham Arthritis and Musculoskeletal Diseases Clinical Research Center and a co-PI on Pathways Linking Education to Health Study with colleagues at the Harvard School of Public Health. She worked with Drs. Kirsch and Yamamoto of the Educational Testing Services (ETS) to develop a Health Activities and Literacy Scale that provides baseline data for health literacy assessment and discussed in a forthcoming ETS policy report. Dr. Rudd authored the action plan for the health literacy objective in Health People 2010.

Susan C. Scrimshaw, Ph.D., is Dean of the School of Public Health and Professor of Community Health Sciences and Anthropology at the University of Illinois at Chicago. Dr. Scrimshaw has worked widely with diverse populations in cross-cultural settings in the fields of medical and applied anthropology, demography, culture change, and population health. An involved IOM Member, Dr. Scrimshaw has served on the IOM Board on International Health and the IOM Panel on Cancer Research among Minorities and the Medically Underserved. She is Member of the Task Forces on Community Preventive Services and on Violence Prevention at the Centers for Disease Control and Prevention, and Member of the Executive Council of the Illinois Department of Public Health. Dr. Scrimshaw has worked extensively with city, state, governmental, national, and United Nations agencies. She has been honored by the American Anthropological Association and the Society for Applied Anthropology with the Margaret Mead Award for outstanding achievement in bringing anthropology to a wider audience.

William Smith, Ed.D., is Executive Vice President and Senior Social Scientist of Development Program Services at the Academy of Educational Development (AED). Dr. Smith supervises programs of communication and marketing for social change, and serves as senior scientist for the development of behavior change programs at AED, publishing and speaking to policy-making audiences around the world. He often acts as consultant to international organizations including UNICEF and WHO, as well as national departments of health and the Centers for Disease Control and Prevention. Dr. Smith is recognized as one of the leading specialists in the application of social marketing to social change, and he is co-founder of the Institute for Social Marketing. He has designed, supervised, and evaluated social marketing and communication campaigns on HIV/AIDS prevention in 22 countries, and infant and maternal health in 35 countries of the world.

IOM Staff

Lynn T. Nielsen-Bohlman, Ph.D., is a Senior Program Officer in the Board on Neuroscience and Behavioral Health. Dr. Nielsen-Bohlman's research focused on human distributed cortical networks in working memory and attention, and their modulation by arousal, aging, cortical and subcortical degeneration, and cortical lesion. Her studies on the differential involvement of anterior and posterior cortices in working memory provided the first evidence of a distributed working memory network in humans. Dr. Nielsen-Bohlman received her Ph.D. in physiology from the University of California at Davis in 1994. She was a postdoctoral fellow at the University of California, Berkeley, and the University of California, San Francisco, Assistant Professor of Psychiatry at Vanderbilt University, and a Psychology Department faculty member at Belmont University and the University of Maryland University College. She is the Study Director for the Committee on Health Literacy, and has worked in science and education outreach for two decades.

Allison M. Panzer is a Research Assistant in the Board on Neuroscience and Behavioral Health, and has worked on studies of the pathophysiology and prevention of adolescent and adult suicide and how to optimize the public health response to long-term and short-term mental health consequences of terrorism. This work has contributed to two IOM reports: *Reducing Suicide: A National Imperative* and *Preparing for the Psychological Consequences of Terrorism: A Public Health Strategy.* Allison received her Bachelor's Degree from Wesleyan University with coursework in psychology, sociology, and neuroscience, and has pursued postgraduate studies while at the National Academies.

Benjamin N. Hamlin, Research Assistant at IOM, received his bachelors in Biology from the College of Wooster in 1993 and a degree in health sciences from the University of Akron in 1996. He joined the National Academies in 2000 as a Research Assistant for the Division on Earth and Life Studies. His work at IOM has included *Testosterone and Aging: Clinical Research Directions; Review of NASA's Longitudinal Study of Astronaut Health; Health Literacy: A Prescription to End Confusion; Improving Medical Education: Enhancing the Behavioral and Social Science Content in Medical School Curricula;* and *NIH Extramural Center Programs: Criteria for Initiation and Evaluation.*

Allison L. Berger is a Project Assistant in the Board on Neuroscience and Behavioral Health. She is currently working on two IOM studies: *Health Literacy* and *Introducing Behavioral and Social Sciences into Medical*

School Curricula. Before joining the IOM staff, she enjoyed a 5-year tenure as an Administrative Assistant for the American Psychological Association (APA) where she assisted the APA Committee on Psychological Test and Assessment, Committee on Scientific Awards, and the Committee on Animal Research and Ethics. She also worked on several funding and grant programs sponsored by the APA Science Directorate.

Andrew M. Pope, Ph.D., is Director of the Board on Neuroscience and Behavioral Health, and Director of the Board on Health Sciences Policy at IOM. With a Ph.D. in physiology and biochemistry, his primary interests focus on environmental and occupational influences on human health. Dr. Pope's previous research activities focused on the neuroendocrine and reproductive effects of various environmental substances in food-producing animals. During his tenure at the National Academy of Sciences and since 1989 at IOM, Dr. Pope has directed numerous studies; topics include injury control, disability prevention, biologic markers, neurotoxicology, indoor allergens, and the enhancement of environmental and occupational health content in medical and nursing school curricula. Most recently, Dr. Pope directed studies on NIH priority-setting processes, organ procurement and transplantation policy, and the role of science and technology in countering terrorism.

Index

A

AARP, 119, 292–293

ABEL. *See* Adult basic education and literacy system

Aboriginal people, cultural language of, 114–115

Academy for Educational Development, 153

Academy of General Dentistry, 193

Access to health care and preventive services, 179–180
  See also Language access

Accreditation Council for Continuing Medical Education (ACCME), 159

Accreditation of health systems
  Joint Commission on Accreditation of Healthcare Organizations, 14, 16, 55, 199, 228
  National Committee for Quality Assurance, 14, 16, 55, 199–201, 228, 278

Accreditation of medical education
  Accreditation Council for Continuing Medical Education, 159

Ad Hoc Committee on Health Literacy, 36

Adult Basic Education and Literacy (ABEL) system, 10, 154

Adult education system, 154–157
  context of, 154–155
  incorporating health content into, 156–157
  strategies and opportunities in, 155–157

Adult Literacy & Lifeskills Survey (ALL), 62

Adult population groups
  percentage with literacy skills at NALS levels 1, 2, or 3-4, 64
  percentage with literacy skills at NALS levels 1 or 2, 294

Advertising and marketing
  FDA involvement in, 194
  a popular source of health information, 123–124

Advocacy organizations, 292
  for African-Americans, 294–295
  for the elderly, 292–293
  for Hispanics, 293–294
  prison systems, 296
  professional associations, 296–297
  social service agencies, 296

African-Americans
  advocacy organizations for, 294–295
  literacy proficiency among, 63
  National Association for the Advancement of Colored People, 294–295

I